Routledge R

The Prevention of Tuberculosis

First published in 1908, this book presents a study of tuberculosis. It looks first at its causes, before examining how the problem of mortality from illness had already been reduced. The third part of the book then focuses on measures for reducing and annihilating tuberculosis altogether. Being written in the earlier years of the twentieth century, the book will not only be of interest to medical students and practitioners, but also to historians.

The Prevention of Tuberculosis

Sir Arthur Newsholme

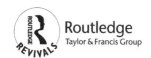
Routledge
Taylor & Francis Group

First published in 1908
by Methuen & Co.

This edition first published in 2015 by Routledge
2 Park Square, Milton Park, Abingdon, Oxon, OX14 4RN
and by Routledge
711 Third Avenue, New York, NY 10017

Routledge is an imprint of the Taylor & Francis Group, an informa business

© 1908 Arthur Newsholme

The right of Arthur Newsholme to be identified as author of this work has been
asserted by him in accordance with sections 77 and 78 of the Copyright,
Designs and Patents Act 1988.

All rights reserved. No part of this book may be reprinted or reproduced or
utilised in any form or by any electronic, mechanical, or other means, now
known or hereafter invented, including photocopying and recording, or in any
information storage or retrieval system, without permission in writing from the
publishers.

Publisher's Note
The publisher has gone to great lengths to ensure the quality of this reprint but
points out that some imperfections in the original copies may be apparent.

Disclaimer
The publisher has made every effort to trace copyright holders and welcomes
correspondence from those they have been unable to contact.

A Library of Congress record exists under LC control number: 08033920

ISBN 13: 978-1-138-90793-5 (hbk)
ISBN 13: 978-1-315-69319-4 (ebk)
ISBN 13: 978-1-138-90810-9 (pbk)

THE PREVENTION
OF TUBERCULOSIS

BY

ARTHUR NEWSHOLME,
M.D., F.R.C.P.

PRESIDENT OF THE EPIDEMIOLOGICAL SECTION OF THE ROYAL SOCIETY OF MEDICINE
LATE MEDICAL OFFICER OF HEALTH OF BRIGHTON

WITH THIRTY-NINE DIAGRAMS

METHUEN & CO.
36 ESSEX STREET W.C.
LONDON

First Published in 1908

PREFACE

THE promise to write this book as one of a series dealing with the public aspects of Medicine was made in 1906. The greater part of it was written over a year ago, Part I. almost entirely so, the quotations from the Second Interim Report of the Royal Commission appointed to inquire into the Relations of Human and Animal Tuberculosis, with such slight modifications of inference as were necessitated by it being added subsequently.

Part II. is a restatement of an investigation of which the results were last set forth in the *Journal of Hygiene* for July 1906. Although necessarily lengthy and full of detail, the argument and conclusion that institutional segregation is the predominant cause of the decline of phthisis in this country has great importance in its bearing on the administrative measures considered in Part III. It is perhaps unfortunate that the argument is continuous from end to end, and that its effect is misconceived when only parts of it are considered disjoined from the remainder. In the absence of this continuity the investigation could have yielded no more than ground for surmise or conjecture. The history of the public health service gives familiar proof of the important place taken by scientific hypothesis among the tools at our disposal. When, however, conclusions can be tested by actual experience, such experience obviously affords a surer basis for administrative action ; and in a matter of such immense importance to public health as the control of tuberculosis, the intricacies of a statistical inquiry embodying historical and international experience are worth undertaking and mastering if, as happens often and is certainly so in the present case, the question cannot be discussed conclusively without it.

The chapters on statistics are indispensable to the main arguments of the book, especially to those in Part II. If, for instance, statistics of phthisis are largely vitiated by transference between this disease and bronchitis, important reasoning as to the course of phthisis can scarcely be based on them. Where not otherwise stated, the English statistics are derived from the Reports of the Registrar-General of Births and Deaths and from Dr. Tatham's letters therein ; some of these tables have been calculated separately, or readjusted for my special purposes.

The bibliography on p. 415 does not pretend to be complete. It comprises only the papers and books actually quoted in this volume. It is hoped that the index of names of places and persons will form a useful supplement to the subject-index.

This volume is written almost solely from the standpoint of the public health administrator, and is intended primarily for medical officers of health. It is believed, however, that it will also be interesting and useful to all medical practitioners, to many members of Sanitary Authorities and Hospital Committees, to patients themselves, and to that increasing proportion of the public who desire to know more of preventive medicine. As therapeutics in the more limited sense of the word has been entirely excluded from its scope, there appears to be no impediment, except, perhaps, lack of interest, to this wider utility of the discussion of tuberculosis here attempted.

I have to thank my friend H. C. Lecky, M.A., M.B., and H. P. Newsholme, B.A., B.Sc., for reading portions of the manuscript, and for valuable suggestions, and the latter for seeing the volume through the press.

A. N.

LIST OF FIGURES

CONTENTS

PART I

CAUSATION OF TUBERCULOSIS

PART I

CAUSATION OF TUBERCULOSIS

TERMS EMPLOYED

TUBERCULOSIS: the general name given to the disease resulting from the invasion of any part of the body by the *tubercle bacillus*.

General Tuberculosis	⎫ Names given to tuberculosis where
Acute Miliary Tuberculosis	⎬ many parts of the body are
Acute Tuberculosis	⎭ attacked simultaneously.
Phthisis	⎫
Pulmonary Phthisis	⎪
Pulmonary Tuberculosis	⎬ Tuberculosis of the lungs.
Consumption	⎭
Tabes Mesenterica	⎫ Tuberculosis of the peritoneum
Tuberculous Peritonitis	⎬ and of the abdominal lymphatic glands.
Tuberculous Meningitis	⎫
Acute Hydrocephalus	⎬ Tuberculosis of the membranes
Brain Fever (in part)	⎭ surrounding the brain.
Lupus	Tuberculosis of the skin.
Caries	,, ,, bone.
Scrofula	,, ,, l y m p h a t i c glands.

Consumption, Tabes (both of Latin origin), and Phthisis (of Greek origin) are all words the literal meaning of which is "wasting."

The term Phthisis has been used sometimes in a sense wider than that of Tuberculous Phthisis or Pulmonary Tuberculosis; *e.g.* miners' phthisis, knife-grinders' phthisis, etc. In most, if not in all such diseases, tuberculosis forms an important, though possibly superadded, cause of death. Possibility of error from this cause will only affect the statistics of special localities.

CHAPTER I

MAGNITUDE OF THE EVIL: *A.* MORTALITY

TUBERCULOSIS is a disease caused by the destructive lesions set up in the lungs or in other parts of the body by a special bacillus or microbe. The disease is infectious, *i.e.* is communicable from man to man and from animals to man ; and it never originates in the body apart from the invasion of the special bacillus.

Being an infective disease, tuberculosis comes into the same category as the infectious diseases enumerated in Tables I. and III. Large sums of money very properly are spent each year in the prevention of these diseases ; hitherto but little has of set purpose been spent on measures for the prevention of tuberculosis. We may, therefore, with advantage consider, in the first place, the relative magnitude of these different causes of death. In Table I. are set out the deaths from the acute infectious diseases and from tuberculosis.

TABLE I.[1]—ENGLAND AND WALES, 1904
Number of Deaths from—

Measles and German Measles	12,341
Whooping-Cough	11,909
Diarrhœa and Dysentery	29,674
Enteric Fever	3,153
Diphtheria	5,763
Scarlet Fever	3,770
Typhus Fever	37
Small-pox	507
	67,154
Pulmonary Phthisis	41,851
All other Tuberculous Diseases	18,354
	60,205

Thus tuberculous diseases in 1904 caused 60 deaths for every

---

[1] All the statistical material relating to England and Wales contained in this volume is derived from Dr. Tatham's valuable annual letters to the Registrar-General of Births and Deaths, unless otherwise stated.

67 caused by the aggregate of the chief acute infectious diseases. These figures do not bring out fully the relative importance and seriousness of deaths from tuberculosis. Although infantile deaths are regrettable, they do not cause so great a loss to the community and so much distress and suffering to the survivors in a bereaved family as do deaths in early and middle life. The following table is important in this connection :—

TABLE II.—ENGLAND AND WALES, 1904

Out of every 100 *Deaths at all Ages the number occurring at different Ages from each Cause of Death was—*

	Under 10.	10–20.	20–45.	45–65.	65 and over.
Measles	99·1	0·5	0·3	0·1	...
Whooping-Cough . .	99·9	0·1	...	...	...
Diarrhœa . . .	93·5	0·2	0·7	1·6	4·0
Phthisis	4·8	10·1	56·5	25·3	3·3

Thus 99 out of every 100 total deaths from measles and whooping-cough, and 94 out of every 100 deaths from diarrhœa, occurred under 10 years of age, while only 5 out of 100 deaths from pulmonary tuberculosis occurred under this age ; and during the working years of life (20–65) 82 occurred out of every 100 total deaths from phthisis, as against no deaths from whooping-cough, less than a half per cent. of the total deaths from measles, and less than 2½ per cent. of the total deaths from diarrhœa.

If we compare the mortality from tuberculosis with that from infective diseases, other than those enumerated in Table I., we have the following result :—

TABLE III.—ENGLAND AND WALES, 1904

Number of Deaths from—

Influenza	5,694 (the highest number in any one year was 13,756, in 1890).
Puerperal Fever	1,654
Erysipelas	1,206
Syphilis and other Venereal Diseases .	1,871 (doubtless understated).
Tetanus (Lock-jaw) . . .	257
Malaria	106
Anthrax	20
Glanders	4
Hydrophobia	0 (in 1885 the number was 60 ; it has not been so high since).
	10,812
All forms of Tuberculosis . . .	60,205

Evidently none of these diseases occupies so important a place as tuberculosis, though in the public administration of the

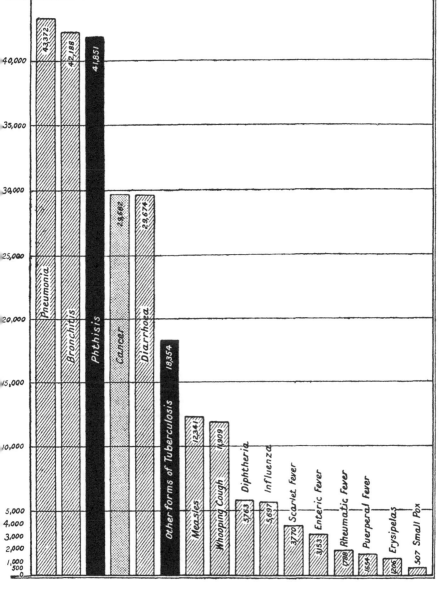

Fig. 1.—Comparative Magnitude of some of the Chief Preventable Causes of Death in England and Wales

country much larger sums are spent in the control of hydrophobia, glanders, anthrax, and puerperal fever than have hitherto been spent in direct measures against tuberculosis.

In the Registrar-General's returns for England and Wales other diseases than those enumerated above are classified as infective, *i.e.* produced by infection received from without. Omitting pneumonia for separate consideration, the number of deaths returned as due to infective diseases in 1904 was 140,431, the total number of deaths from all causes in the same year being 547,784. Of the total (140,431), 60,205 were caused by tuberculosis, 77,966 by the other infective diseases named in Tables I. and III. Rheumatic fever, which is undoubtedly infective, though not classified as such in the official returns, caused 1788 deaths in 1904. Probably most, if not all the diseases of the respiratory organs have an infective origin, and many not recognised as such are tuberculous. Pneumonia in 1904 caused 43,372 deaths, bronchitis 42,188, all other diseases of the respiratory organs excepting pulmonary tuberculosis 8059 deaths. The relative magnitude of the most important preventable causes of death is shown in Fig. 1. The list is not complete, but the most important items are included. Pneumonia and bronchitis have been added, although only partially preventable under present conditions. Cancer has also been added, because, although not directly preventable, many of the deaths from it are pre-

TABLE IV.—ENGLAND AND WALES, 1904

Death-rate from Phthisis per 100,000 *living at each Age-group*

Ages.	Males.	Females.	Persons of Both Sexes.
0– . . .	39	31	35
5– . . .	15	20	17
10– . . .	19	44	32
15– . . .	80	102	91
20– . . .	161	125	142
25– . . .	213	158	184
35– . . .	270	170	218
45– . . .	310	148	226
55– . . .	255	117	182
65– . . .	126	65	92
All Ages . .	146	103	124

ventable by early recognition and removal of the diseased parts.

MORTALITY IN TERMS OF THE POPULATION—DEATH-RATES.— In 1904 the death-rate in England and Wales from phthisis was 1·46 per 1000 of population among males and 1·03 per 1000 among females. The death-rate varies greatly at different ages, as will be seen from the table on preceding page, derived from Dr. Tatham's Report to the Registrar-General. In this table the death-rates are stated per 100,000 living at each age-period separately for the two sexes.

The facts in this table can be more clearly seen when set out graphically as in Fig. 2.

The significance of the different age distribution of the phthisis death-rate in the two sexes will be subsequently considered (p. 168). At present we need only record the fact, as bearing on the value of the lives sacrificed to this disease. The age distribution of deaths from phthisis may be stated in three different ways :—

(1) The *death-rate* from this disease may be given per 1000 or per 100,000 living at each period of life, as in Fig. 2.

(2) The deaths from this disease may be stated in *proportion to the total deaths from the same disease at all ages.*

(3) Or these deaths may be stated in *proportion to the total deaths from all causes at the same age-period.*

The first is the only method which can be employed in comparing the age incidence of the disease in different populations. The second and third methods are useful for special purposes. By means of the second method we can ascertain the proportional incidence of deaths from phthisis at different ages, and by the third we can state its importance in proportion to other causes of death at each age-period. From these standpoints the second and third methods tell us more than the first ; for a high death-rate may occur among a relatively small population. Thus the male death-rate from phthisis of 126 per 100,000 at ages over 65 is higher than that of 39 per 100,000 in male children under 5, but the two rates represent an equal percentage (3·1) of the total male mortality from this disease at all ages. In the following table the second and third ratios mentioned above are given for each sex :—

TABLE V.—ENGLAND AND WALES, 1904

Proportional Mortality from Phthisis

Age.	Males.		Females.	
	(1) In proportion to 100 Deaths from Phthisis at all Ages.	(2) In proportion to 100 Deaths from all Causes in the same Age-period.	(1) In proportion to 100 Deaths from Phthisis at all Ages.	(2) In proportion to 100 Deaths from all Causes in the same Age-period.
0– . . .	3·1	0·7	3·4	0·7
5– . . .	1·1	4·2	2·0	5·7
10– . . .	1·4	9·5	4·3	20·6
15– . . .	5·6	26·1	9·7	35·4
20– . . .	10·8	38·5	11·9	36·7
25– . . .	23·1	37·0	25·3	32·3
35– . . .	22·8	28·1	20·3	21·2
45– . . .	18·9	18·2	13·0	11·2
55– . . .	10·1	7·7	6·9	4·4
65 and upwards .	3·1	1·4	3·2	0·8
All Ages . .	100·0	8·5	100·0	6 0

The same facts are set forth graphically in Figs. 3 and 4. Comparing the three sets of facts depicted in Figs. 2–4, it will be noted that the highest male death-rate from phthisis occurs at the age-period 45–55, the age-periods 35–45 and 55–65 coming next. The highest proportion of the total male deaths from phthisis occurs at the ages 25–35 and 35–45 ; and phthisis bears the highest proportion to deaths from all causes at the ages 20–25 and 25–35.

In the female sex the highest death-rate from phthisis occurs at the ages 35–45, 25–35 coming next, the highest proportion to deaths from phthisis at all ages occurs at the ages 25–35, and to deaths from all causes at the corresponding age-period at ages 20–25.

Of the total deaths from phthisis 91·3 per cent. in males and 87·1 per cent. in females occur at the ages 15–65, the working years of life.

TUBERCULOUS DISEASES OTHER THAN PHTHISIS.—Phthisis is not the only fatal disease due to tuberculous infection. In 1904

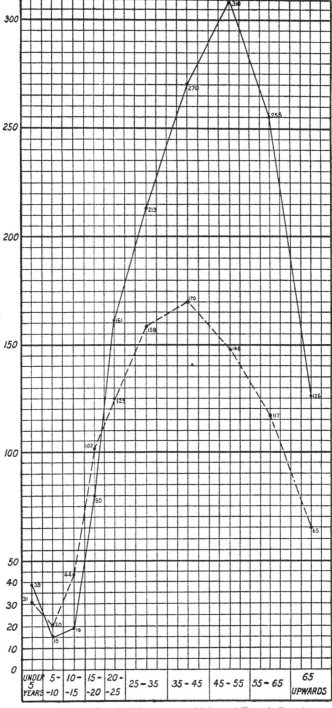

FIG. 2.—England and Wales, 1904.—Male and Female Death-rates
from Phthisis at different Age-periods
(Males—continuous line; females—interrupted line)

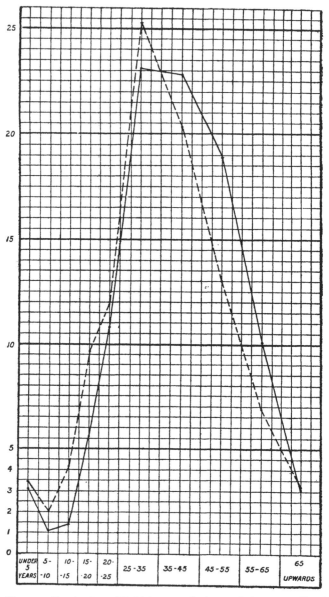

FIG. 3.—Deaths from Phthisis at each Age-period per 100 Total
Deaths from the same Disease at all Ages
(Males—continuous line; females—interrupted line)

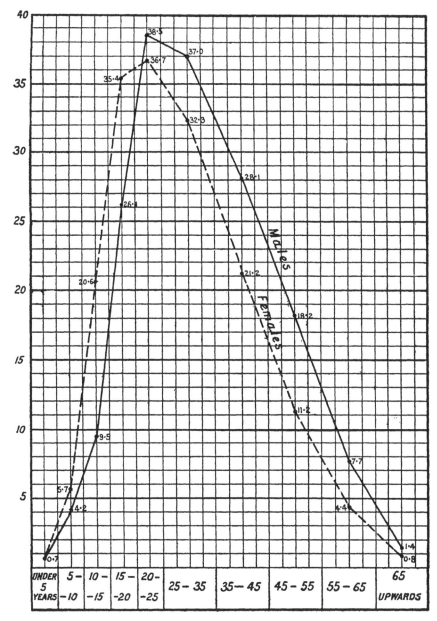

FIG. 4.—Deaths from Phthisis at each Age-period per 100 Deaths from all Causes at the same Age-period

the number of deaths caused by each form of tuberculosis was
returned as follows :—

TABLE VI.—ENGLAND AND WALES, 1904

Number of Deaths caused by various forms of Tuberculosis

	Males.	Females.	Total.
Pulmonary Phthisis	23,850	18,001	41,851
Tuberculous Meningitis . . .	3,359	3,030	6,389
Tuberculous Peritonitis ⎫ . . .	1,994	1,921	3,915
Tabes Mesenterica ⎭ . . .	1,064	834	1,898
Lupus	28	38	66
Tubercle of other Organs . . .	957	705	1,662
General Tuberculosis	2,253	2,062	4,315
Scrofula	47	62	109
	33,552	26,653	60,205

The death-rate in 1904 from all the tuberculous diseases excluding phthisis was 54 per 100,000 persons, 59 per 100,000 males,
and 50 per 100,000 females ; the corresponding figures for all
tuberculous diseases being 178, 205, and 153. Thus phthisis
accounts for 69·5 per cent. of the total deaths ascribed to tuberculosis.

The age distribution of the deaths from tuberculous diseases
other than pulmonary tuberculosis enumerated in Table VI.
will be more conveniently discussed in the chapter on Accuracy
of Certification.

CHAPTER II

MAGNITUDE OF THE EVIL: *B.* SICKNESS AND ECONOMICS

IT has been shown in Chapter I. that 11 per cent. of the total deaths in England and Wales are registered as due to tuberculosis, and that seven-tenths of these are caused by phthisis. Table V. also shows that among males 91 per cent. and among females 87 per cent. of these deaths occur between the ages 15 and 65, and 86 and 77 per cent. in the two sexes respectively at ages 20–65.

ECONOMIC VALUE OF LIVES LOST.—Each child during his years of helplessness and until he is able to support himself by his own exertions is having expended upon him time, money, and effort, which may be regarded as so much capital invested with a prospect of future returns. If he dies in infancy, the measurable loss is much less than if death is postponed until the age of 15. Although it is scarcely necessary to make elaborate calculations as to the expenditure on maintenance, etc., which is lost by death occurring before or during school-life, it obviously represents a considerable capital sum. Between the ages of 15 and 20 it is probably exceptional for the earnings to more than balance personal expenditure, and, if this be so, all deaths up to the age of 20 may be regarded as involving a serious loss of capital expenditure. After this age the problem becomes more complicated. During the next five years a large proportion of the population marry, and thus incur new obligations before the balance against them can possibly have been paid off. It is during the ages from 25–65, and especially during the ages 25–55, that the worker can hope to pay back the value of his own earlier maintenance (*a*) by personal savings, (*b*) by investing capital in the formation of a home and the upbringing of a family in his turn. Each family represents in this respect an investment on the instalment system, and the only hope of completing the investment, and leaving no debt for survivors to redeem or owe to the community, is for the worker to live and to remain able to work, until all his children are able to earn their livelihood, and until his wife and himself can maintain themselves in their old age.   That is the ideal.   It can only be realised when the worker is not cut down by illness or killed by disease or accident.   Hence the immense economic significance of the fact that among men nine out of every ten deaths from phthisis occur between the ages of 15 and 65.   Some data for the determination of this loss have been calculated by Dr. T. E. Hayward (1904).[1]

EFFECT ON THE DURATION OF LIFE OF THE ELIMINATION OF PHTHISIS.—Dr. Hayward calculated by the life-table method what would be the effect of totally abolishing phthisis from the death-returns of England and Wales for the decade 1891–1900.   The main results thus obtained are summarised in the following table :—

TABLE VII.—ENGLAND AND WALES, 1891–1900

Survivors and Future Expectation of Life at Different Ages in Males

Age.	Number of Survivors at each Age out of 100,000 born.		Future Expectation of Life (Mean After Lifetime).		Percentage Increase in the Expectation of Life produced by the Elimination of Phthisis.
	Based on the Mortality from all Causes.	Based on the Mortality from all Causes excluding Phthisis.	Based on the Mortality from all Causes.	Based on the Mortality from all Causes except Phthisis.	
0– . .	100,000	100,000	44·1	46·3	5·0
5– . .	75,093	75,256	53·4	56·2	5·3
15– . .	72,592	72,897	45·1	47·9	6·3
25– . .	69,446	70,654	36·9	39·2	6·3
35– . .	64,716	67,676	29·2	30·8	5·3
45– . .	57,655	62,138	22·2	23·0	3·9
55– . .	47,424	52,742	15·8	16·2	2·3
65– . .	33,163	37,830	10·3	10·4	1·0
75– . .	15,813	18,303	6·1	6·2	...
85– . .	3,121	3,629	...	...	...

[1] It is convenient to note here that when a date is given in brackets after a name, the full title of the paper or book quoted will be found in the bibliography at the end of this volume.   The same remark applies when a name and a page reference are given in brackets.

It will be observed that the number of survivors from infancy to the age of 15 out of a given number born is not materially increased by the elimination of phthisis. From this point onwards the elimination of this disease would steadily increase the number of survivors. At the age of 55, for instance, the number of survivors would be 11 per cent. greater than under the actual conditions holding good in 1891-1900, while the mean expectation of life would be increased by 2·3 per cent.

FINANCIAL GAIN BY THE ABOLITION OF PHTHISIS IN MEN.—Some conception of the financial gain that would be secured were pulmonary tuberculosis abolished is given by Table VII., which shows that, judging by the experience of 1891-1900 in England and Wales, the abolition of phthisis would increase the expectation of life of every male aged 15 years by 2·8 years, and of every male aged 25 years by 2·3 years. Taking the average increase of expectation for the 3,080,166 males aged 15-25 at the last census (1901) to be 2·5 years, it follows that these males who, in 1901, were at or near the beginning of their working life would, but for phthisis, live in the aggregate 7,700,315 years more than under present conditions they can expect to do. A reference to Table VII. shows that the greatest part of this increase of life would be in the working years of life before 65 ; and if we assume that the average wage of each is 20s. a week, a possible gain of over £400,000,000 might be obtained on the above lives, or not far from ten millions sterling annually. And this makes no allowance for the loss sustained by protracted sickness ; nor for the further loss from premature death of women from the same cause.

ILLUSTRATIONS OF FINANCIAL LOSS BY PHTHISIS.—(1) The experience of Friendly Societies throws light on this point. Mr. A. W. Watson (1902) has published an investigation of the experience of 819,716 members of the Oddfellows Society during the years 1893-97. These members represented persons exposed in the aggregate for 2,995,724 years to risk of sickness, and for 3,180,378 years to risk of death. During these years the average annual death-rate per 1000 members was 12·3. This Society has not published any results as to causes of mortality, but the Ancient Order of Foresters has published (1903) a report summarising for the five years 1897-1901 the number of total deaths and deaths from consumption which occurred among its

580,405 benefit members, equivalent to 2,721,822 years of life. The following table summarises the results for them and for 224,374 wives and widows of members during the same period :—

TABLE VIII.—FORESTERS

Death-rates from all Causes and from Consumption, 1897–1901

	Benefit Members.		Wives and Widows of Members.	
	Death-rate per 1000 from—		Death-rate per 1000 from—	
	All Causes.	Consumption.	All Causes.	Consumption.
England	13·2	1·8	12·1	1·5
Ireland .	12·1	2·7	12·0	3·3
Scotland	9·6	2·6	10·1	1·8
Wales .	12·7	1·8	12·8	1·7
United Kingdom .	12·9	1·9	11·9	1·5

It is evident that the experience of the Foresters and the Oddfellows as regards general death-rates is very similar, and it may be assumed that this is so also for consumption, and that in both Societies this disease causes at least 15 per cent., or about one-seventh of the deaths from all causes. Returning for a moment to Table V. and Fig. 4, it will be noted that the proportion of deaths from phthisis to total deaths from all causes is greatest from 20 to 45 years of age, at which ages it varies from a third to a fourth of the total number. At ages 55–65 it has declined to one-twelfth of the total deaths from all causes. In the total experience of the Foresters the proportion is, as we have seen, one-seventh, and the proportion must be higher than this in the working years of life 15–65. Further allowance has to be made for the fact that consumption only causes death after prolonged disablement, and almost certainly causes a higher proportion of the total sickness than of the total mortality. Assuming that it causes one-fifth of the total disablement at ages 15–65, we can calculate what this meant for the 819,716 members of the Manchester Unity of Oddfellows during the years 1893–97. According to Mr. Watson's tables, these men experienced in these years 4,707,680 weeks of sickness, of which 941,575 must be attributed to consumption. The expense to the Oddfellows of this amount of sick relief, and of the deaths associated with it, must have been at least half a million sterling, and the loss of wages to the men themselves at least double this amount.

At a time when Friendly Societies are finding that the claims on their funds are necessitating higher contributions or smaller benefits, their wisest policy evidently is to aid by every means in their power in diminishing this serious drain on their resources.

(2) As bearing on the éxperience of English Friendly Societies, facts given by Mr. Hoffman (1901) relating to the experience of the Prudential Insurance Company of America may be given. He shows that " at the ages of most importance for Industrial insurance purposes almost one-half of the entire mortality is due to consumption." His statistics, unfortunately, do not give the number of lives at risk, but his facts are nevertheless most suggestive.   He says :—

The annual cost of deaths from tubercular diseases to the Prudential Insurance Company of America is approximately, on the basis of three years' experience, the sum of $800,000.   Over 6000 deaths are annually due to this cause in our experience at the present time. . . . While on the average we have received $24.00 from those who died from consumption, we returned to the beneficiary under Industrial policies over $134.00, a net loss of about $110.00 on every case, or more than half a million dollars during the course of a year.   Of course, there is a great difference as to the losses sustained at different age-periods, and naturally the income is least at the younger ages.   As age increases, the average duration of insurance increases, and the amounts paid in premiums to the companies tend more to approach the amounts paid out in claims, but the fact remains, that taking the business as a whole we lose about $110.00 on every death from consumption which occurs in our experience at the present time. If you examine these facts closely you will realise the great interest of the Industrial companies in the problem of diminishing the mortality from tuberculosis, especially at the early ages when, as for instance at 25–29, we will have received $18.00 in premiums to every $150.00 paid out for losses.

(3) Dr. Hermann Biggs (1903) after a careful estimate places the expense of tuberculosis to the people of the United States at $330,000,000 (£66,000,000).   He first calculates the loss to New York City by putting a value of $1500 (£300) upon each life at the average age at which deaths from tuberculosis occur.   This gives a total value of £3,000,000 for the lives lost annually.   To this has to be added the loss due to the fact that

for at least nine months before death these patients cannot work; and the loss of service at $1 a day, and the cost of food, nursing, medicines, attendance, etc., at $1.50 a day results in a further loss of $8,000,000 (£1,600,000), making a yearly loss to the city from tuberculosis of $23,000,000 (£4,600,000). The estimated annual total of 150,000 deaths from tuberculosis in the United States represents in the same way a loss of $330,000,000 (£66,000,000). He further points out that the total expenditure in the City of New York in the care of tuberculous patients is not at present over $500,000 (£100,000) a year—that is, it does not exceed 2 per cent. of the actual loss by death, etc. " If this annual expenditure were doubled or trebled, it would mean the saving of several thousand lives annually, to say nothing of the enormous saving in suffering."

(4) The experience of the German Imperial Insurance Office ascribes a much higher proportion of the total sickness to consumption than the one-fifth which I have tentatively given on the basis of the one-seventh proportion of deaths in the experience of the Foresters. Bielefeldt reports that of every 1000 German workmen aged 20–25 who are rendered unfit for work, 548 owe their sickness to tuberculosis, while at ages between 25 and 30 the proportion per 1000 is 521. At the higher ages, as the amount of non-tuberculous sickness increases, the proportion of tuberculosis becomes less.

(5) In publications of the National Association for the Prevention of Tuberculosis, it is estimated that one-eleventh of the total cost incurred in the relief of pauperism in England and Wales is caused by consumption. The total expenditure in poor-law administration in the year ending Ladyday 1907 was £14,035,888, so that on this basis considerably over a million sterling is annually spent on paupers who were made such by consumption.

(6) The experience of the workhouse infirmary of Brighton gives some insight into the immense cost incurred in the support of parochial consumptive patients. That part of the borough of Brighton comprised within the parish of Brighton has a population of about 102,000. During the eight years 1897–1905, 372 consumptive patients were treated in its infirmary. The average and total stay of these patients in the institution is shown in the following table :—

TABLE IX.—PHTHISIS

Brighton Workhouse Infirmary Statistics from July 15, 1897, *to May* 23, 1905

	Total Number of Days spent in Workhouse by Patient before—		
1. Patient only Once in Workhouse.	Leaving Workhouse.	Death.	May 23, 1905. (Still In).
Number of days under each heading.	11,128	21,306	9133
Number of patients under each heading.	98	148	18
Average number of days for each patient.	114	144	507
2. Patient Twice in Workhouse.	Leaving Workhouse 2nd Time.	Death during 2nd Stay.	May 23, 1905. (Still In).
Number of days under each heading.	2998	5883	5521
Number of patients under each heading.	17	12	4
Average number of days for each patient.	176	490	1380
3. Patient Three Times in Workhouse.	Leaving Workhouse 3rd Time.	Death during 3rd Stay.	May 23, 1905. (Still In).
Number of days under each heading.	2146	2874	261
Number of patients under each heading.	3	6	1
4. Patient Four Times in Workhouse.	Leaving Workhouse 4th Time.	Death during 4th Stay.	May 23, 1905. (Still In).
Number of days under each heading.	966	3217	924
Number of patients under each heading.	3	3	1
5. Patient Five Times in Workhouse.	Leaving Workhouse 5th Time.	Death during 5th Stay.	May 23, 1905. (Still In).
Number of days under each heading.	613	...	...
Number of patients under each heading.	2	...	...
6. Patient Six Times in Workhouse.	Leaving Workhouse 6th Time.	Death during 6th Stay.	May 23, 1905. (Still In).
Number of days under each heading.	337	...	3259
Number of patients under each heading.	1	...	2

N.B.—The word " Workhouse " is used to include Infirmary.
The average stay of each patient was 221 days, including those still in.

This on the basis of 14s. a week[1] means a total cost for maintenance and treatment of £8221, or an annual cost of over £1000 a year. If we assume that the expenditure per 1000 of population is the same in other parts of the country as in Brighton, this implies that on the indoor relief, *i.e.* on the institutional treatment of consumptives in workhouse infirmaries, an annual sum of about £331,000 is spent in England and Wales. This estimate makes no allowance for the large sums given in relief of the relatives of consumptives both before and after their death, and in relief of consumptives who are allowed to remain at home instead of going into infirmaries. If these items be added together, it is likely that they would exceed the annual sum of a million sterling, and would confirm the estimate quoted in paragraph (5).

(7) Farr (1885) stated that the number constantly sick to one annual death was 2·8 in the police and in some friendly societies. According to the experience of the Manchester Unity of Oddfellows during 1893-97 there were 3·35 years of sickness for every annual death at ages 20-65. Although consumption is more chronic than most disabling forms of disease it is doubtful if it causes on an average 3 years of disabling sickness. Doubtless in the above average (3·35 years for every death) is included much sick-leave for minor complaints; and it appears likely that the amount of sick-leave given for comparatively slight ailments has increased. If, however, we assume that only one year's disablement is caused by every fatal case of consumption, then the direct loss per annum in England and Wales produced by the death of men aged 20-65 from consumption, reckoning wages at £50 a year, judging by the experience of 1904, amounts to £1,015,400. This is the loss in wages, reckoned at the above rate. No allowance is made for the cost of the illness, for the interference which every sickness involves with the work of others, or for the infection of others and resultant further loss of health and money.

The preceding calculations are merely given as illustrations of the terrible national loss of money and efficiency caused by tuberculosis. They fail to show the full extent of the mischief wrought. Looking at the subject from the standpoint

[1] This is about the average cost in an infirmary calculated separately from the workhouse.

of national economics, it is not open to dispute that the most elaborate and complete measures of every description against tuberculosis would only cost a fraction of the present total loss inflicted by this disease, and that this expenditure would as time goes on be paid for many times over in the prevention of sickness and increase of efficiency of the community.

CHAPTER III

ARE THE STATISTICS RELATING TO TUBERCULOSIS TRUSTWORTHY?

HAVING obtained some idea of the amount of havoc at present wrought by tuberculosis, we must—before considering the changes in this respect in this and other countries—ascertain what degree of confidence can be placed in the official statistics of this disease.

COMPLETENESS OF CERTIFICATION OF CAUSES OF DEATH.— In drawing deductions from our national statistics, it must be borne in mind that, although national registration of births and deaths was inaugurated in 1837, it was not until January 1, 1875, that it became compulsory for medical practitioners to give certificates of the cause of death of each patient dying under their care. Before this duty became compulsory, medical practitioners certified the majority of deaths, but Farr (1885, p. 523) notes that in 1871 about 8 per cent. of the total deaths were not medically certified. The proportion in 1904 had declined to 1·4 per cent.

There is little doubt that the incomplete medical certification of deaths must affect the trustworthiness of the statistics for phthisis for years before 1875, though to what extent cannot be stated. It is not likely that it does so to such an extent as to make the figures before and after 1875 incomparable. This appears to follow from the regularity of the fall in the death-rate from phthisis before and after this year; but the gradually increasing completeness in medical certification of causes of death needs to be borne in mind.

Beyond this there is the further point as to the gradually increasing accuracy of medical certificates. There can be little doubt that deaths certified at the present time in this country to be due to phthisis are, as a rule, correctly returned. The following exceptions to this rule require to be noted :—

(a) *Inaccurate Diagnosis in Children.*—In children, the term broncho-pneumonia not infrequently conceals acute tuberculosis, especially when the " broncho-pneumonia " occurs after imperfect recovery from such diseases as whooping-cough and measles. Coates (1891) has drawn attention to the frequency of errors of diagnosis in children. He quotes the figures of the Great Ormond Street Children's Hospital, London, for 1877, which showed that of 77 deaths from all causes 35·5 per cent. were due to tuberculosis ; and he considers that we may safely affirm that of the total deaths under 10 years of age among the masses of the people, one-third are due to tuberculosis. In Paris, according to Landouzy (*Trans. Tuberc. Congr. Paris,* 1888, p. 202), one-third of the deaths under 2 are due to tuberculosis. Compare these statements with the experience shown by our national returns for 1904, as given in Table X.

TABLE X.

Percentage at each Age of the total Deaths from all Causes in England and Wales in 1904, *which were returned as caused by Tuberculosis* (*all forms*)

Aged			All Ages under 5.	Aged 5-10.
0-1.	1-2.	2-5.		
4·2	11·9	9·2	6·2	19·1

Table V. gives similar facts for phthisis alone. In explaining the discrepancy between the percentages in early life given in Table X., and the statements made by Coates and Landouzy, it has to be remembered that the latter are dealing only with hospital statistics, and both probably have included deaths in which tuberculosis was secondary to other diseases (*e.g.* whooping-cough), whereas in the Registrar-General's returns these would be entered under the heading of the primary disease. When allowance is made for these facts, there remains, probably, in the national returns considerable understatement of the mortality from tuberculosis in early life, which is not completely counterbalanced by the return of many deaths as " tabes mesenterica," in which there is no tuberculosis. There is no evidence that recent statistics of tuberculosis in early life are not fairly comparable with those of past years, and there is some evidence to the contrary.

(b) *Inaccurate Diagnosis in Old Age.*—Concerning the other extreme of life Dr. Glover Lyon has expressed the belief that " if all the deaths from senile phthisis were properly registered, the registered mortality from phthisis would increase right up to the end of life, as is the case in New York." The diminution of mortality from phthisis after the age of 60 he believes is entirely due to erroneous certification. Dr. Lister also has drawn attention to the fact that in cases in which there is senile emphysema and bronchitis, great difficulty is often experienced in diagnosing phthisis clinically. Error may therefore creep in at these old ages. There is no internal evidence to show that in our national statistics these possible sources of error have been acting at different periods to a markedly varying extent.

(c) *Inaccurate Diagnosis at all Ages.*—1. *Confusion between Phthisis and other respiratory Diseases.*—The most likely sources of error in phthisis statistics are deaths returned under the headings of bronchitis and pneumonia. In the following table the comparative death-rates from these diseases are given for a series of years :—

TABLE XI.—ENGLAND AND WALES

Death-rates per 100,000 of Population in successive Periods from—

Period.	Bronchitis.	Pneumonia.	Bronchitis and Pneumonia.	Phthisis.
5 years, 1866–70 . . .	191	107	298	245
5 ,, 1871–75 . . .	222	103	325	222
5 ,, 1876–80 . . .	238	100	338	204
5 ,, 1881–85 . . .	215	100	315	183
5 ,, 1886–90 . . .	214	113	327	164
5 ,, 1891–95 . . .	207	125	332	146
5 ,, 1896–1900 . . .	156	120	276	132
4 ,, 1901–04 . . .	168	121	289	123

The question arises whether the rates in Table XI. for years before 1875 are comparable with the later rates. Comparing 1871–75 with the two succeeding quinquennial periods, no change in the pneumonia death-rate is visible, and little, if any, change in the death-rate from bronchitis. The following

diagram shows the difference in the course of phthisis and of
bronchitis and pneumonia together (thus combined because

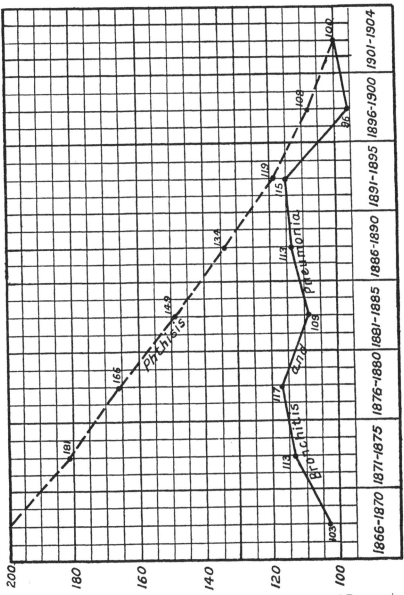

FIG. 5.—Relative Death-rates from (a) Phthisis, (b) Bronchitis and Pneumonia
in England and Wales, the rates for 1901-04 = 100

there may have been transference between these two, especially between capillary bronchitis and broncho-pneumonia). The death-rates from phthisis and from bronchitis and pneumonia respectively in 1901–04 are stated as 100, and earlier rates given in proportion to this figure. By this method, which is adopted in several other instances throughout this work, the items compared start from a point of the same magnitude, and the variations under each heading are comparable on the same scale.

There is no evidence in Fig. 5 that phthisis has declined in consequence of transfer of deaths from that heading to bronchitis and pneumonia. The possibility of confusion between pneumonia and bronchitis and phthisis can be further tested by a comparison of the age distribution of the death-rates from these diseases in 1861–70 with that of 1901. This is done in the table on next page for males, and in Fig. 6, which sets out the same facts graphically.

It will be noted that in Fig. 6, and in each of the columns of comparative figures in Table XII., the death-rate at all ages in the aggregate is stated as 100, and the rates for different age-periods are stated in proportion to this. It has not been thought necessary to reproduce the table and diagram for the female sex, as the result is the same as for males. By means of Fig. 6 we can compare for each age-period the relative incidence of fatal phthisis and of fatal bronchitis *plus* pneumonia at each age-period in 1861–70 with that in 1901. The comparison is interesting, as it affords no evidence that there has been any considerable transfer between bronchitis *plus* pneumonia and phthisis. Some postponement of the maximum death-rate from phthisis is seen in Fig. 6 to have occurred in males, and the same change has occurred for females.

So far, then, as confusion with other diseases is concerned, it does not appear likely that the phthisis statistics of recent years are to any serious extent incomparable with those of earlier years. Phthisis when a fatal disease is easily recognised, and the official figures within a limited margin may be regarded as approximately true.

2. *Return of Phthisis as " Tuberculosis."*—Nor does it appear probable that the tendency on the part of doctors which has shown itself in recent years, to return deaths as " tuberculosis " without any statement of organ affected, has caused a serious

TABLE XII.—ENGLAND AND WALES, MALES

Death-rates per 100,000 of Population at different Age-periods

Ages.	Bronchitis.				Pneumonia.				Bronchitis and Pneumonia.				Phthisis.			
	Death-rates.		Comparative Figures.		Death-rates.		Comparative Figures.		Death-rates.		Comparative Figures.		Death-rates.		Comparative Figures.	
	1861–1870.	1901.	1861–1870.	1901.	1861–1870.	1901.	1861–1870.	1901.	1861–1870.	1901.	1861–1870.	1901.	1861–1870.	1901.	1861–1870.	1901.
0–	512	489	280	355	582	535	462	391	1094	1024	354	373	99	32	40	22
5–	16	8	10	5	28	29	22	21	43	37	14	14	43	15	18	11
10–	4	2	2	1	10	8	8	8	14	13	5	5	61	20	25	13
15–	6	2	3	1	17	24	13	18	23	26	8	10	219	80	89	54
20–	11	3	6	2	27	36	22	27	38	39	12	14	388	168	157	113
25–	25	6	14	4	39	53	31	39	63	59	20	22	409	216	166	145
35–	67	25	37	18	61	103	49	75	128	128	47	47	417	291	169	195
45–	174	99	96	72	89	164	71	120	263	263	85	96	386	315	156	212
55–	448	324	245	235	132	233	105	170	580	577	188	210	330	253	134	170
65–	1009	828	551	600	193	326	153	238	1202	1154	389	420	202	159	82	107
75–	1981	1940	1080	1410	234	439	186	320	2214	2379	717	865	66	61	27	41
All Ages	183	138	100	100	126	137	100	100	309	275	100	100	247	149	100	100

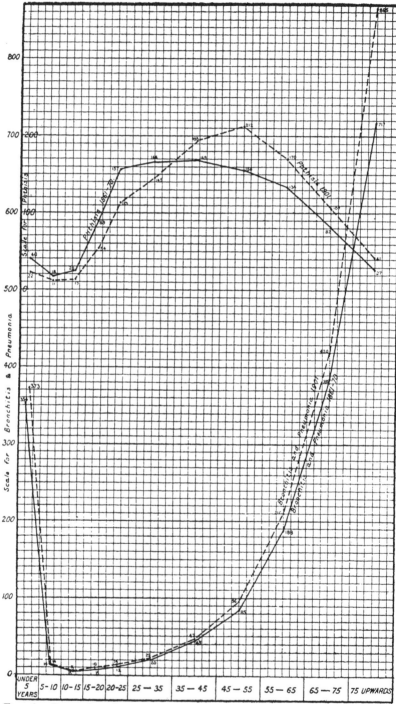

Fig. 6.—Comparison between 1861–70 and 1901 of relative Death-rates at different Age-periods from Bronchitis *plus* Pneumonia and from Phthisis

transfer from phthisis. When checking the mortality returns of Brighton for three years, I found that 496 deaths were returned as phthisis and 39 as tuberculosis, acute tuberculosis, or miliary tuberculosis. Many of these, doubtless, had not had recognisable pulmonary tuberculosis, and were properly returned ; and the residuum would only slightly reduce the great decline in the death-rate from pulmonary tuberculosis which has occurred. Thus, if in the figures for the whole of England and Wales, given in Table VI. on page 12, half of the 4315 deaths from general tuberculosis were transferred to phthisis, the phthisis death-rate would only be changed from 1·24 to 1·30 per 1000 of population.

TUBERCULOUS DISEASES OTHER THAN PHTHISIS.—Tuberculous diseases other than pulmonary in 1904 caused 29 per cent. in males and 33 per cent. in females of the total deaths from tuberculosis. We must next inquire into the validity of the death-returns under these headings.

TUBERCULOUS MENINGITIS.—We may adopt the same method of age comparison as for phthisis ; only in this instance 1871–80 must be compared with 1901, because in 1861–70 the decennial supplement of the Registrar-General did not separately tabulate this disease.

TABLE XIII.—ENGLAND AND WALES

Annual Death-rate from Tuberculous Meningitis per 100,000 Persons of both Sexes at each Age-period

Age-period.	1871–80.	1901.
0–	190	109
5–	30	27
10–	12	12
15–	5	6
20 and upwards	1	2
All Ages	32	18

There has been a reduction in the death-rate from tuberculous meningitis (acute hydrocephalus), which corresponds roughly with that from phthisis (Table XVI.). Tuberculous meningitis is nearly always secondary to other tuberculous diseases, as of the glands or joints. Apart from the presence of such other diseases, and unless an autopsy is made, tuberculous cannot with certainty be distinguished from other forms of meningitis.

Most of the deaths from tuberculous meningitis occur at ages under 5. In the following table the death-rates at each individual year of the first five years of life at the earliest period available in the Registrar-General's reports are compared with those for 1901.

TABLE XIV.—ENGLAND AND WALES

Annual Death-rate from Tuberculous Meningitis per 100,000 Persons of both Sexes at each Age

Period.	Ages.					All Ages under 5.	All Ages.
	0–	1–	2–	3–	4–		
1871–80	368	301	125	76	59	190	32
1901	178	144	83	67	50	109	18
Percentage Decline of Death-rate from Tuberculous Meningitis . . .	52	52	34	12	15	43	47
Corresponding Percentage Decline of Death-rate from Phthisis between 1871–80 and 1901	65	62	51	46	50	60	41

It will be noted that both in 1871–80 and in 1901 the death-rate from tuberculous meningitis at ages under 5 was about six times that at all ages. This appears to indicate that the statistics of the two periods are comparable. Of course it does not follow that they are accurate, and the comparisons given in the two lowest columns of Table XIV. of percentage declines in the death-rate for each of the first five years of life with those of phthisis, throw further doubt on this point. The statistics of tuberculous meningitis in the first year of life are especially open to doubt. H. Armstrong (1902) states that the post-mortem records for eighteen years at the Liverpool Infirmary for Children contain particulars of 85 necropsies in which tuberculous meningitis was found. Of these 10 were in the second year,

18 in the third year, and not one in the first year of life.
Fagge states that only three cases of tuberculous meningitis
in the first year of life were verified in Guy's Hospital in forty
years.

TABES MESENTERICA AND TUBERCULOUS PERITONITIS.—
Tabes mesenterica is a name which should correctly be applied
only when it is clear that the patient has tuberculous disease of
the abdominal lymphatic glands.   Unfortunately it is often used
in death certificates when the patient has died from a slow
wasting disease accompanied or not by abdominal symptoms
such as diarrhœa.   As Drs. Ashby and Wright state in their
work on Diseases of Children, " Mesenteric disease is much
more frequently diagnosed than discovered post-mortem."
Similarly, Dr. Donkin (*Brit. Med. Journ.*, vol. ii. p. 1046, 1899),
says, " All kinds of intestinal and other disorders are constantly
styled tabes mesenterica by those who fail to cure them."   The
usual condition mistaken for it is wasting or marasmus caused
by chronic gastro-intestinal catarrh.   In the great majority of
fatal cases of tabes mesenterica, this disease is accompanied by
general tuberculosis.   Tabes mesenterica is seldom and tuberculous peritonitis still less frequently a direct cause of death.
In the following tables these two diseases are included together.
The separate tabulation of tuberculous peritonitis in the Registrar-
General's returns was not begun till 1901.

TABLE XV.—ENGLAND AND WALES

*Annual Death-rate from Tabes Mesenterica and Tuberculous Peritonitis
per* 100,000 *Persons of both Sexes at each Age-period*

Age-period.	1871–80.	1901.
0–	203	125
5–	13	10
10–	8	7
15–	6	5
20 and upwards	3	3
All Ages	32	19

Here again there has been a reduction in the death-rate

similar to that in phthisis.   The comparison for each of the first
five years of life is shown in the following table :—

TABLE XVI.—ENGLAND AND WALES

*Annual Death-rate from Tabes Mesenterica and Tuberculous Peritonitis
per 100,000 Persons of both Sexes at each Age*

Period.	Ages.					All Ages under 5.	All Ages.
	0-	1-	2-	3-	4-		
1871–80	533	296	88	36	21	203	32
1901	364	138	47	25	17	125	19
Percentage Decline of Death-rate from Tabes Mesenterica . . .	32	53	47	31	19	38	41
Corresponding Percentage Decline of Death-rate from Phthisis between 1871–80 and 1901	65	62	51	46	50	60	41

It will be noted that under 1 year of age the death-rate
from tabes mesenterica declined 32 per cent.   This should be
especially noted because Thorne in his Harben Lectures for 1895,
comparing 1891–95 with 1851–60, showed an increase in the
infantile death-rate under this head of 27·7 per cent, and founded
on it an important inference as to the importance of bovine milk-
supply in the causation of tabes mesenterica.   In view of the
opposing experience when 1871–80 is compared with 1901, the
only inference justifiable is that the statistics of infantile tabes
cannot be trusted.   The general experience of pathologists is
that the number of deaths from tabes increase as the end of the
first year of life approaches.   Compare with this the fact that of
the 2977 deaths registered in 1901 as caused by tabes mesenterica,
594 were at ages under 3 months, 1036 at ages 3–6 months, and
1347 at ages 6–12 months.   Evidently many of the deaths
returned as tabes mesenterica would be found to be due to causes
other than tuberculosis were all death certificates verified by
autopsies.

Although there is a close correspondence in the aggregate
for all ages between the declines in the death-rates from phthisis

and from tabes mesenterica, this is not consistently so at the earlier ages, and we must regard the statistics of this disease as on a plane of trustworthiness much inferior to that occupied by the statistics of phthisis.

COMPARISONS OF DECLINE IN DIFFERENT TUBERCULOUS DISEASES.—Mention has been made of the parallelism of movement of the death-rates from each of the forms of tuberculosis which are tabulated separately by the Registrar-General. This point is worthy of further study, in view of the side-light thrown by it on the trustworthiness of the statistics.

TABLE XVII.—ENGLAND AND WALES

Annual Death-rate per 100,000 *Persons of both Sexes from each of the chief Forms of Tuberculosis*

Period.	Phthisis.	Tuberculous Meningitis.	Tabes Mesenterica.	Scrofula.
5 years, 1850–54	281	43	27	15
5 ,, 1855–59	265	39	26	15
5 ,, 1860–64	257	37	27	16
5 ,, 1865–69	253	35	32	14
5 ,, 1870–74[1]	228	32	30	12
6 ,, 1875–80	208	28	34	14
5 ,, 1881–85	183	26	29	16
5 ,, 1886–90	164	24	27	18
5 ,, 1891–95	146	23	24	19
5 ,, 1896–1900	132	21	20	18
4 ,, 1901–04	123	19	17	17

If we reduce the four columns of death-rates to the same scale by giving each rate for 1901-04 as 100, and state all the other rates in each column in proportion to this, a more exact comparison can be made. The result is shown in Fig. 7. Evidently the somewhat less trustworthy rates for tabes have not consistently followed the law of decline which is shown to an almost equal extent by phthisis and tuberculous meningitis.

[1] The figures up to 1879 are taken from the Annual Report of the Registrar-General of Births and Deaths for 1880, p. lxxix. The classification was altered in 1881, and the returns for scrofula before and after 1880 are not comparable. After 1880 the last column in Table XVII. includes lupus, tubercle of other organs, and general tuberculosis as well as scrofula.

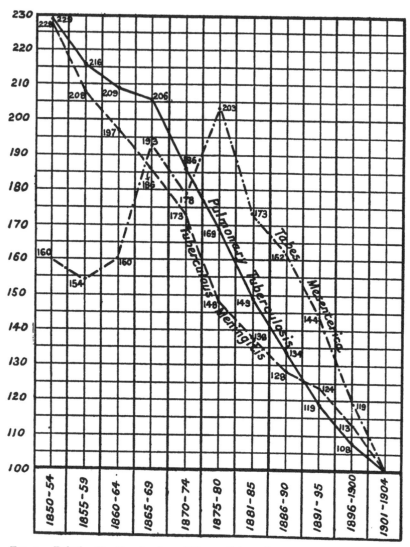

FIG. 7.—Relative Death-rates from different Tuberculous Diseases from 1850–54 to 1901–04, the Death-rate in the most recent period in each instance being stated as 100

CHAPTER IV

THE HISTORY OF PHTHISIS

UNTIL the eighteenth century medical men confused under the names of phthisis or its English equivalent consumption all the acute and chronic diseases of the trachea, bronchi, lungs, pleuræ, and lymphatic glands when these were accompanied by progressive debility and emaciation. In reading the old descriptions of phthisis it is not difficult, however, to recognise that pulmonary tuberculosis formed a large portion of this congeries, and it is not without interest to trace, however sketchily, the views as to the nature of phthisis which have been held in different generations. We may deal first with what may be described as the PRÆ-ANATOMICAL PERIOD, in which post-mortem dissections were rare, and in which views as to the nature of phthisis were based almost solely on the symptoms recognised during life.

Hippocrates (460–377 B.C.) described the disease, ascribing it to a suppuration of the lungs, which may arise in various ways. Galen (130–200 A.D.) also described it, and believed it so infectious that it was dangerous to pass an entire day in the company of a phthisical person (Walshe, p. 459). Hippocrates, Galen, Aretæus (*circa* 50 B.C.), and Celsus (*circa* 30 B.C.) all described the disease, but not one of them appears to have recognised the existence of the tuberculous nodules which form its char-acteristic lesion. With the discovery of these we arrive at the

ANATOMICAL PERIOD.—Franciscus D. Sylvius (1614–1672 A.D.) was the first to recognise the causal relation of these nodules to phthisis, so that the first step towards accurate knowledge of its pathology may be said to have been due to the making of autopsies, which became fairly frequent in the seventeenth century. Sylvius thought the nodules to be the lymphatic glands of the lungs, and thus to be analogous to scrofulous growths. Much speculation was devoted to these nodules ; and in the year 1700 Magnetus first described the more minute nodules known as miliary tubercles, comparing them to millet seeds, and showing their presence in the kidneys, liver, and spleen, as well as in the lungs. Morgagni (1682–1772) disputed the glandular nature of tubercles; Thomas Reid (1778) wrote of them as being not enlarged glands, but the products of exudation. Matthew Baillie (1793) gave the following description of tubercles :—

Tubercles are firm white bodies interspersed through the substance of the lungs, and apparently formed in the cellular structure ; for nothing like a gland is to be discovered in the cellular membrane of the lungs in a healthy state; and the follicles of the bronchi are not converted into tubercles; they are first very minute; the clusters probably unite and form larger masses; the most common in size is that of a garden pea ; they are firm in their consistence, and often contain a portion of thick curdy pus. . . .

Thus Baillie recognised that the large nodules in tuberculosis are produced by fusion of smaller tubercles. He described the cheese-like substance of these large nodules as scrofulous matter, recognising it and pus as the two characteristic products of advanced tuberculosis. At the same time he attempted to distinguish between caseating pneumonia and tubercles in a condition of caseation.

Bayle (1774–1816), the precursor and teacher of Laennec, published in 1810 the records of 109 autopsies on tuberculous patients, and traced the minute tubercles through the subsequent stages of suppuration and caseation. He was of opinion that phthisis was a disease not peculiar to the lungs but dependent on a tuberculous diathesis or special constitutional tendency.

Laennec (1781–1826) made investigations and published teaching on tuberculosis which has been well described as a *tour-de-force* of objective analysis. He taught that every phthisis develops from tubercles, and that phthisis and tuberculosis are interchangeable terms, the tubercle being a new product which appears either in isolated nodules or infiltrated through the tissues. In both forms, he showed that it was first grey and hyaline, gradually becoming opaque and very dense, and later softening and discharging its contents through the bronchi, leaving cavities in the substance of the lungs.

Scrofulous glands were merely tuberculosis confined to the lymphatic glands. Laennec denied the inflammatory origin of tuberculous matter, and especially the transformation of pneumonia into tuberculosis. He was very sceptical also as to the causation of tuberculosis by bronchial catarrh. In these respects modern pathology has in the main confirmed his marvellous insight.

Although Laennec's views were adopted by Louis in France and by Hughes Bennett and others in Great Britain, the tyranny of error gradually overshadowed Laennec's teaching, and what is known as the dualist theory prevailed. According to this theory, which cannot even now be said to be entirely abandoned, most of the lesions of tuberculosis are not due to the tubercles, but are primarily inflammatory in origin, the tubercles being secondary to the inflammatory changes. Niemeyer formulated this view in the words, " The greatest danger to which a phthisical patient is exposed is that of becoming tuberculous."

The PERIOD OF MICROSCOPICAL INVESTIGATION began about 1840, and although it did not solve the problem of the pathological unity between caseous pneumonia and miliary tuberculosis, it was not fruitless. In 1844, Lebert thought he had found distinctive tubercle corpuscles in the tubercles. Rokitansky, whose book on Pathological Anatomy first appeared in 1842, declared that tubercles were new growths composed of inspissated proteins. The doctrine of " dyscrasia " or evil constitutional conditions was then to the fore, and as a follower of this teaching Rokitansky considered the " tuberculous habitus " to be very important.

In 1847, Reinhardt showed that the so-called tubercle corpuscles may originate from pus cells, thus diminishing their importance. In the same year Virchow did much to buttress the dualist theory by teaching that the process of caseation is not peculiar to tuberculosis. In 1852 he limited the term " tubercle " to miliary tubercles, which he described as new growths subsequently changed by caseation, calcification, or fatty degeneration followed by absorption. He is chiefly responsible for the dualist theory which has done much to hinder the progress of investigation.

A step towards unlearning this erroneous teaching was taken when Buhl in 1857 showed that in at least 90 per cent. of his cases of tuberculosis in the lungs pre-existent caseous masses were present somewhere in the body. He attributed the tuberculosis to these cheesy foci, infective products from which had gained admission to the blood and then formed tuberculosis in the lungs or disseminated miliary disease in various organs. Here we have the first clearly expressed conception of miliary tuberculosis as a self-infection caused by the absorption and distribution of infective material derived from older foci in the patient himself.

Although Laennec's teaching led to scrofula being commonly regarded in France as the same disease as tuberculosis, in other countries the belief in its separate origin has only recently disappeared.

The adoption of EXPERIMENTAL METHODS OF INVESTIGATION of tuberculosis led to further advance towards precision of knowledge. From remote times the view that phthisis was an infectious disease had occasionally been taught (p. 55). Some early attempts at producing artificial infection were not successful, and Klencke's successful experiments in 1843 were overlooked. He injected tubercle cells taken from miliary tubercles into the jugular vein of rabbits, and twenty-six weeks later at the autopsy found widespread tuberculosis of liver and lungs.

Villemin's epoch-making experiments were published on December 5, 1865. He inoculated rabbits subcutaneously behind the ear with matter taken from grey and yellow human tubercles, and found that (1) animals thus inoculated developed pulmonary tuberculosis, (2) control animals which had not been inoculated remained free from tubercle, and (3) other animals similarly inoculated with pus from non-tuberculous patients did not develop tuberculosis. Later on he obtained results similar to those given under (1) by inoculating with caseous material from tuberculosis, with the sputum of consumptives, and with tuberculous material from a cow. Villemin summed up the contents of his note to the Académie de Médecine in the following words: " (1) Tuberculosis is the effect of a specific causal agent, in short of a virus. (2) This agent must reside like its congeners in the morbid products formed by its direct action on the normal elements of the affected tissues. (3) Introduced into an organism susceptible to its action, it must continue to reproduce itself, and at the same time to reproduce the disease of which it is the essential principle and the determining cause. Experiment has confirmed these results of induction." He added: " Tuberculosis is a specific affection, caused by an inoculable agent. Tuberculosis belongs then to the class of virulent diseases, and in the nosological scheme must take its place beside syphilis, but closer still to glanders."

The Académie de Médecine was not convinced. During the following year Villemin worked continuously on new experiments, and on October 30, 1866, reopened a discussion on the same subject. Having been accused previously of experimenting on rabbits already tuberculous, he took in his new experiments animals of different species. His inoculation experiments succeeded in nine out of nine rabbits, in two guinea-pigs, in a dog and in a cat. A sheep, a cock, and a pigeon remained immune. Having by his extended basis of operation eliminated the element of chance, he reaffirmed his conclusions, and a commission under Colin was appointed by the Académie to investigate his results. In its report of July 1867 it refused to accept Villemin's conclusions.

They were true notwithstanding; and to Villemin belongs the immortal fame of being the first to show the essential *distinction* in tuberculosis *between the virus causing the disease and the lesions produced by it*. In 1868 he published his *Etudes sur la Tuberculose* in which he further answered objections, vigorously defended the idea of contagion, and argued against the existence of a special tuberculous diathesis, a view which at that time dominated and still influences medical minds to a great extent.

Villemin's experiments were repeated by others with varying results. Progress was retarded by the fact that in some experiments tuberculosis followed the inoculation of pus, particles of sponge, and other apparently non-tuberculous materials. Burdon Sanderson in 1868–69 confirmed Villemin's work, and the following extract from one of his reports to the Medical Officer of the Privy Council shows the stage to which he had brought the investigation :—

As regards the question of a specific contagium of tubercle, we think it very important to note that this is not as yet disproved by the facts of traumatic tuberculosis. It still remains open to inquiry whether or not injuries which are of such a nature that air is completely excluded from contact with the injured part are capable of originating a tuberculous process. The results of the following experiments undertaken at the instance of Mr. Simon, with special reference to this question, seem indeed to suggest that they may not be so. Setons steeped in carbolic acid were inserted in ten guinea-pigs on the 24th of September 1868, each animal receiving two. At the same time extensive fractures of both scapulæ were produced on five others, care being taken not to injure the integuments. No tuberculosis or other disease of internal organs resulted in either case : these facts certainly point to the necessity of further investigation in this direction.

In 1876, when Simon ceased to be Medical Officer to the Local Government Board, the specific infectivity of tuberculosis, and the question whether this infectivity was dependent on a specific organism, were matters which occupied the attention of pathologists in all parts of the world ; but neither question had been settled experimentally. Further trials by Chauveau and Klebs in 1873 and by Baumgarten and Cohnheim in 1880 showed that the discrepant results referred to above were caused by faulty experimentation involving accidental infection of the animals. Thus Cohnheim had in the first instance concluded that tuberculosis is not a specific process. In a second series of experiments, however, he inoculated animals in the anterior chamber of the eye. By this means he was able to follow each stage of evolution of tuberculosis of the iris and cornea, and to establish fully its specific character. On the strength of these experiments he foretold the early discovery of the parasitic agent of tuberculosis. Before this discovery was made H. Martin showed that the nodules produced by foreign bodies were not inoculable in other animals, whereas true tubercles were re-inoculable without any diminution in virulence. Thus the specificity of tubercle was further demonstrated by its continuous inoculability in a series of animals. William Marcet repeated Villemin's results by inoculation of guinea-pigs with tuberculous sputum, and failed to produce similar results with bronchitic sputum ; and he stated rightly that an inoculated guinea-pig might thus serve as a means of diagnosis in doubtful phthisis.

Before the final proof of the specificity of tuberculosis was given, much advance was made in our knowledge of its methods of spread. Chauveau proved that tuberculosis could be produced by eating meat, etc., containing tuberculous material, and concluded that human and bovine tuberculosis were identical.

He also showed that it was the particulate part of morbid secretions which was capable of spreading infection. Villemin had made the statement that tuberculosis could be spread by inhalation of the virus, and pointed out the rôle of dried expectoration in its dissemination ; and Tappeiner was the first to demonstrate on dogs the possibility of dissemination of infection in this way.

Pasteur's work rendered it likely that tuberculosis was due to bacteria. It was found that the basic aniline dyes had a special elective affinity for bacteria, staining them deeply. Ordinary staining by this means failed to show bacteria in the morbid growths of tuberculosis, but after various attempts Robert Koch succeeded in staining the bacilli of tuberculosis by first adding a small quantity of an alkali to the aniline stain, and thus rendering it capable of penetrating the resistant outer membrane of the tubercle bacillus. Other means of obtaining the same result were subsequently discovered ; and a distinctive fact of great importance was discovered, when it was found that even strong mineral acids, which decolorised other stained bacilli, failed to discharge the colour from the tubercle bacillus.

On the 24th March 1882, Koch contributed to the Physiological Society of Berlin his note on " The Discovery and Cultivation of the Bacillus of Tuberculosis." He isolated, cultivated outside the body, described, and differentiated the infective organism of tuberculosis, and proved that it could continue to produce the same lesions indefinitely. By a method of double coloration, he showed the bacilli coloured blue on a brown ground of vesuvin. He showed their presence in all known tuberculous lesions and in tuberculous expectoration, and demonstrated the virulence of the tubercle bacillus in expectoration which had been dried for eight weeks.

Having thus traced the steps by which the crowning demonstration of the infectivity and of the infective agent of tuberculosis was obtained, it will be convenient to summarise briefly the pathological and clinical features of the disease produced by the bacillus, and next to describe its biology, before dealing more fully with the questions of infectivity and the conditions governing the spread of infection.

In looking back on the history of tuberculosis, three names stand out pre-eminently—Laennec, Villemin, and Koch. It is chiefly to these three men,—the last of them aided by the wonderful work of Pasteur and his followers,—that we owe the discovery that tuberculosis is an entirely preventable disease. On their work is based our exact knowledge of the nature of tuberculosis, and the more accurate means for its prevention which we now possess.

The history of phthisis since statistics became available is given in the course of the argument of Part II. (p. 212 *et seq.*).

CHAPTER V

THE MORBID ANATOMY AND SYMPTOMS OF PHTHISIS

THIS work deals solely with tuberculosis from the point of view of preventive medicine and public health. Even when we come to consider the sanatorium treatment of consumptives, this will be chiefly considered as a means of preventing others from becoming consumptive. Notwithstanding this intentional limitation, the subject cannot be discussed fully unless a short description of the pathology and symptoms of tuberculosis is given. Such a description is necessary not only before we can estimate the value of sanatorium treatment, but also in order that the means of spreading and preventing the spread of infection, and particularly the phenomenon of latency, may be understood and their importance appreciated.

Pulmonary tuberculosis is caused by the invasion of the lungs by the tubercle bacillus. The terminal bronchioles ending in the minute air vesicles or alveoli have a diameter of from 3 to 4 tenths of a millimetre, while the tubercle bacillus measures from $1\frac{1}{2}$ to 3 thousandths of a millimetre in length. So far therefore as size is concerned, there is no difficulty in the tubercle bacillus being drawn by inspiration into the air vesicles, where it produces its evil results.

THE COMMENCEMENT OF THE INVASION.—The method by which the bacilli reach the alveoli, whether by inspiration, by spread from the lymphatic glands near the root of the lung, by the blood circulation, or in all these ways at different times, will be considered subsequently.

From the very commencement of the attack the tubercle bacillus meets with resistance. Its opponents are some of the wandering or patrol cells of the body ; in the earlier stages they consist almost entirely of amœboid cells or leucocytes, derived from the blood and the marrow ; at a later stage larger wandering amœboid cells are produced by the rapid proliferation of ordinary non-wandering connective tissue cells and of the cells lining the alveoli or air vesicles. Both kinds have the power of ingesting foreign substances, and are called *phagocytes*.

Attracted chemically by soluble substances produced by the bacilli, phagocytes migrate into the invaded area, and there attack the invaders in two ways. (1) Under the irritation due to bacterial toxins they throw off into solution complex substances called antibodies. These may act either by neutralising the toxins, in which case they are called antitoxins ; or by destroying the bacterium itself. (2) The phagocytes push delicate fingers of protoplasm round the bacteria, which are thus enveloped and afterwards absorbed. The importance of this process of *phagocytosis* was first emphasised by Metchnikoff. Sir Almroth Wright has recently shown that phagocytes cannot absorb bacteria unless the latter have been acted on previously by specific substances present in the fluid part of blood. These substances he has called *opsonins*. They are, like other antibodies, produced by the tissue cells and leucocytes. In normal blood they are present in approximately constant proportion, but great variations occur in disease. The bacillus therefore is opsonised by the surrounding exuded plasma ; its vitality is not affected, but it is in some unknown way rendered absorbable by phagocytes.

THE PROGRESS OF THE INVASION.—If the invasion is small and the leucocytes lusty, the invaders are vanquished. But otherwise the invasion progresses. Leucocytes are killed by the bacterial toxins, and their dead bodies accumulate as pus. The leucocytes may even be a source of danger to the body. They may pass with their load of bacteria into the surrounding tissues, and here, owing to their supply of intracellular antibodies being insufficient, they may be destroyed by the living bacteria within them, so that the bacteria are again free, like the Greeks from the wooden horse in the siege of Troy. It is at this point that we have to take up our description of the lesions produced by tuberculosis.

THE LESIONS IN TUBERCULOSIS.—The tubercle bacilli have entered the body and the leucocytes have failed to kill them. The earliest and most characteristic lesion produced is the *grey tubercle.* Its size varies from a pin's point to a pin's head, or occasionally it may be as large as a small pea. It is grey and slightly translucent. Under the microscope it is seen to consist of a group of small and large cells containing tubercle bacilli. The grey tubercles gradually become converted into *yellow tubercles*, which are opaque, slightly granular, dry and friable. They increase in size by coalescence, and then further changes occur. Both grey and yellow tubercles are destitute of blood vessels, but their presence causes inflammatory changes in the surrounding vascular tissues. This often ends in suppuration with the formation of an abscess, whose contents find their way into the nearest bronchiole and are expectorated. The cavity thus produced in the lung may go on discharging muco-pus for years. It may join with other cavities to form larger cavities ; the discharge from which produces gradual exhaustion of the patient, while the toxic products absorbed from them into the circulation produce the characteristic hectic temperature of phthisis. Occasionally severe hæmorrhage (hæmoptysis) occurs owing to the bursting of a blood vessel. The cavity, if single, may gradually contract and heal. Many consumptives with such cavities in their lungs have under favourable conditions survived and worked for many years.

The change from grey to yellow tubercle is due to caseation, a process so called because the diseased part has a cheesy appearance and consistence. In chronic cases the caseous material may become calcified, and at this stage the process may stop. In small tubercles fibrous changes may occur, the diseased part being converted into fibrous tissue.

Three figures in Hughes Bennett's *Lectures on the Principles and Practice of Medicine* (ed. 1859) so clearly illustrate the three stages of tuberculosis of the lungs that I have reproduced them here. Fig. 8 shows the formation of grey tubercles and some yellow tubercles. At the apex of the lung some of the latter have broken down into an imperfect cavity.

In Fig. 9 a lung is shown in a more advanced condition of disease. Tuberculosis is extensively infiltrated in the upper lobe, and a considerable cavity has formed.

In Fig. 10 the third or last stage of pulmonary tuberculosis is shown. The upper half of the lung is occupied by an enormous cavity, and a smaller cavity has been excavated in the lower lobe. Very often the patient does not survive long enough to show such extensive disease. Happily the history of a large number of cases of pulmonary tuberculosis is not correctly depicted in Figs. 8 to 10. There may be only one or a few of the white dots (grey tubercles) shown in Fig. 8, and these may completely heal by calcification or fibrosis. In fact in very few cases of phthisis is the destructive process continuous. As Hughes Bennett (p. 715) puts it :—

It is continuously checked, and for a time slumbers; and all morbid anatomists have recognised, even in the worst specimens of tubercular lungs, numerous cicatrices and evidences of attempts to heal. These attempts are more or less perfect, and when ineffectual, it is owing to the circumstance that as one portion of lung cicatrises, another becomes the seat of recent tubercle.

In Fig. 11, taken from the same source, the upper portion of a right lung is shown, in which are calcareous masses occupying the place where formerly was active tuberculous disease.

As a rule, except in children, the top of the lung is first and chiefly diseased. The explanations given of this fact are not altogether satisfactory, but it is probable that the anatomical distribution of the bronchial tubes gives the key to the problem. The apical bronchi take a very steep direction upwards ; and this implies that in expiration there is a dead point here, and that in coughing a backward air current may easily drive foreign matter into these relatively inactive regions. The fact that in children apical phthisis is less common may be due to the fact that in them the upper part of the lung is relatively short and the apical bifurcation of bronchi less steep ; but it is also explicable on the supposition that in children invasion of the lungs from the lymphatic glands at their root is more common than in adults.

How Tuberculosis spreads in the Lungs.—This occurs often (a) *through the air passages*. When a cavity is formed and its contents are being expectorated from any one point, it is easy to understand how some of the semi-purulent expectoration can be drawn into the tubes of healthy parts of the lungs. Here it sets up caseating broncho-pneumonia, the lesion which predominates when animals are rendered artificially tuberculous by the inhalation of tuberculous spray. Such cases in man usually progress rapidly. Disease also commonly spreads (b)

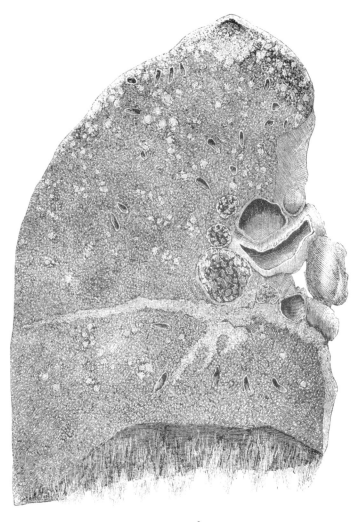

FIG. 8

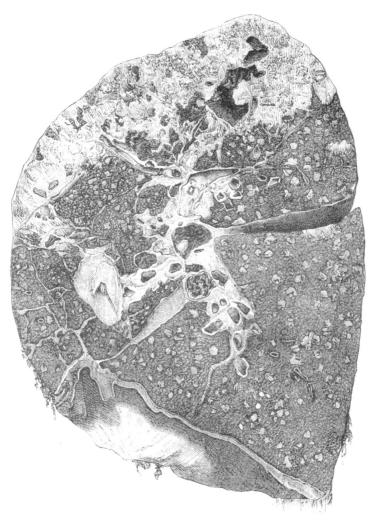

FIG. 9

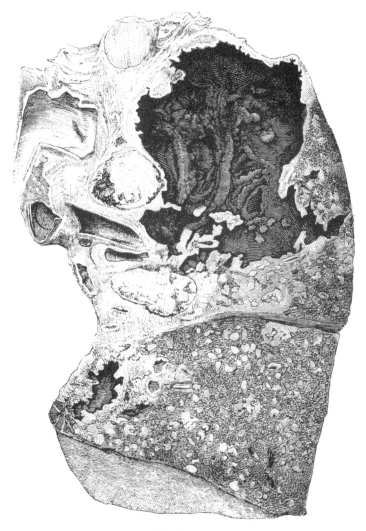

FIG. 10

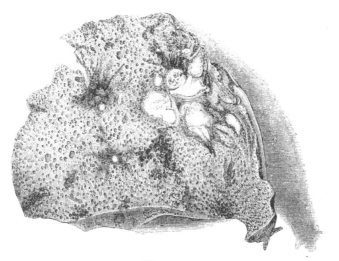

FIG. 11

by infection of the lymphatics. Phagocytes ingest tubercle bacilli from the yellow tubercles, and then pass on into the neighbouring lymphatic vessels. In these vessels or in the glands fed by them such phagocytes as perish release the contained tubercle bacilli, and thus infect neighbouring parts. Hence around a caseous mass are often seen more recent grey and yellow tubercles. The lymphatic glands at the root of the lung are also involved early. (c) If the infective material gains access *to the blood vessels*, as when a tuberculous growth erodes the coat of a vessel, bacteria are disseminated by the circulation of blood either to other parts of the same lung or throughout the body, producing general tuberculosis.

Symptoms of Phthisis.—From the preceding description of the lesions found in fatal cases of phthisis the symptoms of the fully established disease may be gathered. An irritating cough, accompanied by abundant expectoration of muco-purulent material, in which tubercle bacilli can usually be found ; hectic fever ; copious cold sweats at night ; and rapid emaciation.

The *symptoms of onset* are commonly very insidious. The patient is languid, suffers from increasing weakness, and is often thought to be suffering from " anæmia." Anæmia with a dry cough in most instances means early phthisis. Sometimes profuse hæmoptysis is the earliest symptom recognised, and it is often the first symptom which induces a patient to consult a doctor. This symptom always means that an already formed tubercle, usually a caseous mass, has ulcerated into a blood vessel, and indicates therefore older tuberculous disease.

At certain stages of phthisis there may be no expectoration, and this does not always imply that active mischief is in abeyance. Cases with expectoration are described by German doctors as " open," those without as " closed " ; the distinction is important, as the latter are relatively non-infective. Progressive cases all become " open " sooner or later.

Varieties of Phthisis.—The great majority of cases belong to the chronic variety. Some are very *acute*, the whole case only lasting from a few weeks to three or four months. Such cases often resemble pneumonia, and some are so acute as to simulate enteric fever. Of the *chronic form* of disease, some show progressive deterioration, ending fatally in from six to twelve months; others have repeated acute attacks, with intervals of apparent recovery and quiescence, the intervals becoming shorter as time progresses ; in others a sharp attack occurs, and the patient then permanently recovers. To these must be added a large number of unrecognised cases, in which recovery occurs, and in which it is difficult to obtain any history of lung disease. The patient may have been " off colour " for a time, may have been anæmic, and may have had a slight cough. He then " recovers by encapsulation, unaware that the shadow of the black hawk's wing had rested upon him " (Allbutt, p. 1152). Further particulars of such cases are given, pp. 82 to 84.

THE CURABILITY OF PHTHISIS. — The vast majority of attacks of phthisis are followed by recovery. This fact cannot be too strongly emphasised. It is not a new fact discovered since the open-air treatment of the disease came into vogue, but has been known to pathologists and physicians from time immemorial. Hippocrates taught that " phthisis, if treated early enough, gets well." In modern times Carswell (quoted by Brouardel, p. 66) wrote in 1838 : " Pathological anatomy has never, perhaps, given a more decided proof of the cure of a disease than it gives in cases of pulmonary phthisis."

Hughes Bennett (p. 716) says :—

In 1845, I made a series of observations with reference to the cretaceous masses and puckerings so frequently observed at the apices of the lungs in persons advanced in life. The conclusion arrived at was, that the spontaneous arrestment of tubercle in its early stage occurred in the proportion of from one-third to one-half of all the individuals who die after the age of forty. The observations of Rogée and Boudet, made at the Salpêtrière Hospital in Paris, amongst individuals generally above the age of seventy, showed the proportion in such persons to be respectively one-half and four-fifths.

According to Charcot, " phthisis is susceptible of cure completely and definitely even at the period of cavities." Brouardel quotes Laennec, Nat. Guillot, and Letulle as showing that in more than half the post-mortem examinations made by them old healed tuberculous lesions were to be found.

Commenting on these results Dr. Ribard says :—

These figures, from the similarity even of their results, are striking. They show very clearly that half the men, said to be well and non-tuberculous, dying of old age or fortuitous causes, have at a certain time in their life been attacked by tuberculosis but have recovered. Many are therefore affected, and many recover, if half the human race have tubercle and go on living without discovering them. Such is the truly reassuring result of autopsies.

Dr. Thomas Harris of Manchester (1889) taking the deaths of persons over 20 years of age who died in the Manchester Royal Infirmary found healed phthisis ("involuted tuberculosis ") in about 38 per cent. of the post-mortem examinations made by him.

Coates (1891, p. 351), after giving an account of 131 consecutive autopsies at the Glasgow Royal Infirmary, says : " It appears that, taking even the most serious forms of internal tuberculosis, such as consolidation of lungs, tuberculous disease of the verte-bræ, tuberculosis of the peritoneum, there is evidence that spontaneous recovery takes place in a proportion equal to that in which death occurs."

Austin Flint (1882), after analysing 670 cases of phthisis in his practice, concluded that " in a certain proportion of cases this disease ends favourably irrespectively of any ap-preciable extrinsic agencies." He draws attention as follows to the self-limitation which is exemplified in the majority of fatal cases (p. 617) :—

The disease, as a rule, advances not by a continuous progress, but by a series of successive. invasions separated by variable intervals. After each invasion, or as it has been termed tuberculous eruption, there is a temporary self-limitation of the disease.

The continuous advancement of the disease as an exception to the rule is the pathological feature of the so-called " galloping consumption " or phthisis florida.

DURATION OF PHTHISIS.—From the preceding pages it is evident that the duration of phthisis is very variable. It is interesting to note the estimates of its duration given by different authors. According to Austin Flint it may vary from three weeks to forty years. Similarly Portal said " eleven days to forty years." Laennec gave its average duration excluding miliary tuberculosis as 24 months, Louis and Boyle on the strength of 314 cases said 23 months, Audral 24 months, Sir J. Clark (from patients in private practice) 36 months. C. J. B. Williams and C. T. Williams (Quain, 1894) give an average duration in 198 fatal cases of $7\frac{3}{4}$ years, and in 802 living cases of $8\frac{1}{8}$ years. All these cases had been over a year under observa-tion, which necessarily excludes some acute cases ; but with this exception they state that these figures " may be taken as a correct average for the duration of the disease among the upper classes under modern treatment, especially as 72 per cent. of the living had recovered sufficiently to pursue their usual avocations, and many among them had already lived upwards of 20 years since their first attack."

Walshe (1871) gives the average duration for hospital cases in Paris as 23·5 months. He speaks of a case lasting 22 years, and of cases frequently lasting from 5 to 10 years. Dettweiler gives the average duration of life of the middle-class consumptive as 7 years, but Cornet (p. 250) says that the average duration in adults cannot be placed higher than 3 years, and in children even less. He also quotes Leudet's data, which comprise 48 cases, among whom the average duration was 5 years for those in good circumstances, 3½ years for those in hospitals. All the figures show a shorter duration among the poor than among the well-to-do.

If the average duration of phthisis could be worked out separately for patients whose illness started at different ages some light would probably be thrown on the varying estimates given above. As a general rule, it is a more acute illness in the young, and becomes more chronic with advancing years, though there are many exceptions to this rule. A further point doubtless has affected the estimates of its duration quoted above. It is well known that in the less acute cases the course of the disease is not uninterrupted. There are attacks of " bad colds," of " influenza," or of pleurisy, or of actually recognised phthisis and then occur intervals in which all symptoms are in abeyance these intervals shortening if the case progresses. The intervals may sometimes extend over many years. Is the duration of such cases to be reckoned from the first occurrence of recognisable symptoms to the end of the case ? If so, many months and even years in which the patient is apparently well will be included. Until these points are settled, statements as to average duration of phthisis should only be accepted when accompanied by information as to the intervals during which symptoms were in abeyance.

CHAPTER VI

THE TUBERCLE BACILLUS

THE tubercle bacillus (or bacillus of tuberculosis) is a non-motile organism, rod-like in shape, with rounded ends. Its length is from 2 to 5 μ (μ = one-thousandth of a millimetre), that is, from one-half to one-third the diameter of a red blood corpuscle, whilst its width is about one-sixth of its length. When stained with aniline dyes the bacilli often show a beaded appearance, which Koch regarded as indicating the presence of spores ; but this point is doubtful. We have already seen (p. 41) that Koch succeeded in staining the bacilli after long soaking of cover-slip preparations in alkaline methylene-blue and then using vesuvin as a brown contrast stain. Ehrlich soon made known a more certain and more convenient procedure. He first stained for fifteen to twenty minutes with an aqueous solution of aniline methyl violet or fuchsin, and then decolorised with dilute nitric acid, which eliminated the colour from everything except the tubercle bacilli. Other methods have been since devised, of which the following is the most convenient, especially for the examination of suspected sputum.

THE ZIEHL-NIELSEN METHOD OF STAINING.—A small solid bit of sputum is taken, spread on a clean cover-glass and allowed to become dry. The cover-slip, held in a forceps, is then passed three times through the flame of a spirit lamp, holding the sputum-spread side uppermost. This fixes the film. A watch-glass is partially filled with a solution composed of fuchsin 1 part, absolute alcohol 10 parts, and carbolic acid (5 per cent. aqueous solution) 100 parts. The cover-slip is placed film downwards on this solution, which is heated until it steams slightly. The cover-slip after three to five minutes is removed, the excess of dye washed off with water, and the slip then dipped in a 1 in 4 solution of sulphuric acid. As soon as all visible colour has disappeared from the film, it is rinsed with several portions of a 60 to 70 per cent.

alcohol, and finally with water. The film is then counter-stained with a 1 per cent. aqueous solution of methylene-blue. On miscroscopic examination the specimen thus prepared shows the red bacilli on a blue background.

The above staining reaction is almost specific for the tubercle bacillus, since the leprosy bacillus and the few others which act somewhat similarly in resisting the decolorising effect of acids are very rarely found under circumstances in which confusion would be likely to arise. When bacilli in human expectoration answer to the above test it is practically certain that the expectoration is derived from a tuberculous patient.

It must be remembered that negative results from single examinations of suspected sputum carry little weight. Three specimens at least should be mounted from each sputum, and in each of these a large field, spread over the slide in preference to the cover-slip, should be examined before a negative certificate is given.

BIOLOGY OF THE TUBERCLE BACILLUS.—For more complete study of the biological relations of the tubercle bacillus it is necessary to cultivate it on or in artificial media in the laboratory. Koch ascertained that it would not grow on the ordinary laboratory media, gelatine, agar, etc., because these did not remain unaltered at the body temperature. He finally hit on coagulated blood serum as a suitable medium, because it remained solid and moist at the body temperature. Having obtained tuberculous material from newly killed animals suffering from recent tuberculosis, he successfully grew tubercle bacilli by rubbing this material thoroughly on the blood serum by means of a platinum loop, and then placing in an incubator at blood heat (37° C.). After the fifth day dull white specks appeared on the surface of the serum, and these gradually increased in size, producing small dry scales, which subsequently became confluent, forming a greyish-white covering to the serum, the latter not being penetrated or liquefied. He subsequently succeeded in obtaining similar growths from the cavities of tuberculous lungs, from lupus, etc. From observations on such cultures, and on cultures in glycerine bouillon agar, have been deduced certain facts as to the persistence of the life of the tubercle bacillus which have important bearings on the prevention of tuberculosis.

RANGE OF TEMPERATURE.—The tubercle bacillus of mammalian tuberculosis ceases to grow below 29° C. and over 42° C., of avian tuberculosis below 25° C. and over 45° C. The best temperature for the growth of the mammalian tubercle bacillus is 37°–38° C. As these temperatures are not common in the external world, it is important to note that, as Cornet (p. 42) remarks, the tubercle bacillus does not meet with the conditions of growth " except solely and exclusively within the animal organism with its constant and equable temperature of 37°–39° C." Or as Dr. Moxon (1885) put it : " The life of the bacillar parasite is difficult, easily discouraged by unfavourable circumstance, like an aphis by an eastern wind." Beevor, Delépine, and Kanthack have succeeded in obtaining growths of the tubercle bacillus on potato at room temperature ; but this is difficult, and there is no evidence that it occurs frequently. Extreme cold does not kill the bacillus. There is considerable discrepancy in the evidence as to the *thermal death-point* of the tubercle bacillus. Probably different strains of bacilli vary in this respect, and much will depend on the medium surrounding them. Further details on this point will be found on page 409. Generally the tubercle bacillus is destroyed after 4 to 6 hours' exposure to a temperature of 55° C. ; after 15 minutes at 65° C. ; after 5 minutes at 80° C. ; after 2 minutes at 90° C. ; and in a less time at the temperature of boiling water. In a dried condition its vitality may survive higher temperatures than the above.

The RESISTANCE TO DESICCATION shown by the tubercle bacillus is its most significant biological feature. It appears to owe this resistance to the fact that it contains more fat than other bacilli. Koch found that phthisical expectoration which had been allowed to dry and been kept at room temperature for five to eight weeks was still virulent at the end of the time. Schill and Fischer found dried expectoration still virulent on the 95th day, dead on the 179th day. Toma found dried expectoration virulent up to ten months (Cornet, p. 43). The duration of vitality is much less when the tubercle bacilli are exposed to SUNLIGHT. Koch found that in direct sunlight they died after an exposure varying from a few minutes to several hours, according to the thickness of the layer exposed. Diffuse light has the same effect after an appreciably longer time. Strauss found that flourishing cultures of mammalian tubercle bacilli perished completely on exposure for two hours to the rays of the summer sun, while cultures dried in thin smears on glass plates had lost their virulence under similar conditions in half an hour. More recently Mitchell and Crouch (quoted by Lartigau, p. 29) from a study of the influence of sunlight on tuberculous expectoration at Denver concluded that the tubercle bacillus as expectorated on a sandy soil is still virulent after thirty-five hours' exposure to the direct rays of the sun, the virulence becoming lost soon afterwards.

Where there is no free access of air or sunlight the retention of virulence in deposited tubercle bacilli has been observed at the end of 130 days by Ransome and of 184 days by Fischer. It may be added that Cadeac and Malet have produced positive results by inoculation of material from tuberculous lungs which had previously been buried for 167 days.

It must be noted that the fact that a tubercle bacillus takes and retains the specific stain, does not prove it to be alive. A bacillus heated to the temperature of boiling water will take the stain equally well. This remark is important in view of the enormous numbers of tubercle bacilli daily expectorated by consumptives (p. 104). It is probable that the majority of them are non-virulent, though in phthisis generally the infectivity probably is proportional to the total number of bacilli discharged. The infectivity although great must not be exaggerated. The tubercle bacillus grows with exceptional slowness both inside and outside the body. It has a feeble vitality under both conditions, and is easily rebuffed. The one circumstance under which the extra-corporeal life of the bacillus is prolonged is desiccation in places not exposed to sunshine. Such dry expectoration will contain numerous living bacilli.

CHAPTER VII

INFECTIVITY OF TUBERCULOSIS: *A*. HISTORY OF VIEWS HELD

THE belief in the infectivity of phthisis is as old as any extant account of the disease. Hippocrates said that it was of all diseases the most dangerous, and fatal to the greatest number of mankind. Galen believes it to be dangerous to pass a single day in the company of a consumptive. Avicenna the Arabian (A.D. 1037) referred to diseases which are " taken from man to man like phthisis." Ballonius, a physician of large practice in Paris in the fifteenth century, noted the frequent occurrence of phthisis in those who tended consumptives. Both Morgagni and his teacher Valsalva (seventeenth century) asserted that they objected to conduct autopsies on consumptives on account of the danger of infection. In Italy the belief in the infectiousness of phthisis took practical form in legislative enactments. In 1746, Ferdinand VI. issued to the medical men in charge of the various districts an instruction which ran as follows :—

Experience having shown how dangerous is the use of linen, furniture, and articles which have been used by persons afflicted with, or who have died of hectic, phthisical, or other contagious diseases, we enjoin on all physicians to give notice of those persons who are sick with or who have died of phthisis, so that the Alcade may cause the linen, clothing, furniture, and other objects used personally by the patient, or which have been in his department, to be burned ; so that the Alcade may also order the apartment in which the patient died to be replastered and whitewashed, and the flooring or flagging of the room or alcove in which the patient's bed was placed to be changed. Besides, a registration must be kept of places from which clothing found in the shops of second-hand clothes dealers comes, with information as to the names and residences of the vendors, as well as the persons who have used the linen and garments, and dealers in old clothes ordinarily doing business in infected clothes. The Alcade shall issue a paper attesting that the said goods are free from contagion ; this paper shall be the sole authorisation by which dealers in second-hand goods will be allowed to keep or sell such goods. Any physician who will not give notice of consumptive patients, or those who have died of consumption, to the Alcade of his quarter, shall incur, for the first offence, a fine of 200 ducats and suspension from the practice of his profession for one year ; and for repetition of the offence a fine of 400 ducats and the punishment of exile for four years. All other persons (infirmarians, domestics, attendants on the sick) who will not report the case shall incur a penalty of thirty days in prison for the first offence, and four years in the galleys for the second offence. Civil, religious, and military authorities shall cause to be burned in civil and military hospitals all linen which shall have been used by phthisical civilians or soldiers.

In 1754 the members of the College of Physicians of Florence pronounced themselves as on the whole favouring the conclusion that phthisis is communicable. In 1782 the city of Naples, warned of the infectivity of phthisis by the Medical College of its University, enforced a law for the isolation of consumptives and the disinfection of their homes and belongings.

Nor were such views confined to Italy. In a letter to the *Lancet* by Dr. Stretton (December 17, 1898), the following quotation is given from a book written by Gideon Harvey, M.D., about 1660, in which consumption is described as an endemic and epidemic disease :—

And considering withal its malignity and contagious nature, it may be numbered among the worst Epidemicks or popular diseases, since next to the Plague, Pox, and Leprosie, it yields to none in point of contagion ; for it's no rare observation here in England, to see a fresh coloured lusty young man yoake to a consumptive female, and him soon after attending her to the grave.   Moreover nothing we find taints sound lungs sooner, than inspiring or drawing in the breath of putrid ulcered consumptive lungs ; many having fallen into consumptions, only by smelling the breath or spittle of Consumptives, others by drinking after them ; and what is more, by wearing the Cloaths of Consumptives, though two years after they were left off.

In *The Expedition of Humphry Clinker*, written by Smollett in 1771, the same notion of infectiousness finds laughable expression. Writing from a fashionable inland health-resort, he says :—

I wish I had not come from Brambletonhall, after having lived in solitude so long.   I cannot bear the hurry and impertinence of the multitude ; besides, everything is sophisticated in these crowded places. Snares are laid for our lives in everything we eat or drink ; the very air we breathe is loaded with contagion. We cannot even sleep, without risk of infection. I say, infection. This place is the rendezvous of the diseased. You won't deny, that many diseases are infectious ; even the consumption itself is highly infectious. When a person dies of it in Italy, the bed and bedding are destroyed ; the other furniture is exposed to the weather, and the apartment whitewashed before it is occupied by any other living soul. You'll allow, that nothing receives infection sooner, or retains it longer, than blankets, feather-beds, and mattresses— 'Sdeath ! how do I know what miserable objects have been stewing in the bed where I now lie ? I wonder, Dick, you did not put me in mind of sending for my own mattresses; but, if I had not been an ass, I should not have needed a remembrancer. There is always some plaguy reflection that rises up in judgment against me, and ruffles my spirits ; therefore let us change the subject.

The experience of George Sand is also interesting. In 1839 she wrote from Spain as follows concerning Chopin, her travelling companion, who was already consumptive, although he did not die until ten years later :—

Poor Chopin, who had a cough since leaving Paris, became very ill. I called in a doctor—two doctors—three doctors, each more stupid than the other, and soon it was spread abroad that he was in the last stage of consumption. There was great alarm, phthisis being rare in these climates, and regarded as contagious. We were regarded as pest-breeders; and furthermore as heathens, as we did not go to Mass. The owner of the small house which we had rented turned us brutally out of doors, threatening furthermore to bring an action against us compelling us to limewash his house, which he said we had infected. We were plucked by the law like chickens.

At Barcelona later on the landlord demanded to be paid for the bed on which Chopin had slept.

Medical men gradually tended towards the opinion that tuberculosis was non-infectious, and began to explain it as a manifestation of a special constitution or diathesis, while public opinion in many countries still regarded it as infectious, this belief being carried in some instances to foolish extremes. The histories of cholera and influenza present similar anomalies. Thus the Royal College of Physicians of London in 1854 reported that " the theory that cholera is propagated and diffused by means of human intercourse, receives no support from the facts relating to variations in the intensity of cholera epidemics, and the circumstances determining these variations." In another part of their report they quoted the extraordinary rapidity of the increase of cholera in a town as " an additional reason for believing that the diffusion of cholera in a town is independent of contagion." In the same report they record their impression that "the share borne by human intercourse in the dissemination of the disease is larger" than the statistical facts seem to indicate. A joint inquiry was made by the Provincial Medical Association of England into the contagiousness of influenza in the epidemic of 1836–37, the medical answers to the questions on this point being "of an almost uniform tenour, the opinion of nearly all those who had the most extensive opportunities of investigating the disease, and the best means of arriving at a definite conclusion, being that there is no proof of the existence of any contagious principle by which it was propagated from one individual to another."

And yet more exact information and more accurate medical investigations have proved that infection is the sole means for the spread of these two diseases. Tuberculosis differs from them in infectivity chiefly in its longer latency and more protracted course.

CHAPTER VIII

INFECTIVITY OF TUBERCULOSIS: *B.* EXPERIMENTAL EVIDENCE

INFECTION BY INOCULATION. — Villemin's experiments (p. 38) gave the first positive evidence of infectivity. Previous conclusions to this effect were of the nature of surmises, and naturally liable to exaggeration and misconception. Villemin's experiments undoubtedly did much to popularise the idea that tuberculosis is an infectious disease. Koch's experiments demonstrated this fact, and placed Villemin's induction on a solid foundation.

Koch's experiments may be briefly summarised, as they illustrate admirably the process used to prove the causal relation between a given microbe and the specific disease caused by it.

(1) He took as seed material the tuberculous lymphatic glands from freshly killed guinea-pigs which had been inoculated about three or four weeks previously with tuberculous material. (2) This material was smeared on blood serum and incubated at 37° C. until a sufficient growth of tubercle bacilli had slowly occurred. (3) From this test-tube cultivation other tubes of blood serum were similarly smeared, by rubbing some of the small scales from the first tube over the serum in them. Koch cultivated the tubercle bacilli in test tubes in this way through as many as seventy generations. (4) The inoculation of guinea-pigs and other susceptible animals with such cultures was followed by the appearance of tuberculous nodules and other lesions identical with those found in the animals which produced the original tuberculous material. (5) Tubercle bacilli were found in these experimentally produced lesions as in the original lesions of the first animals, and these tubercle bacilli showed the same cultural characters, and when inoculated into animals produced similar lesions to those of the original

disease. Similar experiments made with tuberculous expectoration from human consumptives, and with tuberculous meat and milk, gave the same results. The proof is rendered complete by the further fact that tubercle bacilli are not found in any diseased conditions other than tuberculosis.

This is a convenient point to revert to the instances in which apparently tubercles had been experimentally produced by non-specific inoculation (p. 39). Klebs suggested that extraneous infection was the cause of these anomalous results, and Fränkel and Cohnheim showed that this was the correct explanation. Watson Cheyne (1883) proved the same thing by a series of carefully checked experiments on rodents. Wilson Fox in 1867–68 had apparently produced tuberculosis in twenty-three out of 117 animals inoculated with such materials as pus, putrid muscle, seton, etc., which were supposed to be non-tuberculous. At his suggestion the experiments were repeated some years later by Dawson Williams, under conditions which prevented the occurrence of external infection, and in each case a negative result was now obtained.

The evidence that tuberculosis is infective is not confined to experimental inoculation. Were it so, it might still be reasonably contended that tuberculosis is only communicable like tetanus or hydrophobia by introduction of the infective material (contagium) under the skin. Experimental observations, however, have proved that it can be spread either by the inhalation or the ingestion (swallowing) of tuberculous material.

Infection by Inhalation. — Tuberculosis has frequently been induced in guinea-pigs by making them breathe in an atmosphere containing dust contaminated by tubercle bacilli. The lungs in such animals become tuberculous in two or three weeks, the extent of the lesions depending on the duration of life before the animal is killed or dies. The lungs present the same appearances of caseous pneumonia as do the lungs of man in ordinary phthisis. The liver and spleen of the infected animals also become tuberculous, and the bronchial glands appear to be affected as soon as the lungs.

Infection by Ingestion.—Experimental tuberculosis of the intestine has been produced in guinea-pigs, rabbits, dogs, cats, calves, sheep, monkeys, etc., by feeding them with tuberculous material. Pigs are readily susceptible to such infection, and frequently become infected through being fed on skimmed milk derived from tuberculous cows. In these cases the small lymphatic follicles in the wall of the intestine are commonly infected first, followed about four weeks later by the mesenteric and cæcal glands. Out of twenty animals examined after experimental feeding with tuberculous material Sidney Martin found the small intestine to be involved in all but one, and the cæcum in all but three. Intestinal lesions may be absent, especially when the dose of infection is small ; and in this case the first lesions are in the lymphatic glands. From the mesenteric and cæcal glands the infection passes to the cœliac glands, the liver and spleen, the bronchial and posterior mediastinal glands, and the lungs. Baumgarten, Fisher, and others have shown that tubercle bacilli can pass through the mucous membrane of the intestine without producing any local ulcer.

CHAPTER IX

INFECTIVITY OF TUBERCULOSIS: *C*. STATISTICAL AND CLINICAL EVIDENCE

O N the strength of the statements given on pp. 8 and 49, it has been assumed by some that phthisis is so common and so often a non-fatal disease that everyone is more or less exposed to infection, and that consequently infection can play only a very minor part in its causation. The evidence as to the percentage of the total population (say roughly one in every two) showing evidence of old tuberculous lesions is derived from hospital practice. Persons belonging to this type possibly form a majority of the total population, and although the proportion probably is smaller in other grades of life, we may assume for present purposes that the same proportion holds good for the general population in England and Wales. But it by no means follows that one-half of the total population at any given time is actively tuberculous and discharging tuberculous material. The fact that recovery has occurred and the patients have died from other diseases or from accident, shows the absurdity of such an assumption. It is highly probable that the vast majority of those showing post-mortem these healed lesions were " closed " cases, in which the micro-organisms could not escape ; so that the patients were not infective even during a few months of their life. Further light is thrown on the point by a comparison between the deaths from phthisis and the population at each five- or ten-yearly period of life. In Table XVIII. the deaths from phthisis have been multiplied by three, on the commonly accepted supposition that for each death from phthisis during a given year, three other patients have been constantly ill with the same disease. On this basis it will be seen that the proportion òf consumptives in the general population is 1 for every 263 persons, varying from 1 in 1881 at ages 5–10 to 1 in 141 at ages 35–45. At the working years of life, 20–65, on the same assumption it is 1 in 168.   Probably the number actually phthisical at any given time exceeds this proportion; but it is equally probable that *the number at any given time capable of imparting infection* is not greater than these figures would

TABLE XVIII

At Ages—	Population of England and Wales at the Census 1901.	Deaths from Pulmonary Phthisis in England and Wales in 1901.	On the Assumption that each Annual Death from Phthisis means the Presence of three Consumptives in the Population, the Proportion of Consumptives in the General Population at each Age-period was—
Under 5 . . .	3,716,708	1,171	1 in 1006
5–10 . . .	3,487,291	623	1 ,, 1881
10–15 . . .	3,341,740	987	1 ,, 1129
15–20 . . .	3,246,143	2,917	1 ,, 371
20–25 . . .	3,120,922	4,590	1 ,, 227
25–35 . . .	5,255,840	9,922	1 ,, 177
35–45 . . .	3,996,005	9,451	1 ,, 141
45–55 . . .	2,902,191	6,653	1 ,, 145
55–65 . . .	1,943,250	3,459	1 ,, 187
65–75 . . .	1,076,006	1,260	1 ,, 285
75 and upwards .	441,747	193	1 ,, 763
Total—All Ages .	32,527,843	41,226	1 in 263

NOTE.—The above proportions are based on an average duration of three years for each case of phthisis. On page 360 I have assumed an average duration of ten years, which would include also a large number of cases that are never fatal. These estimates must be carefully distinguished from the estimated numbers discussed on page 15, which are concerned with ascertaining in a life-table population traced to death, how many total consumptives there are.

lead one to suppose.   On this point the considerations detailed in Chapter XIII., and particularly on page 101 need to be borne in mind.

CLINICAL EVIDENCE OF INFECTIVITY.—Underlying all investigations of the history of individual cases for evidence of infectivity are certain fundamental data, which may conveniently be summarised here :—

   1. Tuberculosis is due to a specific bacillus.

   2. Tuberculosis has been produced experimentally in animals by the introduction of this bacillus, in inspired air or with food.

3. Man is subject, *e.g.* in infected households and workshops, to the conditions which have been proved experimentally to produce tuberculosis in animals.

It is in the light of these general considerations that the following instances of probable infection are to be judged. They are given as typical of the form of reasoning which in the light of wider investigations is now known to be applicable to such cases, and of the kind of evidence which without such wider investigation could not be regarded as possessing great weight.

All the following cases have been taken from local investigations of notified cases.

CASE 1.—*Domestic infection.   Father to son*

C. P., æt. 25, admitted to sanatorium October 5, died November 22, 1906, of acute phthisis. Was unmarried, and lived with his parents up to the time of his illness. His mother, two sisters, and a brother are alive and well. No tuberculosis known in the family except the father.

Domestic Influences.	Age.	Year.	Extra-domestic Influences.
	0	1881	
	14	1895	Worked as a labourer, "odd jobs," up to 19.
Probably father was ill from this date.	19	1900	Has worked as a general labourer, generally in the shops of the railway works.
In June 1903, father died, æt. 41, death being returned as due to "pulmonary and laryngeal tuberculosis, 15 months."	22	1903	
C. P. says he had no cough until a few weeks before admission to sanatorium.	25	1906	

Comments on Case 1.—There was protracted infection from the father ; also possible industrial infection, but this would be only casual.   A latent period of at least three years occurred between his father's death and his first symptoms.

CASE 2.—*Domestic infection.   Father to son, or brothers to brother. Action of auxiliary influences*

W. O., admitted to sanatorium September 18, discharged

October 25, 1906; had advanced tuberculosis both lungs.   Had cough for four years before admission.   Four sisters and one brother have escaped tuberculosis.

Domestic Influences.	Age.	Year.	Extra-domestic Influences.
	o	1871	
Mother died of phthisis . .	13	1884	
	14	1885	Apprenticed as a gasfitter.
Brother died of phthisis, æt. 22, in Brompton Hospital; had previously lived at home.	19	1890	
Another brother died of phthisis, æt. 27, at W. Until a few months previously had lived with present patient. Domestic infection ceased in 1892.	21	1892	
	28–31	1899–1902	Served in the Boer War. Had enteric fever. *Began to cough while in South Africa.*
Lived in lodgings after returning from South Africa.	33	1904	*Had pleurisy*, and was aspirated.
	33–35	1904–06	Gasfitter.

Comments on Case 2.—In my opinion the protracted domestic infection which ceased nine to ten years before he began to cough caused this patient's tuberculosis, the sickness, exposure, and privations of the Boer War serving to light up latent trouble. The alternative is that more recent infection in South Africa caused his illness.

The same question of domestic or industrial infection is raised in Case 3.

CASE 3.—*Domestic infection from brothers and sisters*

A. G., æt. 32, admitted to sanatorium August 1, discharged September 12, 1906.   The main facts are set forth in the scheme on next page.

Comments on Case 3.—The patient's father and mother are alive and well, and there is no family history of phthisis in past generations or among uncles or aunts.   The patient has been exposed to home infection from childhood until he was 15 years old.   His first symptoms of phthisis occurred ten years later. Several possibilities of casual extra-domestic infection present

5

themselves—(1) when a railway shunter; (2) when a black smith. His work at a music hall was after frequent cough had

Domestic Influences.	Age.	Year.	Extra-domestic Influences.
Excepting the years 1897–1902, has lived at home and been exposed to the following chances of acquiring tuberculosis :—	o	1874	
One brother, æt. 19, died at home of phthisis.	5	1879	
One sister, æt. 21, died at home of phthisis.	7	1881	
One sister, æt. 5, died at home of "congestion of lungs."	8	1882	
	13	1887	Left school.
	15	1889	} In an auctioneer's office.
	17	1891	A railway porter in E. (shunting and lamps—did not clean out carriages).
A sister, æt. 21, died in an asylum of phthisis, 3 years after leaving home.	19	1893	Has worked during these ten years as a striker and black smith in the railway works.
Patient left home and went into lodgings for 5 years.	23	1897	
Began to have a slight cough from this time.	26	1900	
Patient returned home. No known domestic infection from 1890 (the date sister left for an asylum) up to 1906.	28	1902	
A brother, æt. 42 (married, with 4 children), attended Brompton Hospital for a few months with one lung affected. No chance of infection between the two brothers.	30	1904	Worked as an attendant at a music hall. Is somewhat alcoholic.
In July, severe hæmoptysis . .	32	1906	

occurred, and probably the same remark applies to his alcoholic habits.

CASE 4.—*Protracted domestic infection from parents and brothers and sisters*

Florence S., æt. 24, admitted to sanatorium September 3, discharged November 24, 1906; early phthisis, with tuberculous cervical glands.

The main facts are set forth below.

Domestic Influences.	Age.	Year.	Extra-domestic Influences.
Has been exposed to domestic infection probably from early childhood.	0	1882	
Father, a waiter, died, æt. 45, of phthisis.	8	1890	After the father's death in 1890, the mother began a small laundry, and the patient and her two sisters have helped in it. The patient is chiefly engaged at needlework.
A brother, æt. 15, died of phthisis.	11	1893	
A sister died of phthisis . .	12	1894	
Mother died, æt. 48, of phthisis . *First noticed enlarged cervical glands. Axillary glands soon afterwards inflamed and suppurated for two years.*	16	1898	
A brother died, æt. 28, of phthisis .	17	1899	
A brother, æt. 34, died of phthisis.	21	1903	
A sister, then aged 27, was notified as phthisis in June 1903. Tub. bac. present. Was in sanatorium Aug.–Sept. 1903. Is now (Dec. 1906) quite well.	21	1903	
Cough developed a few weeks before admission to sanatorium. Tub. bac. found. Cervical glands still large and indurated, axillary glands the same.	24	1906	

Comments on Case 4.—The patient can scarcely be said to have been free from the possibility of infection during her whole life. She showed tuberculous glands at the age of 16, and signs of pulmonary disease eight years later.

CASE 5.—*Doubtful whether domestic or industrial infection operative*

Clara R., æt. 29, admitted to sanatorium July 16, discharged August 11, 1906.

Comments on Case 5.—This is a good illustration of a large number of cases in which several points are open to doubt. Was the patient infected from her mother, the industrial conditions merely breaking down her resistance ?   Were the " constant colds " only bronchial attacks on which phthisis was eventually engrafted by infection from some of the other work-girls ; or, as is more likely, did she have phthisis from 18 years of age onwards ? If the latter view is taken, two possible sources of

Domestic Influences.	Age.	Year.	Extra-domestic Influences.
Mother died after " breaking a blood vessel." Patient does not know if the mother had a cough previously.	0 10	1877 1887	
	15	1892	Patient went as a dressmaker. Worked with the firm A. for 2½ years, with a friend who died in 1901 of pulmonary tuberculosis, and was delicate in 1892, but is doubtful if she then had a cough.
Began to have " constant colds."	18	1895	Patient went to firm B. for 3 years
Father died of " emphysema."	21 22	1898 1899	Went to firm C. for 4 years. Workroom containing 12 girls was overcrowded.
	24	1901	Often visited the bedridden consumptive friend mentioned above.
	25	1902	Went to firm D. for 2 years. Large workroom here.
At Christmas had a bad cough. *In May 1905 was in bed 5 days, and since then always cough and expectoration.*	27 28	1904 1905	Went to a smaller dressmaker's place for 9 months ; room underground, stuffy and dusty.
Admitted to sanatorium 3 months after tub. bac. were found in sputum.	29	1906	Went to firm F. ; large work-room.

infection are still known, the dressmaker friend or her mother. If the mother died of phthisis, I should lean to the view that she was the probable source of infection, because domestic exposure is generally more intimate and more protracted than occupational exposure to infection.

CASE 6.—*Domestic infection from a non-relative.   Influence of industrial fatigue*

Geo. S., æt. 39, admitted to sanatorium with extensive tuberculosis both lungs, September 8, and discharged November 2, 1906. Father and mother, five brothers, and two sisters all healthy. No tuberculosis known in his or his wife's family except that the latter's father died over twenty years ago of this disease. The main facts of his illness are summarised below.

Domestic Influences.	Age.	Year.	Extra-domestic Influences.
None.	0	1867	
			Has been a house-painter all his working life.
Married	20	1887	
Three children living : two died stillborn, one as shown below.			
Has occasionally sublet part of his house, but not, so far as he or his wife knows, to people with bad coughs except as shown below.			
Had a man named P. and his family occupying part of the house for about a year. P. was then ill with phthisis, and died at Easter 1903.	35–36	1902–03	
G. S.'s child died of "consumption of the bowels" in August 1903. This child was born November 1902, became ill when 4 months old ; never had diarrhœa.			
Cough began late in this year .	37	1904	
	39	1906	

No extra-domestic or family source of infection could be detected. The facts as to the P. family need to be stated in some detail. G. S., his wife, and four children had two rooms for themselves and let off the rest of the house to P. and family, who lived here for nine months. The two families were not very friendly, but there was a common scullery and w.c. P. was very dirty in his habits, and spat about. His spit-cups were often left in the scullery. About six weeks after P.'s death, patient and his family left this house. It should be added that Mrs. P., her son and two daughters were quite well in November 1906.

Comments on Case 6.—It seems likely that G. S. and his child were both infected by P. The escape of the P. family, and of the other members of the S. family, does not exclude this ; similar experiences of escape are not uncommon in the acute infectious diseases. G. S. while living in the same house as P. was working very long hours, and it is likely that this made him more open to infection.

CASE 7.—*Possible public-house infection*

W. W., æt. 42, admitted to sanatorium August 23, discharged October 4, 1906.   No family history of phthisis.

Domestic Influences.	Age.	Year.	Extra-domestic Influences.
No infection known.	0	1864	
	12	1876	Began work as an errand boy.
Father died of asthma, æt. 44 .	18	1882	
Married	23	1887	Worked as a butcher's assistant. Daily frequented various public-houses, and has been a free toper from this time onwards.
	30	1894	Worked as an outside salesman at various butchers' shops.
	39	1903	
Had a bad cough at Christmas time, which got well again.	41	1905	Worked in a baker's shop.
In June severe hæmoptysis, which recurred on four occasions.	42	1906	

Comments on Case 7.—There is no evidence of family or other domestic infection, and none of industrial infection.   The public-house is the most likely source of infection.

CASE 8.—*Possible occupational infection*

W. H., æt. 33, admitted to sanatorium October 3, discharged October 31, 1906.   There is no family history of tuberculosis. Father and mother, three brothers, and three sisters all alive and well.   Married for seven years; two children, both well.

Domestic Influences.	Age.	Year.	Extra-domestic Influences.
No infection known.	0	1873	No definite infection known.
	19	1892	A soldier from 1892–1904, in India and South Africa.
Married	26	1899	
	31	1904	On returning from South Africa was engaged as a cleaner in the P.O. One of chief duties is to sweep out the rooms.
Has had a cough for a year, and expectoration for about 6 months before admission to sanatorium. Never pleurisy or blood-spitting.	33	1906	

Comments on Case 8.—The patient's present occupation—sweeping out public offices—is a possible source of infection, but he may have been infected while a soldier or elsewhere. The case is one of a class in which a probable statement of infection is impracticable.

GENERAL CONSIDERATIONS ON THE STATISTICAL STUDY OF HISTORIES OF INFECTION IN PHTHISIS.—The preceding cases illustrate the types of history often obtained in investigating cases of phthisis. The difficulties in tracing the source of infection in a given case are much greater than in the acute infectious diseases. There is an extremely variable period of latency, and the symptoms of the initial stages of the disease may pass unrecognised. The study of latency is so important a part of the problem that the next chapter is devoted to it ; and all histories of infection should be viewed in the light of the facts there set out. In view of the great prevalence of the disease, there is the further difficulty that the patient probably has been exposed to several sources of infection; and one has to attempt to balance quantitatively the probability of these as the active agent in producing disease. They may, in fact, have all been co-operating in overcoming the patient's powers of resistance.

For many years past I have carefully investigated the history of all cases of phthisis notified in Brighton. From 1902 onwards (p. 341) a large proportion and during the last year over half of these patients have been treated in the Borough Sanatorium. It has been possible in this way to obtain fuller information as to the patients than would have been otherwise practicable ; and this information has convinced me that histories obtained at a single interview with phthisical patients cannot be trusted. My experience is that the inquiries made at the first interview set up trains of thought and recollection, which when followed up at a later interview may completely alter the opinion formed at the first interrogation. For this reason I have preferred to state below a summary of a hundred consecutive sanatorium cases investigated very carefully by Dr. H. C. Lecky, at the Brighton Sanatorium, in preference to a very much larger number, in which less complete information had been obtained. These hundred cases had been exhaustively studied, and for that reason the results obtained respecting them are stated in some detail. The conclusions based on the less completely exhaustive investigation of a much larger number of cases coming under my observation during a series of years, confirm the view that prolonged latency of already existing disease is not so rare as it is often supposed to be.

In the following table a hundred patients, thus fully investigated, are classified according to the history obtained :—

TABLE XIX

		No. of Patients.
A. Definite limited domestic infection and definite onset	.	20
B. ,, ,, ,, ,, indefinite onset	.	12
C. Possible continuing domestic infection and definite onset	.	7
D. ,, ,, extra-domestic infection and definite onset	.	7
E. ,, ,, public-house ,, ,, ,,	.	1
F. ,, ,, domestic ,, indefinite onset	.	4
G. ,, ,, extra-domestic ,, ,, ,,	.	4
H. No exposure known and definite onset .	.	16
I. Suspicion of temporary exposure and definite onset .	.	11
J. No exposure known and indefinite onset .	.	9
K. Suspicion of temporary exposure and indefinite onset	.	7
L. History incomplete after every effort made .	.	2
		100

By limited infection is meant that the exposure to infection is known to have ceased at a given date, as, for instance, at the death of a consumptive mother.

The difficulties of classification of histories of infection are very great ; and the above headings have been adopted after much consideration. Thus it has been necessary to separate cases where the date of onset of symptoms could be definitely stated from others in which this was dubious ; and to separate cases where a definite limit to exposure to infection could be stated from others in which exposure may have continued up to the date of onset of the patient's illness.

The table shows that in 32 per cent. of the cases definite infection could be traced. In a further 23 per cent. there was a possibility of such infection, but the history was not so precise as in the previous group. In 25 per cent. of the total cases no exposure to infection could be traced. In a further 18 per cent. there was suspicion of temporary exposure to infection, but the history was defective or indefinite.

The fact that in 25 per cent. of the cases no source of infection could be discovered is instructive. Even though a considerable number of these are explained probably by the fact that many patients having open tuberculosis are never seen by a doctor and do not die of this disease, it appears likely that in an uncertain proportion of cases of phthisis,—probably among the most susceptible members of the community,—effective infection may be received from merely casual sources of infection.

STATISTICAL STUDY OF LATENCY.—In Table XIX. out of 100 total cases 20 had a definite history of infection ceasing at a known date, followed after an interval by phthisis in persons who had been exposed only, so far as could be ascertained, to this limited infection. Of these 20 patients 11 were men and 9 women. The duration of latency in these cases was as follows :—Under 1 year, 1 ; 1–2 years, 4 ; 2–3 years, 0 ; 3 years, 1 ; 5 years, 2 ; 6 years, 1 ; 9 years, 1 ; 10 years, 3 ; 13 years, 1 ; 15 years, 1 ; 17 years, 1 ; 20 years, 2 ; 22 years, 1 ; 27 years, 1.

Thus of the 20 cases 6 only appeared to have had a latency of less than 5 years ; in 4 the latent period varied from 5 to 10 years ; and in 10 there was a latency of over 10 years.

In the same table 12 additional cases are noted in which infection ceased at a given date, but the date of onset of phthisis in the person exposed to this infection could not be definitely ascertained, though always after the cessation of exposure. In 4 of these the duration of latency could not be stated even approximately ; in one it was probably 2 years ; in one, 3 years ; in one, 5 years ; in one, 7 years ; in one, 8 years ; in one, 10 years ; in one, 14 years ; and in one " many years."

In each of these cases it is possible that more recent casual infection, and not the more remote protracted infection, was responsible for the tuberculosis. The view I have taken throughout is that given one patient in a family the protracted and intimate relationships of domestic life are much more likely than casual extra-domestic infection to be the chief means of spreading tuberculosis ; and that this is so even when the history indicates a period of latency of many years. The possibility of long latency and the importance of protracted duration of exposure in producing efficient infection will be better appreciated when the next chapter and Chapters XIX. to XXVI. have been read.

CHAPTER X

LATENCY IN TUBERCULOSIS

ANALOGY WITH ACUTE INFECTIOUS DISEASES.—Certain features characterise all diseases due to the reception into the body of specific infective material from without. They may be illustrated by the case of small-pox. A person inhaling the contagion or microbes of this disease, unless protected by a previous attack of small-pox or by vaccination, goes through the following stages. There is first a *period of incubation*, or latent period, of about twelve days, in which no symptoms of disease can be detected. Then occur severe initial symptoms which usually consist of vomiting, severe headache and backache, with fever, followed seventy-two hours later by the characteristic skin eruption. After an illness of several weeks, all the symptoms have disappeared, the patient is no longer infectious to those coming into contact with him, and if again exposed to infection he is himself as a rule immune against further attack. That is a typical instance of the course of an infectious disease, and such diseases as whooping-cough, measles, scarlet fever, and typhoid fever conform more or less to the type. Some acute infectious diseases conform less completely to it. Thus in diphtheria the immunity conferred by one attack appears to be less complete than in the diseases just mentioned, and in erysipelas one attack appears to predispose to rather than to protect against a second attack. It is not necessary to enter into the possible causes of lack of immunity in these instances. In diphtheria, and possibly also in erysipelas, it is sometimes associated with the persistence in the patient's body of the bacteria causing the disease. Thus Gresswell in 1886 brought forward certain facts which appeared to show that " diphtheria in certain individuals may become a chronic disease, and from time to time enter upon an active and infectious phase." I have elsewhere collected similar evidence (1904) of cases of diphtheria, and occasionally also of scarlet fever, in which the infection persisted for very long periods, and subsequently reappeared after intervals of considerable length. The analogy between these exceptional conditions and tuberculosis is obvious. In both there is persistence of infection in a more or less latent form, and in both a partial failure to secure by one attack immunity from further attack.

INCUBATION PERIOD OR FIRST PERIOD OF LATENCY.—In the acute infectious diseases this is usually a fixed and somewhat short period, seldom exceeding a few days. In tuberculosis it may be a few weeks or many months, or even many years. There are not wanting illustrations of similar prolongations of this period in other diseases. Thus in pébrine, the silkworm disease investigated by Pasteur, the egg when laid contains the germs of the disease. These do not increase in number in the winter in the eggs, even though the latter are kept at a favourable temperature ; but in spring, with the growth and development of the egg, the disease again becomes fully established. In leprosy, a disease having close affinities to tuberculosis, two to five years is given as the common period of incubation, but a case of probable latency of forty years is described by Abraham (1896). Hydrophobia usually develops, if at all, within six weeks from the time of the bite of a rabid dog. It has been known, however, to remain latent for eighteen months and possibly for several years.

The following illustrations from my case-book illustrate prolonged latency between the last known exposure to infection and the occurrence of an attack of pulmonary tuberculosis. In speaking of *minimum* latent periods in these cases, *it must be understood that every other ascertainable possibility of infection has been investigated with negative result*, and that so far as could be ascertained the patient had only been exposed to the source of infection which is detailed, and to those minor casual infections (p. 73) to which everybody may be exposed.

CASE 9.—Mrs. E. S., æt. 32, was admitted to the sanatorium with phthisis August 13, 1906. She had been exposed to protracted infection as shown in the following scheme, having nursed her father, mother, and two brothers while they were ill and dying with phthisis :—

Domestic Infection.	Age.	Year.	Extra-domestic Infection.
The history makes it probable that during the whole of her childhood her mother and one brother were suffering from chronic phthisis.	0	1874	
In 1891 patient's brother, æt. 21, and mother, æt. 61, died of phthisis at home. Both nursed by E. S. In the same year another brother, æt. 30, died of phthisis in another house. He also was nursed by this patient.	17	1891	No evidence of any obtainable.
Married	19	1893	
Patient's father died of phthisis at E. S.'s house. He was very ill for a year, and in bed for a month before death.	20	1894	
In Nov. E. S. in bed for a week with "influenza and left pleurisy." Some cough ever since.	29	1903	
E. S.'s boy, aged 1½ year, died of acute tuberculosis.	30	1904	
Admitted to sanatorium . .	32	1906	

Comments on Case 9.—First exposure to infection was probably in infancy (1874). The last known exposure was twenty years later. First symptoms of tuberculosis occurred in 1903. The maximum latent period is therefore twenty-nine years, the minimum latent period nine years.

CASE 10.—H. E. G., æt. 25, was admitted to the sanatorium May 28, discharged July 30, 1906.

During his holidays H. E. G. visited his home, but there were no opportunities of protracted infection from the age of 15 to 21, when his cough began. Probably the latent period was much longer than six years, but possibly it was less. There was no family history of tuberculosis on the paternal side ; but the mother's two sisters had died of pulmonary tuberculosis, and the evidence pointed to her having suffered from the same disease at or before the time of her marriage.

The evidence in the preceding cases is purely circumstantial, and when stated in skeleton and apart from a knowledge of the intimate detail of each case is relatively unconvincing. The conclusion, however, that the majority of such cases are really

Domestic Infection.	Age.	Year.	Extra-domestic Infection.
	o	1881	
Lived at Ba. until 15 years old, and there all the following cases of tuberculosis occurred.			
Father died of phthisis one year before H. E. G. left home at the age of	14	1895	
	15	1896	Apprenticed to a draper in London.
Probable minimum primary latent period. ⎰Brother died of phthisis.	16	1897	
Mother died of tuberculosis of kidney.	17	1898	
Sister died of tuberculosis of intestine.	18	1899	Became a draper's assistant in C.
	21	1902	Cough began this year, and in consequence he went to sea as a ship's steward.
	22	1903	Had to give up sea-life, owing to an attack of pleurisy.
	23	1904	Began to expectorate.
	25	1906	Has not been working for the last two years.

cases of prolonged latency and not of yielding to casual and undetected more recent infection, is supported by converging lines of evidence, which may next be considered.

(1) There is pathological and experimental evidence of prolonged latency, primary and secondary, both in tuberculosis and in other infective diseases, both in adults and children.

(2) The clinical occurrence, both in tuberculosis and in other infective diseases, of prolonged secondary latency—*i.e.* of a period during which symptoms of diseases previously present are in abeyance—confirms the occurrence of a similar latency before the first clinical symptoms appear.

PATHOLOGICAL AND EXPERIMENTAL EVIDENCE OF PROLONGED LATENCY IN TUBERCULOSIS.—Attention has already been drawn to the frequency with which small tuberculous lesions are found post-mortem in those who have died from diseases other than tuberculosis (p. 49). Thus Stengel (p. 255) says :—

The lesion may become encapsulated and so remain for years without producing manifest clinical symptoms. This encapsulating membrane may subsequently be penetrated and widespread infection occur. Such latent tuberculosis is particularly frequent in the post-bronchial glands. These are often found diseased in autopsies in which no tuberculosis is found elsewhere. In a notable proportion of such cases emulsions of such glands produce tuberculosis in guinea-pigs, showing true latent tuberculous disease. Such lesions explain sudden miliary tuberculosis, in which no primary focus is found during life.

Cornet (p. 449) says :—

It has been shown, by means of inoculation tests, that if these (encapsulated) foci contain caseous material, virulent bacilli are always present. Only absolutely fibroid scars, as well as thoroughly calcified nodules, proved to be sterile (Kurlow, Green). The consumptive may be said to sit upon a volcano. Until the capsules have become absolutely perfect and impervious barriers, every event which tends to weaken them, or to open up the defects in their architecture, may become the occasion of a further dissemination of the bacilli, of a lighting up of a fresh attack.

It should be added that after giving the above evidence of continued virulence of tubercle bacilli incarcerated in old caseous lesions, Cornet makes the following remarks, which appear to be contradictory to his statement quoted above, and, unlike it, are not supported by experimental evidence :—

It seems to me a little far-fetched to attribute a fresh outbreak of the disease, after a quiescence of years, to the resurrection of the bacilli imprisoned in the old focus, since we know that the life period of the bacilli is bounded by certain definite and narrow limits.

The latter statement is based apparently on the assumption that the bacillus will find as great a difficulty in surviving in caseous nodules at the body temperature, as it experiences after having been expelled with the expectoration. Cornet emphasises Kitasato's demonstration that most of the bacilli in the expectoration are already dead ; but such expectoration is still commonly extremely virulent ; and bacilli in the expectoration imply destructive changes of tissues carried to a much further point, than those manifested in chronic caseous nodules. Cornet asks the question (p. 315) : " What biological facts entitle us to assume that the bacillus is capable of remaining latent through decades, for forty or sixty years, in the human body ? " He is answered partially by the preceding quotations, including his own statement. Other experimenters have furnished similar evidence, which, although not absolutely direct and certain, renders very probable the continuance of latency over many years. Thus J. K. Fowler has shown that recrudescence of human phthisis coincides in certain instances with active changes in the old lesions. In one instance the latency had lasted a period of forty years. Hæmoptysis generally indicates fresh mischief lit up in an old focus of disease. It was the association of recent general tuberculosis with recurrence of active trouble in an old focus which led Buhl to his great generalisation as to the origin of general tuberculosis by self-infection (see p. 37). Debove and Achard (p. 271) speak of these old foci as "le feu qui couve, qui peut s'étendre" under the influence of protracted overwork, fatigue, sorrow, or of an acute inflammatory attack.

In the preceding remarks it has been assumed that naked-eye evidence of old disease was to be found in the cases in which old foci produced acute tuberculosis. It may be noted, however, as having a possible bearing on the problem of latency, that lymphatic glands may contain living tubercle bacilli without showing naked-eye signs of implication. The duration of life of tubercle bacilli under those conditions is unknown. Loomis (quoted by H. Walsham, p. 6), on examining thirty cases in which there were no signs of old or recent tuberculous lesions, found that in eight cases the bronchial glands were infective to rabbits.

A. Macfadyen and MacConkey (1903) took mesenteric glands from the bodies of children who, dying of other diseases than tuberculosis, at the autopsies showed no evidence of tuberculosis. From these glands they injected material into guinea-pigs, and tuberculosis was produced in 25 per cent. of these. How long these bacilli had been in the tissues without producing evidence of disease cannot be said, nor can it be said how much longer they would have survived had the children lived; but these interesting observations open up the possibility of prolonged latency of tubercle bacilli in the absence of naked-eye lesions.

Tuberculous lesions may have long periods of latency in animals, as well as in man. Thus Baumgarten (quoted by Washbourne), inoculated tubercle bacilli into the anterior chamber of the eye of a rabbit. A tubercle formed; this was arrested and converted into cicatricial tissue under treatment by tuberculin. Nine months later the apparently cured tubercle started once more into activity. The active phase subsided for the second time, and there was apparent healing. A year later it again became active and now spread rapidly, general tuberculosis being produced. This instance, in which the bacilli remained alive during latent periods of nine months and a year, was carried out under conditions avoiding the possibility of fresh infection from without.

Müller (1906) states that he re-tested with tuberculin two sets of cows which when calves had been fed with infected milk, and which owing to their positive reaction to the first test had been fattened ; the interval between the two tests in one set was a year, in the other two years.   During the interval the cows had been isolated.   In the first set the whole of the ten cows reacted again ; in the second twelve out of fourteen reacted.   Other cases have been observed where calves which reacted to tuberculin first showed symptoms of tuberculosis $1\frac{1}{2}$ to $2\frac{1}{2}$ years later. In one batch of twenty cows the animals were 4 to 5 years old before symptoms appeared.   Then they suddenly in quick succession became ill and had to be slaughtered.   In all of them an advanced and apparently very old abdominal tuberculosis was found, the lesions being large and showing caseation and extensive calcification, with recent tuberculosis of the lungs and other organs.   Müller adds : a few other cases of the same kind have been observed in which entire years elapsed before the symptoms were exhibited, and in which there had been observed a tuberculosis of the udder at the critical time.

LATENT TUBERCULOSIS IN CHILDREN.—Ganghofner of Prague (1905) has recorded as follows the results of 1800 autopsies on children dying in that city from causes other than tuberculosis, and presenting no symptoms of tuberculosis :—

Out of 460 deaths of children in the 1st year of life							latent tuberculosis was found in	$33 = 7\cdot1$ per cent.
,,	536	,,	,,	aged 1–2	,,	,,	,,	$86 = 16\cdot0$,,
,,	476	,,	,,	,, 2–4	,,	,,	,,	$117 = 24\cdot5$,,
,,	271	,,	,,	,, 4–6	,,	,,	,,	$73 = 26\cdot9$,,
,,	123	,,	,,	,, 6–8	,,	,,	,,	$33 = 26\cdot8$,,

English statistics give somewhat similar results.   It has further to be noted that the absence of tuberculous lesions visible to the naked eye does not completely prove the absence of tuberculosis.   Ganghofner in the paper referred to above gives inoculation experiments proving the presence of latent tuberculosis in children in whom ordinary macroscopic and microscopic examination had failed to prove its presence, and similar observations have been made by others (p. 79).

Unless it can be shown to be an exceptional event for living tubercle bacilli to be present in old tuberculous nodules, the facts narrated in this and the preceding paragraph give a *primâ* fac*ie* case in favour of the view that adult tuberculosis may often be due to the recrudescence of the disease established in small foci within the body in early life. This view was emphasised by Marfan (1905), whose conclusions were that (1) the infant is most exposed to tuberculosis at ages 1–6 ; and that (2) in a considerable number of cases showing evidence of tuberculosis at or after adolescence, the disease has not been caused by recent infection, but by an infection acquired in early life and remaining latent in the interval.

The same conclusion is confirmed by the facts relating to prolonged secondary latency as given below.

PROLONGED SECONDARY LATENCY IN DISEASES OTHER THAN TUBERCULOSIS.—There is, as already mentioned, abundant evidence that diphtheria bacilli may in exceptional cases persist in the throat for months, or rarely even for several years, without any evidence of disease, a second attack being then produced without any known external re-infection. The clinical evidence of this phenomenon in tuberculosis and in diphtheria is strongly confirmed by bacteriological evidence concerning other diseases. Thus Washbourne (1896) states that the spores of the hay bacillus have been found alive in the organs 78 days after subcutaneous injection. He quotes an instance given by Schäfer in which diphtheria bacilli persisted in the throat for six months after the attack. I have published (1904) instances of diphtheria in which infection persisted 102 and 170 days after the patient was apparently well, and cases of scarlet fever in which similarly persistent infection was shown.

The typhoid bacillus sometimes persists in the gall bladder, the bones, etc., for a long time after an attack of typhoid fever. Hinze (quoted by Washbourne) gives a case of a periosteal node appearing four months after an attack of typhoid fever ; six months later this became an abscess, which when opened and cultivations taken from it, showed typhoid bacilli. Buschke found living typhoid bacilli in an abscess seven months and Chantemesse and Widal fifteen months after an attack of typhoid fever. A most remarkable case for this disease is recorded by Dudgeon and Gray (1906), in which the discharge from a bone sinus three years after the patient's attack of typhoid fever gave pure cultures of typhoid bacilli, and appeared to be the cause of the same disease in the patient's wife.

6

Syphilis has many points of resemblance to tuberculosis, especially in the slow evolution of its phenomena and the long intervals during which symptoms are absent. In this disease recrudescence of symptoms frequently occurs, when fresh external infection can be excluded with certainty, after twenty or thirty years of freedom from symptoms ; and in such cases it is occasionally noted that, as in tuberculosis, recognisable initial symptoms may have been entirely absent.

CLINICAL EVIDENCE OF PROLONGED SECONDARY LATENCY IN TUBERCULOSIS.—The following cases are typical of a large number in which long intervals elapsed between the first attack of tuberculosis and later attacks, and in which, I think there is strong reason for believing that the later attack was caused by changes in the old foci of disease, freeing the bacill from their incarceration and disseminating disease to other parts.

Domestic Infection.	Age.	Year.	Extra-domestic Infection.
No exposure to infection known.	0	1852.	
	9	1861	M. D.'s schoolmistress at the National School fell ill.
	12	1864	About this year the schoolmistress died of phthisis, after being ill for 2 to 3 years, during the whole of which time M. D. saw her nearly every day, sitting in her room, and generally helping her.
Probable minimum primary latent period. { Family removed from Ch—m to C—n.	15	1867	
	16		M. D. had no symptoms of phthisis for about 4 years after the death of the teacher.
M. D. was treated for phthisis at the Brompton Hospital 6 months as an out-patient and 5 months as an in-patient.	17	1869	
	18		
Secondary latent period. { Father killed in an accident.	25		
M. D. married . .	28		
No cough or expectoration for 33 years, although delicate.			
Came to Brighton .	47		
Cough and expectoration began again.	50	1902	
Admitted to sanatorium . .	54	1906	

CASE 11.—Mrs. M. D., æt. 55, was admitted to the sanatorium August 20, 1906, with chronic phthisis. Her family history shows complete absence of this disease. Her personal history is presented in the scheme on the preceding page.

Comments on Case 11.—The above facts show in this case a primary latent period of about 4 years, followed by an illness lasting about a year; and then a secondary latent period of 32 years.

CASE 12.—Mrs. A. W., æt. 24, admitted to sanatorium May 12, discharged June 9, 1906. Increase of weight from 8 st. 5¼ lb. to st. 3 lb. Signs of disease at left apex. Has been married 6 years, and done only domestic work since that time. Has had two children, one well, one died aged 3 years of " bronchitis." Husband healthy. Patient was a domestic servant before marriage, and did not work for any consumptive family. Patient's father died of phthisis 2¼ years ago after an illness of 4 years. Patient and her husband lived with the father until 3 years ago. in 1904 she had " influenza," and afterwards was fairly well until March of the present year. When aged 14 had (in 1896) gland removed from the left side of the neck, and in 1904 a gland was removed from lower down on the same side of the neck.

Comments on Case 12.—If it be assumed that the first tuberculous gland was the focus of infection of the lung, there was a secondary latent period of about 10 years. It is possible that t.e father of the patient had infected her more recently. This would make the new primary latent period about 2 to 3 years.

CASE 13.—A. B., æt. 49, a policeman, was notified on september 2, 1905. Tubercle bacilli had been found in his sputum in August 31. Had right pleurisy 16 years ago. His cough dates from October 1903, and he had some hæmoptysis early in 1905. He was said by his doctor to have had " bronchial catarrh " in october 1904. Had been in the police service 23 years, and before that had been a seaman. Is an alcoholic subject. He was admitted to the sanatorium September 8, discharged october 6, 1905, and died March 26, 1906.

Comments on Case 13.—If, as is probable, the pleurisy was tuberculous, there appears to have been a latent period of 13 years between it and the subsequent development of cough.

On this supposition, we must assume an earlier infection to which the pleurisy was secondary. The source of infection is undetermined. The opportunities of infection both in his occupations and in connection with alcoholic indulgence were numerous, and the latent period may therefore have been shorter than given above, there being numerous infections at frequent intervals.

CASE 14.—J. M., æt. 29, admitted to sanatorium March 24, discharged April 20, 1906. Has been a house painter for 6 years, before that a soldier for 7 years, of which 6 were spent in India. Has been married 5 years, but has had no children. His wife is healthy. He has had a cough as long as he can remember, and he had hæmoptysis before going to India. The cough ceased while he was in India, but reappeared on his return, and he has gradually deteriorated in health. His father died of phthisis when he was 10 years old. His brother M. M. was admitted to the sanatorium with J. M., having phthisis and renal disease. The brother's first symptoms date from about 4 years ago. The two brothers have not lived together for 6 years, and then only for a short time.

Comments on Case 14.—The father probably infected both these patients more than 19 years ago. In M. M.'s case there was an initial latent period of about 15 years. In J. M.'s case symptoms of phthisis appeared much earlier ; but an interval of 6 years followed, in which all symptoms were in abeyance.

Domestic Infection.	Age.	Year.	Extra-domestic Infection.
None discovered.	0	1885	None discovered.
Was treated in Brixton for disease of the right lung, being under a doctor for several months. Was then sent into the country for three months, and has been well from that time until Easter 1906, when she again began to suffer from cough. Was sent to Brighton on account of this cough ; and when examined shortly afterwards, was found to have a cavity at the right apex.	7	1892	
	21	1906	

CASE 15.—Jessie R., æt. 21, was admitted to the sanatorium July 26, and discharged October 25, 1906. She had disease, including cavitation, of the upper part of the right lung. See scheme on preceding page.

Comments on Case 15.—The first attack 14 years ago was diagnosed as phthisis. From this date to her present attack, the patient had been well. There was no family history of tuberculosis, and the patient, who is in fairly good circumstances, has not been exposed to any known infection.

CHAPTER XI

SOURCES OF INFECTION

SINCE tuberculosis is an infective disease, its prevention evidently must depend upon an accurate knowledge of the sources from which infection is derived. With rare exceptions, tuberculosis in man has been attributed solely to infection derived from other human patients, or to infection from food animals, especially cattle or pigs. The possibility of infection by animal food-stuffs raises the large question of the intercommunicability of human and bovine tuberculosis, which is discussed in Chapters XVI. to XVIII. Tuberculosis from lower animals is only likely to be conveyed to man to any considerable extent by the ingestion of infected foods, especially milk. From human patients infection may be direct, *e.g.*, in kissing or during coughing accompanied by the projection of particles of expectoration into another person's mouth or nostrils ; or indirect, as when the dried expectoration of a consumptive is inhaled. The chief possible means of infection are thus—

1. The inhalation of dried expectoration.
2. The inhalation of particles of wet expectoration.
3. The ingestion of tuberculous milk or other foods.

Of these three it is agreed by most hygienists that only a relatively small part of the total human tuberculosis is due to tubercle bacilli of bovine or other animal origin, though opinions differ as to the size of this proportion. Very few agree with von Behring in considering bovine infection as the sole or even the chief source of human tuberculosis.

Both 1 and 2 named above are concerned with coughing and expectoration, which are the main means of tuberculous infection. Other discharges from tuberculous patients, as from the bowels in tuberculous enteritis,—or even without such enteritis, when tuberculous expectoration has been swallowed, —from the skin in tuberculous abscesses, by the urine in renal tuberculosis, are doubtless infective, but for fairly obvious reasons they seldom have the same opportunities to cause infection as the expectoration.

Expectoration can, as indicated above, spread infection in two ways. Either it is inhaled after having become dried and powdery, or it is inhaled directly in the form of spray or small pellets expelled as the patient coughs. These two chief modes of infection are fully considered in Chapter XII. In this chapter will be considered briefly certain other modes of infection, less important than the inhalation of infective dust or spray, but conveniently disposed of at this stage. These methods consist in (1) inoculation with tubercle bacilli, (2) infection by kissing or by other means of conveying infected saliva, and (3) infection by contaminated hands or by flies.

INOCULATION WITH TUBERCULOUS MATERIAL.—The subcutaneous injection of tubercle bacilli in experimental animals produces tuberculosis which, following the lymphatic tracts, may soon become general. Such a result is rare in ordinary life, probably because the dose of infection received through cuts or abrasions of the skin is usually small. Lupus, a disease eventually causing a disfiguring ulceration of the skin, is a local form of tuberculous infection. It rarely occurs in covered parts of the skin, and is probably caused by accidental inoculation of tubercle bacilli. Local tuberculosis has occasionally been produced at the seat of local injuries, received, for instance, while making autopsies on tuberculous patients. Such cases are rare, and the resulting tuberculosis seldom extends beyond the next chain of lymphatic glands; but in a few instances general tuberculosis has followed.

The possibility of inoculation with tuberculosis during vaccination with bovine lymph has been asserted. It must be regarded as a very remote and almost negligible possibility; and as non-existent, when,—as is always the case in well-regulated vaccine establishments,—the calves from which the lymph has been obtained are killed and minutely examined for tuberculosis, and the lymph never distributed unless complete absence of tuberculosis can be certified.

INFECTION BY SOILED HANDS.—Obviously a phthisical patient who is not cleanly in his or her habits might easily infect hands and fingers during expectoration, and articles of food might thus become infected. Baldwin of Saranac Lake (quoted by Lartigau, p. 121) examined the hands of fifteen consumptives, and of this number ten were found to be contaminated with tubercle bacilli. These facts emphasise the importance of care in the use of handkerchiefs and spitting-cups, and the need for washing the hands after they have become fouled. This source of infection must, however, be regarded as of much less magnitude than others to b' considered subsequently.

INFECTION BY THE SALIVA.—Drinking-cups, spoons, etc., used in common may be a source of infection, and so likewise may kissing, if tubercle bacilli are present in the saliva. On this point divergent statements are made, Cornet (Cornet, p. 187) saying that the saliva is ordinarily germ free ; while several observers have confirmed the frequent presence of tubercle bacilli in the saliva (Lartigau, p. 121). Cornet himself (Cornet, p. 166) minimises the value of the preceding statement by urging that even if the saliva " should contain bacilli, they would be carried into the mouth and the digestive tract of the other person, and not into the lungs " ; although he says that " with children the case is different. Their mucous membranes are far more susceptible to the bacteria, and it may be that kissing is not infrequently of moment in producing scrofulous cervical glands." With his statement that " so far as we are able to judge, this danger does not play an important rôle among adults," I am inclined to agree. Dosage would probably be small in infection by kissing or by drinking-cups, etc., and it is unlikely that a serious amount of infection is often produced by this means alone.

INFECTION BY FLIES.—It is obvious that flies having fed on or having been fouled by tuberculous expectoration might contaminate food and thus convey infection. This possibility has been proved experimentally. Thus Spillmann and Haus- halter (Cornet, p. 82) found tubercle bacilli in the abdominal cavity and in the fæces of flies which had sucked at the sputum cloths of consumptives. These observations have been confirmed by others. In measuring the relative importance of this method of spreading infection, it has to be remembered that the fæces of flies and the amount of material capable of being carried on their limbs are extremely minute as compared with the material in a single expectoration.

CHAPTER XII

SOURCES OF INFECTION (*Continued*)—DUST AND SPRAY

VILLEMIN (p. 38) appears to have been the first authority to recognise the importance of dried tuberculous expectoration as a vehicle of infection, most previous writers having laid stress on the supposed dangers of direct personal communication, or even of handling tuberculous corpses (p. 35). The deaths from phthisis of Bayle, Laennec, Louis, and several other French physicians who practised much among consumptives, doubtless favoured the view of direct infection from consumptive patients.

Even in recent years the idea that AIR QUIETLY EXPIRED by a consumptive may contain tubercle bacilli has been entertained, and some experiments by Ransome (1882) and by Williams (1883) appeared to confirm it. It is probable, however, that in these experiments insufficient precautions were taken to exclude the possibility of spray or droplets ejected during coughing gaining access to the experimental apparatus. Tyndall has supplied the experimental proof that in quiet breathing expired air is absolutely sterile.

For the rest of this chapter it will be assumed that inhaled dust can penetrate to the air cells of the lungs. The evidence for this statement, and the discussion of the relative share of this and other methods of infection will be given in later chapters. In this chapter we shall discuss the operation of infection by dust and by spray, as far as possible in the historical order of the most important experiments that have been made.

KOCH'S EXPERIMENTS AND CONCLUSIONS.—Koch describes his procedure in experiment 26 of his classical paper as follows :—

A very roomy box, having on one side an opening for the orifice of the spray apparatus, was placed in a garden at a good distance from any habitation. The spray apparatus was placed outside the box, with its orifice projecting into the interior. By means of elastic tubing and a suitable length of lead pipe passing through the woodwork of a closed window, the apparatus was connected with an indiarubber bellows, and so could be worked from the room beyond the region of the spray.

A pure culture taken from a phthisical lung in the human subject, No. 1, and carried through twenty-three generations in fifteen months, was rubbed up with distilled water, and the fluid diluted to such an extent that it looked almost clear. Any visible fragments present in the fluid subsided after standing a short time ; the upper layer, which showed hardly any opacity, was poured off and used for inhalation. Fifty c.cms. were sprayed in the course of half an hour on three successive days, and inhaled by the following animals in the box : 8 rabbits, 10 guinea-pigs, 4 rats, and 4 mice. After the inhalation, the animals were kept in separate roomy cages and well looked after. In some of the animals, dyspnœa appeared after ten days, and 3 rabbits and 4 guinea-pigs died in the course of fourteen to twenty-five days. All the remaining animals were killed twenty-eight days after the last inhalation. All the rabbits and guinea-pigs had numerous tubercles in the lungs, the size of the tubercles being proportionate to the length of time the animals had lived after inhalation.

In this experiment Koch was spraying cultures made from a tuberculous lung, but in his comments on it he says :—

There can likewise be no doubt as to the manner in which the tuberculous virus is carried from phthisical to healthy subjects. By the force of the patient's cough particles of tenacious sputum are dislodged, discharged into the air, and so scattered to some extent. Now numerous experiments have shown that the inhalation of scattered particles of phthisical sputum causes tuberculosis with absolute certainty, not only in animals easily susceptible to the disease, but in those also which have more power of resisting it. It is not to be supposed that man would be an exception to this rule, but, on the contrary, we may surmise that any healthy person brought into immediate contact with a phthisical patient, and inhaling the fragments of fresh sputum discharged into the air, may thereby be infected. But probably infection will not often take place in this way, because the particles of sputum are not small enough to remain suspended in the air for any length of time. Dried sputum, on the contrary, is much more likely to cause infection, as, owing to the negligence with which the expectoration of phthisical patients is treated, it must evidently enter the atmosphere in considerable quantity. The sputum is not only ejected directly on the floor, there to dry up, to be pulverised and to rise again in the form of dust, but a good deal of it dries on bed-linen, articles of clothing, and especially pocket-handkerchiefs—which even the cleanliest of patients cannot help soiling with the dangerous infective material when wiping the mouth after expectoration—and this, too, is subsequently scattered as dust.

It is evident from this quotation that Koch regarded dried sputum as the most fertile source of infection. This view has been confirmed by the experiments of Cornet, Strauss, and many others. We must next consider the experiments and views of the school of Flügge.

FLÜGGE'S EXPERIMENTS AND CONCLUSIONS.—The following summary is made from Flügge's well-known paper (1898). He quotes results previously obtained by Sticker, who failed to infect animals by making them inhale tuberculous sputum mixed with fine sand, and showed that the failure was owing to the fact that although the conglomerate of sputum and sand was driven into the apparatus by a rapid current from bellows used in the experiment, yet it failed to be inhaled by the feeble inspiratory suction of the animal. On the other hand, Cornet succeeded in producing tuberculosis by inhalation in guinea-pigs, by discharging the loaded air direct into the animals' mouths, or by holding them over a carpet while it was swept, so that the sputum particles with which it had been strewn were raised. These experiments in which the sputum is artificially dried and powdered, and the air currents are more rapid than those occurring naturally in a room, are, according to Flügge, not comparable to normal conditions of life.

The important point to settle is whether under natural conditions sputum, as for instance in a handkerchief, ever assumes the degree of dryness requisite for the dust to escape from it and become the source of infection. Experiments were made on this point by Beninde. He showed that weak currents of air would not disperse bacteria from handkerchiefs which had been deprived of 60 per cent. of their moisture by being kept in the pocket for one day. Flügge also states that

sputum on the floor very rarely is left long enough to reach the necessary degree of dryness ; each washing of the floor lessens the danger. In ordinary dwelling-houses it is next to impossible to find dried sputum in the dust, though in workshops, etc., where men may spit on the floor, tuberculous dust can quite well become sufficiently dried to be blown up into the air.

He goes on to say that

sputum is difficult to pulverise finely, and the coarser particles are not dangerous. It is true that sweeping and dusting disturb the coarser particles, but these do not often reach the respiratory passages, and fall so quickly again on to any flat surface, that it is not possible for much to be inhaled ; and as the finer particles, capable of suspension for a long time, are very rarely and sparsely present, the danger is very slight.

Flügge summarises the results of his experiments in the following words :—

> Infection from pulverised dried sputum is doubtless possible, but it occurs relatively seldom, because particles fine enough to be conveyed readily by air can only be formed from completely dried sputum, and then only in very limited quantities.

In his view that the danger from dried sputum has been exaggerated, Flügge in certain particulars was anticipated by Cornet, who, although he is the chief advocate of the view that tuberculosis is spread by infective dust, minimises its operation in the following words extracted from his first work :—

> Any one who has himself tried to rub well-dried sputum into particles and to pulverise it very finely will agree with me that it is no easy task to produce a really fine powder which remains suspended in the air for some time. The strong statements that have been made up to now—that one has only to rub with the foot on the dried sputum to raise immediately a cloud of infectious germs—are absolutely false.

EXPERIMENTAL EVIDENCE OF SPRAY INFECTION. HEYMANN. —Leaving aside experiments under artificial conditions, we may consider those made with the natural spray produced by coughing, sneezing, and speaking. Laschtschenko, after washing his mouth with broth containing *Bacillus prodigiosus*, was able to recover these from agar plates dispersed over a room. Sneezing was most efficient in dispersing the bacteria, coughing next most efficient. He made consumptives cough on to glass, and from four patients he thus obtained abundant tubercle bacilli.

Heymann (1901) carried this further. He first made experiments to determine the local dispersion and limitation of the sputum drops. A patient was placed for 1½ hour in an experimental chamber in which plates were arranged in different positions to receive droplets. After the patient had left the chamber it was carefully closed and protected from sunlight for some hours. The deposits on the plates were then examined by inoculation experiments. In the case of a patient who used a handkerchief before his mouth when coughing, it was found that out of 36 animals inoculated with material from plates taken out of the chamber after its use, 11, or 30·5 per cent., were infected ; and that of 34 animals inoculated from plates taken out of a chamber where the patient did not use a handkerchief, 24, or 70·5 per cent., were infected.

Most of the spray droplets when coughed up by the patient were of a size which made them fall directly on to the glass plates at short range. Some of the finer droplets, however, were easily carried behind the patient by currents of air.

Six experiments were then made, handkerchiefs being held from 5 to 10 cms. (2 to 4 inches) away from the mouth of the coughing patients. Nearly half of the animals inoculated from plates exposed under these conditions escaped infection.

The experiments showed that infective particles are rarely carried more than 1 metre (39·4 inches) beyond the person coughing, so that protection against spray infection is easy to secure by keeping a distance of about an arm's length from the patient, and by the latter using a handkerchief when coughing or sneezing.

Experiments were also made by Heymann on the duration of suspension in air of droplets containing tubercle bacilli. A consumptive was made to cough into an experimental chamber containing twelve covered plates, the covers of which were then by mechanical means removed and replaced at definite intervals. By these and other experiments it was proved that the duration of suspension in air is not great, and consequently the amount of infection thus received—except under conditions of the closest intimacy—must be very small. The larger size of many of the droplets diminishes the duration of suspension in the air. Heymann next draws attention to the adhesiveness of such droplets as have settled. He says :—

If these drops are allowed to dry for a short time on acid plates, they can be rubbed fairly energetically with rough rags without the drops being entirely removed. This fixation would become more definite if the drops had settled on a fairly thick layer of dust ; and with the cleaning methods, *e.g.* damp dusters, etc., employed in sickrooms, it is improbable that much danger exists of infective particles being again raised into the air.

He then investigated the duration of vitality of tubercle bacilli in spray deposited on plates from sputum ejected by an artificial spray apparatus and by patients in coughing. In all, 96 plates were prepared, and were kept from 12 hours to 90 days. It was proved that of the tubercle bacilli from the natural spray those kept in the dark lost their virulence within 18 days at the most, and those exposed to the light within

3 days. The artificially sprayed tubercle bacilli kept in the dark were virulent only for 7 days at the most.

The formation of pulverised sputum and its power of remaining suspended in the air were next investigated. Experiments were made showing that in quiet air after carpet-beating, etc., the suspension of bacilli in the air was very short. In moving air, dust could not be detected ten minutes after the cessation of the beating and brushing. Heymann indicated the defects in Cornet's researches on dust infection. The number of experiments in which droplet infection could be excluded with certainty was, according to Heymann, not great ; and Cornet's technique allowed of the inhalation of coarser particles and of adherent droplets, as well as of the fine dust, which alone would be inhaled under natural conditions. Heymann narrates a number of experiments, in which he claims that these possibilities of error were excluded. The number of tests made was 59, and 5 of the inoculated animals, or 8·5 per cent., were infected with tubercle. Heymann concludes :—

It is consequently demonstrated that dry dust containing tubercle bacilli is only present in slight quantity in rooms of consumptives. The low percentage in his results in comparison with Cornet's was striking, so that a repetition of the experiments using Cornet's spongelet method was thought worth making.

The adoption of this method of collecting the dust gave a greater proportion of positive results, 15·8 per cent. in private rooms, and 40·3 per cent. in hospitals. These results showed Heymann that infective particles may be transported by contact and dust, and deposited at a considerable distance from patients, but that, as a rule, they fall and adhere, being generally too heavy to be blown about.

Adding together Heymann's two sets of dust experiments, the total results were as follows :—

Of a total of 239 dust samples obtained from the sickrooms of consumptives, 44 contained virulent tubercle bacilli (=18·4 per cent.). In the 123 obtained from hospital wards, 30 contained the bacilli (=24·3 per cent.). In the 116 from private houses occupied by consumptives only 14 (=12 per cent.) were infective. The hospital incidence was greater than that in the homes of consumptives, whereas in Cornet's experiments the incidence in the two was nearly equal.

In summing up the conclusions to be derived from his exhaustive investigation, Heymann is of opinion that spray and dust infection are equally important, one form taking precedence over the other, according to circumstances. When spray infection persists for a considerable time, the patient's environment must contain much infective material, but obviously it varies with the stage of disease, and has the limitations of vitality elsewhere indicated (p. 104). As a rule, infective material is not sprayed further than an arm's length. The duration of suspension of droplets in the air is limited, but they have been found as long as half an hour after the last attack of coughing; droplets floating for so long a time as this contain only a few tubercle bacilli. Heymann adds :—

Under natural conditions droplet infection is only operative in circumstances of closest intimacy, in the close intercourse of married people and of mother and child; among attendants on the sick, and in factory-rooms, workshops, and offices.

Tubercle-containing dust particles are produced by the escape of sputum droplets, and by remnants of sputum which may adhere to the hand, pocket-handkerchief, bed-linen, carpets, and furniture, and especially to the floor as the result of spitting. I differ from Cornet in that I do not attribute a greater power to this dust than to spray in producing infection, because to enable infection to be produced the particles of dust should possess an exceedingly fine consistency, enabling them to be moved by even slight air currents. This they do not possess. The closely adhering dust precipitated in sickrooms was found to contain only a few tubercle bacilli; and it may have settled down there in the course of some days, so that these scanty positive results of investigation of the dust afford no positive measure of the danger of inhalation of infective dust. Under special conditions, in factories and workshops and on railways where numbers of human beings crowd together and cause considerable agitation of the air, fine dust is formed, which may produce infection derived from long deposits of phthisical sputum.

INFECTION DURING SPEAKING.—Flügge and others, after rinsing out their mouths with broth cultures of B. prodigiosus, have found that the bacilli could be caught on culture plates in different parts of the room, some of the plates which were placed behind the speaker giving positive results. It would be improper to infer from these experiments that similar dissemination of tubercle bacilli occurs when consumptives are speaking. As Cornet has said (p. 501) :—

When Flügge takes cultures of the prodigiosus into his mouth, determines that the germs are distributed in talking and coughing, and from this argues that the same occurs in the case of the tubercle bacilli, he neglects the most important link in his evidence, the *tertium comparationis*, namely, the proof that the saliva of consumptives contains anything like the same number of germs as when the mouth is filled with a culture of *prodigiosus*. Researches upon this point show that the saliva is either free from the bacilli or contains them in rare cases and in small numbers.

Tubercle bacilli are few in number or absent from the mouth of a consumptive except when coughing. Furthermore, the viscous expectoration is much less easily scattered than watery saliva.

CORNET'S EXPERIMENTS AND CONCLUSIONS.—According to Cornet (Cornet, p. 98), Tappeiner first showed conclusively that infection occurs by means of dust. Tappeiner infected dogs by submitting them to the inhalation of powdered tuberculous expectoration. Koch, Cornet, and others repeated these experiments, substituting pure cultures of the tubercle bacillus for dried expectoration. Other investigators with similar methods failed to infect the animals experimented on. Hence Baumgarten and more recently Flügge have minimised the importance of infection by the inhalation of dried expectoration. Their failures, however, in the opinion of Cornet (Cornet, p. 102) were due to a technique, faulty in departing from the natural conditions governing infection by inhalation. The animals in their experiments had been placed in closed cages, in the air of which dried powdered expectoration was made to circulate by mechanical means. But, as pointed out by Cornet, expectoration is very hygroscopic, and at once under the above conditions absorbs the respiratory moisture, becomes heavy, and is no longer borne along in the inspiratory current of air.

In a series of experiments made in 1898 Cornet set himself to imitate experimentally the conditions which would be found in the dwelling of an unclean consumptive. In a room containing about 99 cubic yards of space he scattered over the carpet dried tuberculous expectoration mixed with dust, and placed guinea-pigs, some on the floor, and others upon stages 2 to 3 inches, 16 inches, and 4 feet above the floor. Then the floor was swept in the usual way with a stiff broom, so that a dense dust was produced. Cornet protected himself by wearing an overall coat, and over his face a complete hood with protected glass openings. A second group of animals was subjected to direct inhalation of infected dust. Of 48 guinea-pigs used, 46 became infected. Neisser (Lartigau, p. 130) showed by other experiments that mild currents of air can carry tubercle bacilli from place to place, and that dried tubercle bacilli can be held for some time in the suspended dust of ordinary rooms.

Cornet (Cornet, p. 502) quotes B. Fränkel's proof that the number of bacilli disseminated by coughing is insignificant as compared with the number released by the drying of expectoration. He let a number of consumptives wear masks for twenty-four hours at a time, and with 219 of these masks he caught 2600 tubercle bacilli in 32 days. Compare with this the 300 million bacilli which Heller estimates to be present in a single pellet of expectoration. This would mean 7200 million in one day, assuming the expectoration to occur only once an hour. Thus one consumptive in one day may discharge *in expectoration* 7,200,000,000 bacilli ; a number of consumptives in 32 days discharged *by coughing* 2600 bacilli. It does not follow that the relative danger from dust and from spray is in the proportion of these figures ; the proportion of each which, while still virulent, reaches the mucous surface of a susceptible person has to be considered. There are no means of stating this ; it will vary with circumstances. Probably dust infection is greater than spray infection in industrial and social life ; dust infection bears a smaller proportion to spray infection in domestic than in extra-domestic life; but the evidence does not show with certainty that under either set of circumstances spray infection operates to a greater extent than dust infection. Whatever be the proportion between the two, practical precautions must take cognisance of both methods of spread.

IMPORTANCE OF DUST INFECTION.—Whatever be the proportionate share of infective dust and infective spray, it is certain that dust plays an important part in spreading tuberculosis. There is abundant evidence that the dust in the vicinity of consumptives contains frequently, while that from other localities seldom contains, tubercle bacilli. Cornet in 1888 (Cornet, p. 86) first clearly established these important facts. Having carefully excluded the possibility of infection from other sources, he inoculated guinea-pigs with the dust obtained from the walls and floors of sickrooms occupied by consumptives. His results were as follows :—

7

In 7 hospitals 38 tests were made, 94 animals being inoculated with dust. Of this number 52 died from diseases other than tuberculosis, 22 remained healthy, and 20, or 21·3 per cent., became tuberculous. In 3 asylums 11 tests were made, 43 animals being employed, of whom 16 died from other diseases 14 remained healthy, and 13, or 39·4 per cent., became tuber culous. In 2 prisons 5 tests were made on 14 animals, all with a negative result as to tuberculosis. In the dwellings and workplaces of consumptives 62 tests were made, 170 animals being employed, of whom 91 died from other disease 45 remained healthy, and 34, or 20 per cent., became tube culous. In a surgical ward 3 tests were made, 8 animal being employed in each instance, with a negative result as to tuberculosis. In certain streets 14 tests were made ; 41 animals were employed, and here again a negative result as to tuberculosis was consistently obtained.

The dust of rooms occupied by consumptives was regularly virulent in the instances in which the patient had been in the habit of spitting into his handkerchief or on the floor ; it showe no evidence of virulence when the spittoon or spit-bottle had been regularly used. Cornet also found virulent tubercle bacilli in the dust of a room in which a consumptive had died six weeks previously. It should be carefully noted that the samples of dust were taken by Cornet from places where they had settled by gravity from the air, and in which direct pollution by tuberculous matter, either coughed up or expec - torated, or by means of dirty fingers, cups, cloths, or otherwise was practically impossible.

Other observers have confirmed these results. Dr. H. Coates researches, carried out under the direction of Professor Delépine at Owens' College, are especially valuable. He found that in only two out of a large number of film preparations of dust prepared by him were tubercle bacilli discoverable. Cultiva - tion methods were obviously out of the question, as other organisms grow so much more quickly than the tubercle bacilli. Cornet's inoculation test was therefore used. Samples of dust were collected from situations in which dust had settled naturally from the air, and where there would be no likelihood of direct contamination with expectoration or by infected articles. Samples of dust were taken from each house from the floor, skirting-boards, walls, shelves, mantelpieces, etc. Three classes of houses were examined.

I. Houses which were in a dirty condition, and in which a consumptive patient was living who was taking no precautions to dispose of his expectoration so as to prevent infection of the atmosphere, but who spat freely on to the floor, or into his pocket-handkerchief, etc.

II. Houses which were in a very clean condition, but in which a consumptive patient was living who was not sufficiently careful as to the disposal of his expectoration.

III. Very dirty houses, in which there had been no case of tuberculous disease for at least three years past.

The following table shows the results obtained :—

TABLE XX

Class I. Dirty Houses containing Consumptives who Used no Precautions.		Class II. Clean Houses containing Consumptives not sufficiently Careful.	Class III. Dirty Houses in which Consumptives had not Lived.
The number of houses from which dust was examined was . . .	23	10	10
The number to be excluded because the inoculated animals died rapidly after inoculation was . . .	2	0	0
The number found infective by inoculation (one by microscopic examination only) was	14	5	0
Thus the percentage of infected houses was	66·6	50·0	...
The average size of the infected rooms was	475 c. ft.	336 c. ft.	...
The average size of the non-infected rooms was	368 c. ft.	506 c. ft.	...
The lighting and ventilation was— Good in 5 positive and 7 negative cases		In 1 positive and 5 negative cases	...
Fair in 1 positive and 1 negative case		In 2 positive and 0 negative case	...
Bad in 8 positive and 1 negative case		In 2 positive and 0 negative case	...
Samples were taken at different levels in	16 houses	...	...
Of these samples the number found infective was	13	...	...
Of the infective samples the number near the floor was . . .	9	...	...
4 to 6 feet above the floor was . .	13	...	...

The preceding results indicate that there is no necessary

relationship between cubic space and the number of tubercle bacilli in a room.   The second series shows that ordinary cleanliness does not alone suffice to prevent the accumulation of infectious material in the rooms occupied by a consumptive. The third series shows, so far as a short series of experiments can, that tubercle bacilli are not present except in the immediate environment of consumptives.   The results obtained in further experiments are interesting.

Five specimens of dust were collected at various elevations from the walls of the waiting-room of the out-patients' department of the Hospital for Consumption in Manchester.   This waiting-room is a lofty, well-lighted, and well-ventilated hall, used by 180 patients every morning.   Ten guinea-pigs were inoculated and killed five weeks afterwards.   None of them showed any signs of tuberculosis.

Five samples of dust were also examined from the waiting-room of one of the large general hospitals, and here also the results were negative.

Dust taken from railway carriages failed to produce tuberculosis, but two samples taken from a general waiting-room at a railway-station both produced tuberculosis.

Tubercle bacilli have been frequently found in the dust of railway carriages, omnibuses, and tram-cars.

CHAPTER XIII

CIRCUMSTANCES LIMITING THE AMOUNT OF INFECTION BY DUST AND SPRAY

1. LIMITED OPPORTUNITIES FOR INFECTION.—We have seen that on the assumption that each annual death from phthisis implies the constant presence in the general population of three infective cases of the same disease, one in every 263 of the population of England and Wales is infective, the highest proportion being at ages 35 to 55 (p. 63). Even if we assume that ten instead of three infective phthisical patients are constantly present in the population for every death from phthisis, the proportion will only be 1 in 79 of the total population. Probably from the point of view of active infectivity three years is a much more likely duration than ten years.

There is little if any foundation for the loose statements as to the ubiquity of the tubercle bacillus. It is true that one-twelfth of the total deaths from all causes are due to phthisis (p. 8), and that at certain ages as many as half the bodies of persons having died from other diseases have been found to present old healed or latent tuberculous lesions (p. 48). One cannot, however, argue from these data that *at any given time* a large proportion of the population are capable of infecting others with tuberculosis. The figures need to be considered, not in relation to deaths from other causes, but in relation to the total population ; and when this is done, the proportion of phthisical persons, on the three years' basis stated above, is only 1 in 1881 of the children aged 5-10 years, 1 in 1129 of the children aged 10-15, and 1 in 141 of adults aged 25-35.

2. NOT EVERY CONSUMPTIVE IS INFECTIOUS, AND A CONSUMPTIVE IS NOT INFECTIOUS THROUGHOUT THE WHOLE OF HIS ILLNESS.—Careful patients do not endanger those with whom they live or work. The experiments recorded on pp. 98 and 100 show that in rooms where consumptives use the simple pre-

cautions required, the dust is free from infective material. (On this point see also pp. 91 and 92.) The experience of hospitals for consumptives appears to confirm the same conclusion. Those patients who habitually swallow their expectoration—and this includes nearly all children and lunatics—are relatively harmless except to themselves, assuming that the excreta are properly disposed of.

Many consumptives again have no expectoration during a large part of their illness ; and in many others repeated examination fails to detect tubercle bacilli. Thus of 326 undoubted cases of phthisis treated in the Brighton Borough Sanatorium during the three years 1903–05, 195, or 59·8 per cent., had tubercle bacilli in their expectoration during their stay in the sanatorium ; 80, or 24·5 per cent., had throughout expectoration showing no tubercle bacilli ; and 51, or 15·7 per cent., had no expectoration at all. Most of these cases had either consolidation or cavitation of the lungs. Of course the failure to find tubercle bacilli in the expectoration of one-fourth of the total patients does not prove their entire absence in these cases ; and it is likely that in some of these cases inoculation experiments would have given positive results. It is almost certain, however, that a considerable proportion of the total cases, in addition to the sixth part who had no expectoration, were not a source of infection while under treatment, and probably not in a large part of the rest of their illness. It should be added that in nearly all the above cases three specimens of expectoration were examined before a negative return was made. On the other hand, Sir Hugh Beevor (1905), when examining the expectoration of 100 cases of phthisis (32 cavity cases and 68 without discoverable cavity), found that tubercle bacilli were absent in only about 15 per cent.

The annual report of the Mount Vernon Hospital for Consumption for 1907 contains valuable data as to examination of sputum of patients, from which the table on the following page has been prepared.

Thus of the total 678 patients 10 per cent. had no sputum while in the hospital, and of the 608 who had sputum 33 per cent. while in the hospital had no tubercle bacilli on repeated examination.

3. CONSUMPTIVES DIFFER GREATLY IN INFECTIVITY.—It has already been mentioned that when there is no expectoration

the danger of infection is absent, whilst when the expectoration is swallowed the danger is only to the patient himself.   It may be taken as a rough guide, that (1) *the danger varies with the amount of expectoration.*   This is not certainly true, and not always true.   Abundant purulent expectoration may show no tubercle bacilli, and scanty expectoration may teem with them.   The rule may, however, be taken as a useful practical guide, and it follows that advanced cases of phthisis in which expectoration is abundant present greater possibilities of infection than early cases (see also p. 394).   It appears probable that the danger from advanced cases may be greater than is implied by the above rule.   Advanced patients are weak and may be bedridden, and under these circumstances are less able carefully to control the hygienic disposal

TABLE XXI

(See p. 102 for Reference to this Table.)

Condition of Patients.	Number of Patients.	Number having no Sputum.	Percentage of Total having no Sputum.	Number of Patients having Sputum.	Number whose Sputum showed no Tubercle Bacilli on Repeated Examination.	Percentage of Expectorating Patients in whom no Tubercle Bacilli were discovered.
Infiltration of one lobe only . .	198	35	18	163	93	57
Infiltration of more than one lobe, but no cavitation	277	25	9	252	54	22
Cavities present .	203	10	5	193	11	5

of their expectoration than if they were less enfeebled.   The importance of careful and cleanly nursing at this stage needs to be emphasised.

(2) *The danger is great in proportion to the frequency of expectoration,* infrequent expectoration being much more likely than frequent to be carefully deposited.

(3) *The number of tubercle bacilli in the expectoration is not a certain guide as to degree of infectivity.*   Dead tubercle bacilli take the stain for microscopic examination as well is living bacilli.   Kitasato (quoted by Cornet, p. 83) proved experimentally that the majority of tubercle bacilli in expectoration or in cavities are already dead.   When therefore Cornet gives a calculation showing that a single patient may expectorate

daily 7200 million bacilli, and Nuttall that a patient with moderately advanced disease and expectorating from 70 to 130 c.c. daily may discharge daily from 1½ to 4½ billions of bacilli, and when Bollinger estimated that 1 c.c. (about a quarter of a teaspoonful) may contain 810,000 to 960,000 bacilli, it must not be assumed that these are all living bacilli. Living bacilli will probably be present, quite sufficient to do mischief if the opportunity arises, but the possibilities of mischief are not so great as might at first be supposed.

4. Virulent Bacilli have a Limited Extra-Corporeal Existence even when left alone.—In streets they cannot (p. 331) be found except in expectoration itself. In dwellings they have a more prolonged vitality, but according to Cornet infective material has usually disappeared from a dwelling after about six months. It is therefore, in all probability, an exaggeration to speak of a house as being saturated with the infection of years. One scarcely needs to add that it would be folly to trust to the slow processes of nature for removing infection, when by disinfection and cleanliness this can be secured at once.

5. Only a few Bacilli reach the Experimentally Determined Duration of Extra-Corporeal Existence.—Direct sunlight kills them quickly (p. 53), being a disinfectant without peer. The dispersion produced by air currents minimises any subsequently received dose of infection, while street cleansing and the more effective scavenging produced by rain sweep infectious material into the sewers. It must be repeated that these factors are mentioned, not with the idea that we can afford to rest content with their operation without stopping indiscriminate expectoration, but to prevent exaggerated notions as to the possibilities of infection.

6. The Dissemination of the Infectious Material discharged by Consumptives is Limited by its Physical Character.—If the patient and his attendants and friends take the simple precautions required to prevent spray infection during the act of coughing, no immediate danger attaches to the expectoration. A lump of expectoration in its wet condition is absolutely incapable of spreading infection, except in the unlikely events of its smearing the hand, or being carried by flies or otherwise, and thus leading to the infection of food or of the cavity of the mouth directly. The tubercle bacilli are as safely imprisoned

in the lump of expectoration as they would be in a bottle. Evaporation of the watery part of the expectoration is not accompanied by any escape of tubercle bacilli.   Currents of air similarly have no effect.   The bacilli cannot leave the expectoration so long as it is moist.   Expectoration is not only moist but also viscid, and thus the tubercle bacilli often remain imprisoned, even after all moisture has evaporated; and sweeping or rubbing with boots, etc., is required to convert the expectoration into a condition of such dryness that its dissemination as dust becomes practicable.   (On this point, see p. 92.)

Even when expectoration becomes dust, and the particulate infective material can be scattered, it obeys the laws of gravity and tends to sink again after being disturbed.   Hence a room which is very infective while sweeping is going on or soon afterwards may be occupied with relative safety an hour or two later. Tyndall's experiments demonstrating how particles of dust settle out of quiet air have clearly shown this.   It must be repeated that it would be unreasonable to trust to the physical laws which minimise the risk of infection, and not to insist on the cessation of indiscriminate expectoration and on the wet cleansing of all occupied rooms and public places.

7. THE AIR EXPIRED BY CONSUMPTIVES IN ORDINARY BREATHING IS ABSOLUTELY STERILE (see also p. 89).

8. The circumstances which limit the amount of infection by presenting opposing forces to the invading bacilli will be considered later.   (Chapters XXII. to XXVII.)

CHAPTER XIV

THE PORTALS OF INFECTION: *A*. INFECTION BY INHALATION

APART from the ingestion of infected food, to be considered later, the predominant means of infection are the spray produced by the consumptive as he coughs or sneezes, and the dust of his powdered expectoration. Where do the tubercle bacilli thus received take root, and how do they reach those parts of the body in which the main lesions of tuberculosis are found ?

They enter the body by the mouth or nostrils, and either (*a*) are passed through the mucous membrane of the mouth or naso-pharynx into the adjacent lymphatics; or (*b*) are swallowed and lodge in the intestines and the mesenteric glands connected with them; or (*c*) are inhaled into the lungs. From any one of the points thus reached the tubercle bacilli may and commonly do pass on to other parts of the body. Lesions thus occur at definite points, but there is no need for the supposition that one part of the body is more susceptible than another to tuberculosis. The lungs and the mesenteric glands, so far as we know, suffer more than other parts only because they are more exposed to invasion.

That tubercle bacilli are inhaled by persons in contact with consumptives, or by animals subjected to experiments with tuberculous dust, has been repeatedly shown. Strauss found tubercle bacilli in the nasal cavities of various healthy persons frequenting the wards of the Charité and Laennec Hospitals in Paris; of 29 persons employed in consumptive wards 9, of whom 6 were orderlies, gave positive results when tested by inoculation on guinea-pigs. St. Clair Thomson (1901) showed that in the healthy nose most of the bacteria inhaled are immediately stopped at the nostrils (see also p. 110). He quotes Liaras as having repeated Strauss's experiments under similar conditions on eighteen persons, but with precautions to secure cultures in each case from the interior of the nose and not from the nostril; the results were negative in each case. Notwithstanding the discrepant result of these observations, there is overwhelming evidence, both clinical and experimental, that tubercle bacilli may be inhaled and find their way by direct or indirect routes to the lungs. The subject may be conveniently discussed under the following heads :—

   1. By what means can the inhaled bacilli be checked?

   2. At what points do the bacilli enter the tissues of the body?

   3. What is the evidence that in phthisis the infection sometimes reaches the lungs by inhalation, and not always indirectly by the lymphatic or blood circulations?

The general rule is that at whatever spot on or in the tissues of the body tubercle bacilli succeed in resisting phagocytic and other inimical agencies, there or in lymphatic glands connected therewith will tuberculosis develop. The usual course is for the tubercle bacilli to pass through the surface on which they have become deposited, and to be carried thence by the lymph stream. The lymphatic glands may act as filters preventing the tubercle bacilli from spreading to other parts of the body; just as glands in the armpit may prevent general blood poisoning from a whitlow. Such carriage by the lymph stream is slow and largely barred by the glands. Rapid transport to more remote parts of the body can occur only when the bacilli have gained access to the blood vessels and are carried with the blood circulation. Then general or so-called miliary tuberculosis occurs, a relatively rare and late phenomenon in the disease.

MEANS BY WHICH THE INHALED BACILLI CAN BE CHECKED.—

1. *The Complexity and Shape of the Respiratory Passages.*—Angles are met with in the nostrils, nasal cavity, pharynx, glottis, trachea, and bronchi, and at every successive angle the inhaled dust is filtered off. With quiet breathing, the greater part is stopped in the nostrils.

2. *The high Reflex Irritability of the Nasal and Pharyngeal Mucous Membrane.*—The irritation produced by the presence of foreign particles may be so great as to cause sneezing and consequent expulsion of the offending particles, together with others too small to offend.

3. *The respiratory passages* are lined with a *coat of mucus*; and the individual *cells are provided with cilia* flicking all particles upwards towards the outlet. By this means a steady flow of mucus towards the pharynx is maintained, and a similar flow along the nose. Accumulated dust is thus swept into a position from which it can readily be ejected. Should the bacilli, notwithstanding the preceding impediments, succeed in obtaining lodgment in any part of the mucous membrane, they have then to do battle with the phagocytes of the body and the antibodies formed in connection with them. If victorious, the bacteria work their way into the underlying lymphoid tissue and along the lymph channels, and establish a primary focus of infection.

POINTS OF ENTRY. — If infective dust or droplets have passed the guarded portals of the mouth and nose, tubercle bacilli may penetrate the mucous membrane of the back of the nose, of the tonsils or larynx, of some lower part of the respiratory tract, or through decayed teeth. An obvious lesion may not develop at the point of penetration. This has been shown by Sidney Martin in the case of animals fed with tuberculous milk, a local ulcer being developed only when massive infection has been received; while only the subjacent lymphatic grands showed disease when the dose of infective material was more minute.

ADENOID GROWTHS, so common in the post-nasal cavities of children before puberty, favour the occurrence of infection; for they narrow the passage for air and hinder the expulsion of particulate matter. Naked - eye evidence of tuberculosis in adenoids is seldom seen ; but many observers have shown by microscopic examination or inoculation that tubercle bacilli are often contained in adenoids. Thus G. Morgan (1899) found tubercle bacilli in from 12 to 15 per cent. of his cases of adenoids in the substance of the morbid structure. Thomson (1901) gives a tabular statement of 1427 microscopic examinations of adenoids, in 5·1 per cent. of which tuberculosis was found. Dieulafoy similarly found tuberculous changes in 5·7 per cent. of his case of adenoids ; and the proportion was increased by inoculation experiments to 20 per cent. It seems likely, therefore, that tubercle bacilli may enter at this point more often than is ordinarily supposed.

The TEETH possibly may also be the point of invasion. Thus G. W. Cook (quoted by Squire, 1906) found tubercle bacilli in the pulp of decayed teeth and in scrapings taken from and around the teeth, especially of the young.

The TONSILS probably play a considerable rôle as a primary site of tuberculous infection. The act of swallowing tuberculous dust or spray or food presses infective particles against the tonsils, in the crypts of which the infective matter may lodge. Like all lymphoid tissue, the tonsils are " on outpost duty, to arrest the invading bacilli," and it is rather remarkable that active tuberculous disease of the tonsils is so seldom seen. Tubercle bacilli are often present in the tonsils without any naked-eye evidence of disease. On this point Latham (1900) has confirmed by the inoculation method the work of Woodhead and many others. He proved that the central portions of the tonsils of forty-five consecutive children aged from 3 months to 13 years showed evidence of tuberculosis in seven instances. Infection through the tonsils is common in pigs. It is probably more common in children than is usually supposed.

The LARYNX is only exceptionally the seat of primary tuberculosis, laryngeal implication being more often a symptom of advanced pulmonary tuberculosis. The trachea and bronchi are also seldom attacked, the inhibitory influences enumerated on page 107 rendering the infection of these parts infrequent.

INFECTION OF THE SUBSTANCE OF THE LUNGS BY DIRECT INHALATION is usually taught to be a frequent occurrence. We must now consider in detail the evidence for and against such direct inhalation.

1. *The Intricacies of the Respiratory Passages.*—It is not surprising in view of these intricacies, and of the moisture and other influences tending to deposit dust during inspiration, that Cohnheim (1890) describes the air passages as forming a comparatively long and narrow, closed and protected tube system ; while Virchow long upheld the view that dust could not find its way into the ultimate lung substance (quoted by Arlidge, 1892), arguing that the black pigment found in miners' lungs was due to altered blood pigment and not to carbon. In 1866, however, he was convinced that his former views on this point were incorrect.

Against these mechanical difficulties must be set the facts

that during hard work breathing becomes more rapid and more laboured, and that the mouth is apt to be open; furthermore, that inspiration takes place over 20,000 times in the twenty-four hours, and often occurs in a very dusty atmosphere. Under these circumstances it need not be the subject of surprise that the defensive arrangements are occasionally overworked and fail to prevent invasion by infective dust.

2. *Experimental Evidence.*—St. Clair Thomson and Hewlett (1895) having ascertained that at least 1500 organisms are inhaled into the nose every hour, and that in London it must be common for 14,000 to enter in an hour of quiet breathing, nevertheless found that the interior of the great majority of normal nasal cavities is perfectly aseptic (p. 106). They also confirmed Hildebrandt's experiments made in 1888, in several instances the trachea of animals killed in the laboratory being found on opening to be free from bacteria.

On the other hand, Zenker (quoted by Arlidge, p. 246) produced red colouring of the substance of the lungs of animals by causing them to inhale a red dust ; and Knauff (quoted by Buck, p. 29), after inhaling particles of ultramarine for only ten minutes, found that the cells of his expectoration contained blue particles in their interior. In ultramarine workers the coloured dust has been recognised in expectoration fourteen days after cessation from work. Rabbits confined in a smoky atmosphere can be shown to have fine particles of carbon in their bronchi. Knauff (quoted by Greenhow, 1869) placed dogs for from one day to three months in a roomy chest, into which the fumes of a smoking oil-lamp were conveyed by a flue opening through the floor. One dog killed after a single day in the smoke chest had the whole surface of the bronchial mucous membrane even to the alveoli of the lungs covered with a deposit of carbon mixed with mucus. Animals kept there for some weeks showed similar deposits throughout the lungs ; the lymphatic glands were very early affected. In animals confined for several weeks in the experimental chest there was almost invariably a deposit of carbon below the pleura. Control animals showed no similar appearances.

It must be admitted, however, that none of these experiments is quite inconsistent with the view that the particles of pigment had been swallowed and reached the lungs by means of the lymph stream ; and the view that the pigment in miners' lungs and similar diseases owes an intestinal origin has in recent years been revived by the French school, especially by Villoret. Van Steenberghe and Grysez fed guinea-pigs and rabbits with food containing mixed coal dust and particles of Indian ink, finding at the autopsy on these animals pigment in the lungs only, the abdominal organs and mesenteric glands being free. Schultze (1906, *Münch. med. Woch.*, liii. 1702) repeated these feeding experiments with similar results, but he is convinced that in feeding experiments, even when undertaken with the aid of a tube, inhalation cannot be excluded, and he explains in this way the deposit in the lungs. That this may be the correct explanation is supported by the fact that in a rabbit having a gastric fistula, through which he introduced pigments into the stomach daily for two months, no deposit was found post-mortem in the lungs. The experimental evidence, in short, cannot be said to have settled the question.

3. *Microscopic Evidence.*—According to Rindfleisch (1875, p. 649), the first lesion in pulmonary tuberculosis occurs at the angles and projections situated where the smallest bronchioles become continuous with the acini. This can be readily understood from Fig. 12, if it be assumed that the tubercle bacilli have been inhaled into the acini. During coughing they will become lodged in the crannies around the opening of the bronchiole (*a*), and disease consequently may start here. The diameter of a minute branch of the bronchus at *a* is from 0·3 to 0·4 mm., as compared with ·0015 to ·004 mm., the size of a tubercle bacillus.

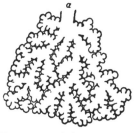

FIG. 12. — Acinus of the Lung, enlarged ten times ; at *a* is the junction of the bronchiole with the acinus

4. *Clinical experience* supports the view that direct inhalation of infective particles into the lung substance is at least exceptional. In 1868 Mr. (now Lord) Lister showed that suppuration did not follow when air had escaped into the pleura through injury of a lung by a fractured rib, thus indicating that the inspired air is probably sterile. His exact words are as follows:—

Why air introduced into the pleura through a wounded lung should have such totally different effects from that entering through a permanently open penetrating wound from without, was to me a complete mystery till I heard of the germ theory of putrefaction, when it at once occurred to me, though we could not suppose the gases of the atmosphere to be in any way altered in chemical composition by passing through the trachea and bronchial tubes on their way into the pleura, it was only natural that they should be filtered of germs by the air passages, one of whose offices is to arrest inhaled particles of dust, and prevent them from entering the air cells.

5. *The relative infrequency of tuberculosis of the larynx* is adduced as evidence of the completeness with which filtration of the inspired air is effected in the naso-pharynx. St. Clair Thomson (1901) found in 100 autopsies in pulmonary tuberculosis that only 30 had laryngeal disease; and in another series that only 1 in 450 had tuberculous nasal disease. But, as already explained, the relative immunity of the larynx is probably due to the freedom of movement of its parts, the violent coughing accompanying local irritation in it, and the active secretion of fluid washing away invading particles. Primary tuberculosis of the larynx occurs sometimes, but it is the exception.

The evidence briefly summarised above is conflicting. In view of what we know to occur in knife-grinders and in lead and slate miners, as well as of the evidence given above, the balance leans to the conclusion that direct inhalation of dust into the lungs occurs. Such dust, if it carries with it the tubercle bacillus, may be regarded as an inoculating needle, securing a firm foothold for the bacillus in the pulmonary tissues.

INFECTION OF THE LUNGS OTHERWISE THAN BY DIRECT INHALATION.—Though it be agreed that the lungs may be invaded directly during inhalation, this is certainly not the only means of infection. The lungs may also be infected secondarily through the following channels :—

(a) *Through the bronchial glands.* Tuberculous material is arrested at the tonsils or elsewhere, and the bacilli pass to the cervical and bronchial glands by the lymph stream. Sims Woodhead's experiments (1898) on a series of pigs fed with milk containing tubercle bacilli throw light on this question. The line of invasion could be traced in these pigs from the tonsils and lymphoid tissues of the throat to the neighbouring lymphatic glands along the neck ; thence to the upper part of the chest, to the glands at the root of the neck and the pleura. In this connection must be noted the frequency with which, in man, pleurisy precedes other signs of pulmonary tuberculosis. Woodhead's conclusion is as follows :—

> I am driven to the conclusion that this method of infection of the glands of the neck through the tonsils must be a comparatively frequent occurrence, especially in children under insanitary conditions, and subjected to various devitalising influences.

There can be little doubt that the infection may spread downwards to the bronchial glands and then into the lungs, and that this is a fairly common method of infection, especially in children. That this is so is confirmed by the fact that in children the parts of the lungs near their roots are often most affected by tuberculosis. According to H. Walsham (1904),

> it is still an open question whether or not the lung can be infected by the gradual extension of the bacilli downwards with the lymph stream. I think in these cases where we find tuberculous change in the cervical glands further advanced than in the bronchial, we may assume that the lung has been infected in this manner.

Case 4, p. 66, is probably one of phthisis originating in this way. It is not unlikely, however, that as in the case of intestinal infection (p. 116) the first chain of glands, in this case the cervical, may escape obvious involvement, the bronchial glands suffering most.

The bronchial glands themselves may be infected from two sources : (a) from the cervical glands, and probably from the tonsils, as indicated above ; (b) from the alimentary canal. Thus Woodhead has traced tuberculosis from a caseous or old calcareous mesenteric gland through the chain of retro-peritoneal glands up through the diaphragm to the posterior mediastinal and bronchial glands, and thence to the lungs. According to Guthrie, to the above methods of access to the mediastinal and bronchial glands must be added the possible passage of bacilli, swallowed with mucus or food, through the œsophageal lymphatic plexus to the posterior mediastinal glands. Squire (1906) believes that the implication of the bronchial glands is oftener produced in the reverse direction, from lungs to glands, than is usually accepted.

(b) *Through the alimentary canal.* This will be considered separately in the next chapter.

(c) *Through the blood stream.* The lungs may be infected

by tubercle bacilli carried in the blood circulation. This circulation of infective products undoubtedly happens in general tuberculosis, as Buhl showed in 1857 (p. 37). A caseous nodule breaks down, its contents enter the blood vessels, are carried to the heart and thence in the round of the circulation. It is likely that a more localised distribution of infection occurs by the blood vessels, when tuberculous material ulcerates into a blood vessel in the lung, and the disease spreads with the blood current to other parts of the lung. According to Volland (Cornet, p. 182), pulmonary tuberculosis is produced by bacilli which have entered the cervical glands and are carried thence within the leucocytes by way of the lymph stream and the lesser circulation to the lungs. We shall discuss later what means, if any, can be used to determine whether a given fatal case of tuberculosis has been caused by inhalation or ingestion ; and, if the latter, whether through the ingestion of human or of bovine infectious material.

CHAPTER XV

THE PORTALS OF INFECTION: *B*. INFECTION BY INGESTION

THE arguments for and against the direct invasion of the lungs by inhaled particles have been given in the last chapter. If direct infection by way of the lungs is escaped, it does not follow that no infection occurs. As we have already seen, the individual may be infected through the mouth, naso-pharynx, or œsophagus. The next possibility of infection is through the stomach. Little is known of this, as separate from intestinal infection, and the subsequent course of the bacilli would be almost the same in both instances. In passing we may note

THE EFFECT OF THE GASTRIC JUICE ON SWALLOWED TUBERCLE BACILLI.—Falk and Wesener exposed tuberculous material to the action of an artificial gastric juice for some hours, and showed that it had not lost its virulence when tested by inoculation on animals. Strauss and Wurtz subjected pure cultures of the avian tubercle bacillus to the action of a dog's gastric juice, and found that at the end of eight to twelve hours the bacilli were still able to produce local tuberculosis when inoculated on animals. It must be remembered, however, that the fat-splitting enzyme of gastric juice is very sensitive to its environment, and is destroyed quickly when the juice is used *in vitro*. Probably the fatty envelope of the tubercle bacillus would be more readily dissolved within the stomach than in an experiment under artificial con-ditions. Nevertheless in the stomach the digestive or inhibitory effect of the gastric juice would be diminished by dilution with food and fluid, and many tubercle bacilli would doubtless pass on unharmed into the small intestine.

THE LESIONS PRODUCED BY INGESTED TUBERCLE BACILLI.—Most of these follow on the passage of the bacilli through the intestinal mucous membrane. The local effect on the mucous membrane varies with the dose and the virulence of the bacilli, and possibly with the age of the patient. Sidney Martin's experiments in feeding pigs with tuberculous material showed that there need not be a local development of tuberculosis at the point of entry of the bacillus (see also p. 113), but that such lesions occurred when major doses of a more virulent strain were given.

It might be argued that in these cases infection had not come *via* the intestine. Thus Cadeac (quoted by Müller, 1905) believes that in most feeding experiments, the tubercle bacilli enter in the region of the mouth and pharynx. Having fed guinea-pigs with material rich in bacilli, he killed them at the end of seven days, and tested the glands of the head and of the mesentery by inoculation, obtaining a negative result in the latter, a positive in the former case. Müller has found that in guinea-pigs fed with infected milk the mesenteric glands may be primarily affected.

A. Calmette and A. Guérin experimented on young goats suckled from their mothers' teats, which had previously been made tuberculous by the artificial introduction of tuberculous material into the mammary gland. They all acquired intestinal tuberculosis, followed by mesenteric disease. Then a number of adult goats were fed with tuberculous material by means of an œsophageal tube. These all contracted grave and rapidly fatal pulmonary tuberculosis, without obvious intestinal and with only a few mesenteric lesions. They concluded that in adults tubercle bacilli pass easily through the mesenteric lymphatic glands to the thoracic duct, and thence through the heart and pulmonary arteries of the lungs.

The Second Interim Report of the Royal Commission on Tuberculosis (1907) gives the details of experiments in which calves were fed with the milk of cows whose udders had been made tuberculous by intra-mammary injection. It was found that in only one out of six calves thus fed was general tuberculosis produced, the tuberculosis in the others being confined chiefly to the intestines and mesenteric glands. Fourteen cows fed with tuberculous milk from various sources showed chiefly mesenteric lesions. On the other hand, generalised progressive tuberculosis was readily produced in monkeys by feeding them with tuberculous milk.

The experiments of Calmette and Guérin indicate that tuberculosis of the bronchial glands and of the lungs may be the result of feeding with tuberculous material, with or without mesenteric disease ; but it appears likely that in human tuberculosis due to ingestion, implication of the mesenteric glands is generally more abundant and more severe than that of other parts of the body.

The age of tuberculous lesions is judged by the presence or absence of caseation or calcification ; these signs being taken to indicate an older lesion than tuberculous disease in which these degenerative changes have not occurred. On the value of such evidence in experimental animals, Professor Delépine (1898, p. 734) may be quoted :—

There are very often clear indications in the body of the victim showing the channels through which the bacilli have penetrated. We have seen how the bacilli infect first the lymphatic glands nearest to their point of entrance. The lymph coming from the intestine passes first through the mesenteric glands. The lymph from the lungs passes in the same way through the bronchial glands. It is therefore evident that in the event of the bacilli penetrating through the intestine the mesenteric glands would be chiefly affected, and in the case of lung infection the bronchial glands would be most involved. There are cases in which death occurs before any other glands than those first invaded have had time to become diseased ; in such cases the state of the glands will clearly indicate the channel through which the bacilli have entered.

In a series of over 300 experiments I have found that tuberculosis of the mesenteric glands occurs extremely late in guinea-pigs infected through other channels than the intestinal canal and the peritoneal cavity, and am absolutely convinced of the value of lymphatic glands as indicators of the path followed by tubercle bacilli in cases which have died before the disease has become too advanced. According to Dr. Woodhead, the post-mortem examinations of the bodies of tuberculous children who had died before the age of five and a half years show that in the large majority of them the intestine and mesenteric glands were affected, and that in 14 per cent. of those cases the mesenteric glands alone were tuberculous.

Notwithstanding somewhat discrepant results from experiments, we may, I think, assume that the evidence of death-returns and still more of post-mortem examinations, gives some indication of the relative frequency of intestinal and of more direct pulmonary infection.

AGE INCIDENCE OF DEATH-RATE FROM THE DIFFERENT FORMS OF TUBERCULOSIS.—The following table, which I have calculated from the Registrar-General's returns, shows the age incidence of the death-rate from the three chief forms of tuberculosis :—

TABLE XXII.—ENGLAND AND WALES, 1901

Death-rate per 100,000 *Persons living at each Age-period*

	0–5.	5–10.	10–15.	15–20.	20 and upwards.
Pulmonary Tuberculosis . .	31	20	41	90	176
Tuberculous Meningitis . .	109	27	12	6	2
Tabes Mesenterica . . .	125	10	7	5	3

Even if a large deduction be made for errors of diagnosis and certification in the returns of tuberculous meningitis and tabes mesenterica, it still remains true that there is an inverse relation between the age incidence of death from those two diseases and that of death from phthisis. Whether, as adults take much less uncooked cows' milk than children, it may be inferred with safety that respiratory infection is more common in adult life and digestive infection in childhood, is still open to doubt. An *à priori* probability to this effect is created ; but this is somewhat shaken by our knowledge of the different channels through which the lungs may become infected. It is quite possible that phthisis originating *viâ* the digestive tract may be more frequent than the above table would indicate.

EVIDENCE FROM AUTOPSIES.—The evidence from autopsies as to which are the oldest lesions is apt to be disturbed by the fact that, no examination being possible until natural death occurs, the bronchial and mesenteric glands may appear to be implicated equally. Possibly also the changes may occur more rapidly in certain lesions than in others. Thus in guinea-pigs lesions advance more rapidly in lymphatic glands than in lungs. Furthermore, as pointed out by H. W. Russell, lesions in lymphatic glands are more easily detected than equally large lesions in a large organ like the lung. These sources of error possibly explain some of the discrepancies in the results of autopsies made at different hospitals, of which the following are examples :—

Dr. L. G. Guthrie (1899) tabulated 77 post-mortem examinations made on tuberculous children at the Paddington Children's Hospital. He found tuberculosis of the various thoracic organs (lungs, pericardium, and pleura) in the aggregate of all the cases examined 105 times, of the various abdominal organs (peritoneum, intestine, spleen, liver, kidneys, and pancreas) 102 times, of the brain and meninges 41 times, and of the bones and joints 6 times. He notes the difficulty in determining the starting-point of infection from the stage of the lesions produced ; but, adopting the usual method of deciding the source of disease, he found that of the 77 cases, thoracic tuberculosis was most prominent and apparently primary in 42 (54·5 per cent.), and abdominal tuberculosis in 19 (24·6 per cent.). In 7 of the remainder (16) the thoracic organs were as much affected as the abdominal. In 6 cases the origin was not discovered, and 3 single cases originated elsewhere. The thoracic glands were found in a state of caseation 46 times, and the abdominal glands 31 times. Both sets were caseous in 15 cases ; in 3 neither set was affected, and in 12 their condition was not noted. Thus the glands were caseous in 62 cases, or 80·5 per cent. of the total. Dr. Guthrie adds that he has not regarded mere caseation as evidence of primary glandular infection, and that he could only trace the origin of tuberculosis with any degree of certainty in 41·5 per cent. of the cases—to the thoracic glands in 17 cases and to the mesenteric glands in 15.

Dr. Guthrie summarises other experiences as follows :—

MM. Rillet and Barthez found the origin in caseous bronchial glands in 79 per cent. and in mesenteric glands in 46 per cent. of cases. Simmonds discovered caseous bronchial and tracheal glands in 73 per cent. and caseous mesenteric glands in 46 per cent., whilst Dr. Walter Colman attributed the origin to caseous thoracic glands in 79 per cent. and to mesenteric glands in 66 per cent. of his cases.

He adds :—

The discrepancy between these statistics and my own may be due to the fact that I have discarded the glands as the primary source of infection unless they have been both obviously caseous, and also associated with miliary, or at all events comparatively recent, tuberculosis elsewhere.

Dr. Still (1899) concluded from post-mortem examinations of 269 children under 12 years of age that the most common channel of infection in children is through the lungs ; that infection through the intestine is less common in infancy than in later childhood; and that milk cannot be the usual source of infection. Dr. A. Latham, tabulating over 3000 post-mortem results on children, says they show that in children tuberculosis of the bronchial glands is the lesion most constantly found, and that disease is in the majority of instances most advanced in these glands. He deprecates the inference that infection has necessarily been conveyed aerially, and considers that infected milk supply plays an important rôle.

Dr. Kingsford (1904) has added further cases and tabulated the results of previous observers in an excellent paper.

It would be easy to give further figures, but they are all inconclusive. It cannot be regarded as settled, to what degree human tuberculosis is due to direct inhalation into the lungs, to entrance of infective material through the tonsils, etc., and to intestinal infection. Much less is this point settled for pulmonary tuberculosis. For a large proportion of intestinal may be and probably is secondary to pulmonary tuberculosis ; and tuberculous meningitis may be secondary to an earlier focus of tuberculosis in any part of the 'body. Conversely, a large, possibly the largest, part of pulmonary tuberculosis may be due not to the direct inhalation of infective material into the lungs, but to secondary implication of the lungs from the neighbouring glands. And these glands or the pulmonary disease itself may furthermore have been the nidus of potential and eventually active pulmonary tuberculosis for many years before the latter disease comes into active existence. The evidence needs to be sifted with the utmost care in each individual case. Even then, the final decision arrived at after a careful balancing of all the available evidence cannot be regarded as certain. But the same remark applies to a large proportion of the broader problems of medicine ; and we are not relieved thereby from the responsibility of adjudicating and of taking practical measures based on our decisions. The obviously safe plan is to guard against all the possible sources of tuberculous infection that have been considered, though the greatest importance must be attached to the prevention of the inhalation or swallowing of dried expectoration or expectoration in the form of spray.

CHAPTER XVI

RELATION OF BOVINE TO HUMAN TUBERCULOSIS[1]

IN the earlier attempts to diminish tuberculosis, the prevention of infection by means of food bulked very largely. The only foods which are of importance in this connection are cows' milk and its products, and the flesh of the ox and pig. Inasmuch as cows' milk is the chief possible non-human source of tuberculosis in man, the question becomes in the main one as to the relation between bovine and human tuberculosis. The earlier view is summarised in the following remarks from the Report of the Royal Commission appointed to inquire into the Effect of Food derived from Tuberculous Animals (1895) :—

Par. 22. As regards man, we must believe—and here we find ourselves agreeing with the majority of those who gave evidence before us—that any person who takes tuberculous matter into the body as food, incurs some risk of acquiring tuberculous disease. . . .

Par. 23. We regard the disease as being the same disease in man and in the food animals, no matter though there are differences in the one and in the other in their manifestations of the disease ; and we consider the bacilli of tubercle to form an integral part of the disease in each, and (whatever may be its origin) to be transmissible from man to animals and from animals to animals.

In Par. 80 of the report of the same Royal Commission it is stated emphatically that " no doubt the largest part of the tuberculosis which man obtains through his food is by means of milk containing tuberculous matter."

The views stated above were generally entertained by Koch among others, judging by his statement in 1882 (*Berliner klin. Wochenschr.*, 1882, p. 230) that " bovine tuberculosis is

[1] This and the next two chapters were written before the appearance of the second Interim Report of the Royal Commission appointed to inquire into the Relations of Human and Bovine Tuberculosis. Any modifications necessitated by that important report are added in footnotes, or in special paragraphs.

identical with human tuberculosis, and is thus a disease transmissible to man."

In 1901, Koch gave his famous address at the meeting of the British Congress on Tuberculosis. In this address he said :—

This manner of infection is generally regarded nowadays as proved, and as so frequent that it is even looked upon by not a few as the most important, and the most rigorous measures are demanded against it. In this Congress also the discussion of the danger with which the tuberculosis of animals threatens man will play an important part.

After excluding the tuberculosis of poultry, which differs so much from human tuberculosis that it can be left out of account as a source of infection for man, he added,

the only kind of animal tuberculosis remaining to be considered is the tuberculosis of cattle, which, if really transferable to man, would indeed have frequent opportunities of infecting human beings through the drinking of the milk and the eating of the flesh of diseased animals.

After indicating the obvious impossibility of investigating the problem by direct experiments on human beings, Koch said :—

Indirectly, however, we can try to approach it. It is well known that the milk and butter consumed in great cities very often contain large quantities of the bacilli of bovine tuberculosis in a living condition, as the numerous infection experiments with such dairy products on animals have proved. Most of the inhabitants of such cities daily consume such living and perfectly virulent bacilli of bovine tuberculosis, and unintentionally carry out the experiment which we are not at liberty to make. If the bacilli of bovine tuberculosis were able to infect human beings, many cases of tuberculosis caused by the consumption of alimenta containing tubercle bacilli could not but occur among the inhabitants of great cities, especially the children.

His remarks on this point will need discussion later (p. 131), but in the meantime we may quote his conclusion, which is that,

though the important question whether man is susceptible to bovine tuberculosis at all is not yet absolutely decided, and will not admit of absolute decision to-day or to-morrow, one is nevertheless already at liberty to say that, if such a susceptibility really exists, the infection of human beings is but a very rare occurrence. I should estimate the extent of infection by the milk and flesh of tuberculous cattle and the butter made of this milk, as hardly greater than that of hereditary transmission, and I therefore do not deem it advisable to take any measures against it.

This important expression of opinion involved a re-testing of the whole question of the relationship between bovine and human tuberculosis, and since Koch's address many have been working at the problem.   In England a Royal Commission was appointed to inquire into the Relations of Human and Animal Tuberculosis, and in 1904 it issued an interim report, from which the following extract is taken :—

We have up to the present made use, in the above inquiry, of more than twenty different " strains " of tuberculous material of human origin, that is to say, of material taken from more than twenty cases of tuberculous disease in human beings, including sputum from phthisical patients and the diseased parts of the lungs in pulmonary tuberculosis, mesenteric glands in primary abdominal tuberculosis, tuberculous bronchial and cervical glands, and tuberculous joints.   We have compared the effects produced by these with the effects produced by several different strains of tuberculous material of bovine origin.

In the case of seven of the above strains of human origin, the introduction of the human tuberculous material into cattle gave rise at once to acute tuberculosis, with the development of widespread disease in various organs of the body, such as the lungs, spleen, liver, lymphatic glands, etc.   In some instances the disease was of remarkable severity.

In the case of the remaining strains, the bovine animal into which the tuberculous material was first introduced was affected to a less extent. The tuberculous disease was either limited to the spot where the material was introduced (this occurred, however, in two instances only, and these at the very beginning of our inquiry), or spread to a variable extent from the seat of inoculation along the lymphatic glands, with, at most, the appearance of a very small amount of tubercle in such organs as the lungs and spleen.   Yet tuberculous material taken from the bovine animal thus affected, and introduced successively into other bovine animals, or into guinea-pigs from which bovine animals were subsequently inoculated, has, up to the present, in the case of five of these remaining strains, ultimately given rise in the bovine animal to general tuberculosis of an intense character ; and we are still carrying out observations in this direction.

We have very carefully compared the disease thus set up in the bovine animal by material of human origin with that set up in the bovine animal by material of bovine origin, and so far we have found the one, both in its broad general features and in its finer histological details, to be identical with the other.   We have so far failed to discover any character by which we could distinguish the one from the other ; and our records contain accounts of the post-mortem examinations of bovine animals infected with tuberculous material of human origin, which might be used as typical descriptions of ordinary bovine tuberculosis.

The result at which we have arrived, namely, that tubercle of human origin can give rise in the bovine animal to tuberculosis identical with ordinary bovine tuberculosis, seems to us to show quite clearly that it would be most unwise to frame or modify legislative measures in accordance with the view that human and bovine tubercle bacilli are specifically different from each other, and that the disease caused by the one is a wholly different thing from the disease caused by the other.

The preceding sketch of a few of the most prominent features in the history of this moot point would not be complete without noting that in 1896 Professor Theobald Smith first drew attention to certain differences between bacilli from human and bovine sources, and in 1898 he classed human and bovine bacilli as separate types or races.   Although the evidence which he advanced had been somewhat neglected until Koch published the results of his limited series of experiments, the idea that there are two types of tubercle bacillus bearing on human disease, the *Typus humanus* and the *Typus bovinus*, is by no means new.

DIFFERENCES BETWEEN HUMAN AND BOVINE TUBERCULOSIS. —1. *Differences in Morphological Characters of the Bacilli.*—The bovine bacillus is more uniform and constant in form than the human bacillus.   It is thick, straight, and short, seldom more than 2 μ in length, and averaging less (Theobald Smith). Human bacilli are larger from the start and tend to increase in length at once in subculture.   They are generally more or less curved.   These morphological differences tend to disappear in the tissues of susceptible animals.   The bovine bacilli stain deeply with carbol-fuchsin, beading being nearly always absent from young cultures and often from old ; human bacilli stain less intensely with carbol-fuchsin, and beading is generally seen, even in early growths.

2. *Differences in Growth in Media.*—Bovine bacilli, according to the same authority, grow more luxuriantly in artificial media than human bacilli, especially in glycerinised broth.

3. *Differences in Reaction.*—Theobald Smith has

called attention to the difference in the movement of the reaction of the glycerin bouillon in which bovine and human bacilli are multiplying. In the case of the bovine cultures this movement leads to a final reaction, either neutral, feebly alkaline, or feebly acid, toward phenolphthalein ; in case of the human cultures to a pronounced acidity to phenolphthalein. In the latter the reaction at first becomes less acid, then either much more acid, or else it remains at a medium level.[1]

---

[1] According, however, to the experimental work done by Dr. A. S. Griffith for the Royal Commission on Tuberculosis (vol. iii. of Appendix to Second Interim Report) these differences appear to be " differences in degree and not in kind, and are attributable to variations in saprophytic power which have been shown to exist on other media."

4. *Differences in Pathogenic Effect.*—The bovine bacillus has a much greater pathogenic power than the human bacillus for all animals with which it has been inoculated ; except that in the pig and guinea-pig 'the susceptibility to both types of bacilli is so great that it is hard to distinguish between them (Ravenel, 1902, p. 26). Koch and Schütz in their experiments found that in pigs also the bovine was much more active than the human bacillus. Rabbits have been found to withstand the injection of doses of human bacilli, when an equal dose of bovine bacilli caused fatal tuberculosis. The difference in pathogenic effect between the human and bovine type is even more obvious in the case of cattle. Thus a subcutaneous injection of 5 cg. of bacilli of the human type caused in cattle only a local reaction at the seat of infection and in the neighbouring glands, the local disease decreasing and not spreading to internal organs, "even after protracted observation," whereas the same dose of bovine bacilli caused disseminated tuberculosis (Kossel, 1905). The difference in the two types is especially marked when animals are fed with pure cultures of the bacilli. When animals have been dosed for three months with cultures of the human type, bacilli are found to have accumulated in the mesenteric glands, without any change there other than calcification, and always without that wider dissemination seen in experiments with the bovine type.

Kossel draws attention to the necessity, in making comparative tests, of taking certain precautions, the ignoring of which may have caused some of the discrepant results published by different experimenters—(1) Comparable material alone should be used,—only young cultures, in which the same nutrient material has been employed. (2) Fresh strains of bacilli must be used, isolated recently from the animal body. (3) Faulty results have ensued from inoculating with pieces of tuberculous organs instead of with cultures. (4) Experiments should be on as wide a basis as possible. Kossel inoculated 27 different strains of bacilli of the bovine type and produced disseminated tuberculosis in 32 out of 33 cattle ; while the inoculation of 38 different strains of bacilli of the human type into 44 cattle produced local lesions only.

The above results can now be checked by the elaborate and protracted experimental observations of the English Royal

Commission given in their Second Interim Report (1907). The experimental results of the work are summarised as follows by Sidney Martin :—

GENERAL SUMMARY OF RESULTS OF THE ROYAL COMMISSION

1. *Bovine Tuberculosis*

(Thirty strains examined)

The bacillus of bovine tuberculosis has been shown by the experiments to have certain characteristics as follows :—

α. It shows some variations in its growth on artificial media, and according to these variations can be arranged into three groups or grades (I., II., III.).

β. When inoculated into bovines, rabbits, guinea-pigs, pigs, goats, monkeys, and the chimpanzee in appropriate doses it produces death by generalised tuberculosis.

γ. It shows stability as regards its cultural characters, both when sub-cultured and when passed through animals. Whether these characters can be altered by prolonged passage in certain animals is still the subject of experiment and cannot now be answered.

δ. It shows great stability in virulence both after long subcultivation and after passing through animals.

2. *Human Tuberculosis*

(Sixty cases examined)

The bacilli of human tuberculosis show a greater variety than those of bovine tuberculosis.

Group I

(Fourteen cases examined)

α. The bacilli obtained from the virus of human beings in this group have all the characters of the bacillus of bovine tuberculosis as regards cultural characters, virulence for the animals previously mentioned, and stability of cultural characters and of virulence.

The bacillus of this group is identical with the bacillus of bovine tuberculosis.

β. The bacillus of these cases was a single bacillus—there was no evidence of a " mixture " of different kinds of bacilli.

γ. The bacillus was the cause of death of the individuals from which it was obtained. This is more particularly shown by the study of Viruses H. 32 " Y.W.," H. 59 " L.B.," and H. 64 " M.G.," in which general tuberculosis was the cause of death of the child. The disease started as abdominal tuberculosis, but became generalised. Culture not only from the mesenteric glands, but also from the bronchial glands and lungs and meninges, had the characteristics of the bovine bacillus in cultivation and in virulence. No mixture of bacilli was here present. The children died of an infection by the bacillus of bovine tuberculosis.

This group includes three cases of cervical gland tuberculosis and eleven cases of abdominal tuberculosis.

Group II

(Forty cases examined)

The bacilli obtained from the virus of human tuberculosis in this group differs from the bacillus of bovine tuberculosis in the following points :—

a. In culture they are more luxuriant and are distinguished as referable to Groups IV. and V.

β. When inoculated into calves and rabbits they do not produce the generalised and fatal disease caused by the bovine bacillus.

The result of inoculation is not a negative one, but varies within certain limits with different viruses, and in rabbits the viruses occasionally kill the animal by producing a generalised disease.

They agree with the characteristics of the bovine bacillus in the following points :—

a. They produce general tuberculosis in monkeys and the chimpanzee.

β. The lesions produced in these animals are the same anatomically as those produced by the bovine bacillus.

γ. The lesions produced in calves and rabbits are histologically tuberculosis, although usually they show retrogression.

This group includes :—

Sputum Culture .	.	.	.	.	2 cases
Pulmonary Tuberculosis .	.	.	.	10 ,,
General	,,	.	.	.	1 case
Bronchial Gland	,,	.	.	.	2 cases
Cervical Gland	,,	.	.	.	6 ,,
Abdominal	,,	.	.	.	8 ,,
Joint	,,	.	.	.	9 ,,
Testicle	,,	.	.	.	1 case
Kidney	,,	.	.	.	1 ,,

The experiments show, however, that this division into two groups of the bacilli found in human tuberculosis is not the whole question.

Group III

(Six cases examined)

The investigation of two viruses, H. 53 " D.H." and H. 49 " T.C." shows that bacilli are obtainable from cases of human tuberculosis which belong to neither group.   The bacilli from the two viruses mentioned showed an irregular virulence in calves and rabbits, and one of them, H. 49 " T.C.," showed also (1) that the culture of the original material lost its virulence after prolonged subcultivation, and (2) that the original virus, although irregularly virulent for calves, became highly and uniformly virulent after being passed through a calf.   The culture of H. 49 " T.C." obtained from the original material has in cultivation the characters of the bacillus of bovine tuberculosis, belonging to Grade II.   There was no evidence of mixture in the case of either virus.

The results of the examination of the bacilli in the case of these two viruses point to the conclusion that the bacilli were bovine in origin and had been altered by residence in the human being.

As bearing intimately on this matter, the question of the transformation of the human bacillus into the bovine as shown in the experiments
previously discussed must be mentioned.

When by passage through calves, the slightly virulent bacillus of
human tuberculosis becomes apparently modified into the bovine bacillus,
it was suggested that it was not a real modification, but that the original
virus was a mixture of bacilli, and that during the passage the bovine
bacillus alone survived. But in these passage experiments there is evidence that at the time when the virus is becoming virulent, the bacilli
separated by culture are " unstable " in virulence for calves and rabbits ;
an instability similar to that of the original virus of H. 49 " T.C."

The consideration of these cases tends to bridge the gap between the
bacilli of Group I. (bovine bacilli) and those of Group II., which they
suggest may only be a form of bovine bacillus, degraded as regards virulence for calves and rabbits, by long residence in the human body.

If bacilli of the bovine and human types have distinctive
characteristics, and differ greatly in their pathogenic effects on
cattle, the answer to the question, is tuberculosis in cattle produced by the bacillus of the human type, must with certain
limited exceptions be in the negative. It does not, of course,
follow from this that human tuberculosis may not be caused
by bacilli of the bovine as well as of the human type. The
results obtained by the Royal Commission as well as by German
and American observers indicate that bovine is at least an
occasional cause of human tuberculosis. There may be said
to be three schools of opinion on the subject :—

1. *Human and bovine tuberculosis are totally distinct diseases,*
and are not to any serious extent intercommunicable. This
appears to be Koch's position, for in his Nobel Lecture (1906)
he says :—

We must attain to absolute clearness as to the manner in which infection in tuberculosis takes place—*i.e.* as to how the tubercle bacilli
get into the human organism, for the sole purpose of all prophylactic
measures against a pestilence must be to prevent the entrance of the
germs of disease into man. Now, as regards infection with tuberculosis
only two possibilities have hitherto presented themselves—namely,
infection by tubercle bacilli emanating from tuberculous human beings
and infection by tubercle bacilli contained in the flesh and milk of tuberculous cattle. After the investigations which I have made hand-in-hand
with Schütz as to the relation between human and bovine tuberculosis,
we may dismiss this second possibility, or at least regard it as so slight
that this source of infection as compared with the other falls quite into the
background. We arrived, namely, at the result that human tuberculosis
and bovine tuberculosis are different from one another, and that bovine

tuberculosis is not transmissible to man. With reference to this latter point, however, I wish, in order to prevent misunderstandings, to add that in saying this I mean only those forms of tuberculosis that have to be taken into account in connection with the combating of tuberculosis as an epidemic disease—namely, generalised tuberculosis and above all pulmonary phthisis. . . . I wish only to add that the testing of our investigations which has been carried out with the utmost care and on a broad basis in the Imperial Office of Health in Berlin has led to a confirmation of my opinion, and that, moreover, the harmlessness of the bacilli of bovine tuberculosis to man has been directly proved by the repeated inoculating of human beings with the material of bovine tuberculosis by Spengler and Klemperer. In connection with the combating of tuberculosis, then, only the tubercle bacilli emanating from human beings have to be taken into account.

2. *The ingestion of bacilli of the bovine type is the essential cause of tuberculosis in the human being.* The chief exponent of this view is von Behring, who, in his Cassel Lecture (1903), says :—

Koch's assertion that there are essential differences between human and bovine tubercle bacilli, and that these differences are not bridged over by any connecting links . . . has since called forth observations from all over the world which positively demonstrate the existence of intermediary stages in the virulence of tubercle bacilli derived from mammals. Generally, tubercle bacilli derived from cattle are more virulent for all animal species thus far examined than are human tubercle bacilli. And the opinion is constantly gaining ground that bovine tubercle bacilli are also more virulent for man.

His own special views are embodied in the following extracts from the same lecture :—

According to my ideas there has not yet been a single well-authenticated case in which pulmonary consumption has originated in adults as the result of a tuberculous infection developing epidemiologically, *i.e.* under conditions essential for infection occurring in nature.

His view is that in all cases in which phthisis is caused, apparently by human infection during adult life, there has been pre-existing tuberculosis of bovine origin, and he holds that

considering the figures . . . showing the enormous diffusion of tuberculosis, the objection is surely justified that the persons thus dying of consumption already had a tuberculous focus in the lungs, and that this pulmonary disease, under a mode of life favourable to tuberculosis, was converted into florid phthisis.

9

It is necessary to give further extracts from this lecture, in order to make von Behring's position quite clear.   He concedes

not only the possibility, but the actual occurrence of pulmonary tuberculosis going on to consumption, as a result of infection of an adult person . . . in the sense that on the basis of an infantile infection a pulmonary tuberculosis has developed, which becomes manifest only through the agency of the additional infection.

His chief contention is contained in the following words :—

I believe I have discovered a new principle which may be expressed thus :

The milk fed to infants is the chief cause of consumption.

3. *Human tuberculosis may be and is caused by bacilli of either the bovine or human type.*   This is the view most generally and justifiably entertained, supported as it is by the balance of all available evidence.   The extracts from the Interim Report of the Royal Commission given on p. 126 show that bacilli of the human type are sometimes very virulent to cattle ; and the practical conclusion given in an earlier report (p. 123) of the same Commission as to the undesirability in the interest of man of relaxing precautions against bovine tuberculosis, must commend itself as reasonable.   Thus Ravenel (1905, p. 147) says :—

Theoretically, there is no reason why the bovine bacillus should not be readily transmitted to man.   It has for all other mammalia on which it has been tried a virulence greatly exceeding that of the human tubercle bacillus.   It would certainly seem a remarkable anomaly for man, who is one of the most susceptible of all animals to tuberculosis, to be immune to the most powerful virus known.   In the whole range of communicable diseases we have nothing comparable to this state of affairs, should we admit it.

These three views will be next considered.

CHAPTER XVII

EVIDENCE OF THE OCCURRENCE OF BOVINE
TUBERCULOSIS IN MAN

THE occurrence of tuberculosis of bovine origin in man to an extent of practical importance is, as we have seen, denied by Koch and those who agree with him. What evidence is there for and against this view? Tuberculosis might conceivably be produced in man by bacilli of the bovine type, (1) if these bacilli were themselves able to cause active disease in him ; or (2) if they were to survive in his tissues in a latent condition for a period sufficient to enable them to become changed into bacilli of the human type.

WHAT EVIDENCE IS THERE THAT BACILLI OF THE BOVINE TYPE CAN CAUSE ACTIVE TUBERCULOSIS IN MAN DIRECTLY, WITHOUT CONVERSION INTO THE HUMAN TYPE ?—The only satisfactory evidence available consists in finding, in the lesions of human disease, bacilli which conform to all the known distinctive tests of the bovine type, including those already given on p. 124. This evidence has been supplied by various workers. Thus Theobald Smith in 1898 made from the mesenteric glands of children two cultures, of which one was of human while the other was pronounced to be of bovine origin. At the same time he supplemented the studies made by Ravenel " upon a presumably bovine culture from a child, by applying a new reaction test " (described on p. 124). " This latter culture had also the characteristics belonging to the bovine bacillus." Later (1904, p. 9), he showed that the bacilli present in three cases of general tuberculosis—a child aged eight months and two adults—did not belong to the bovine type. In a paper published in 1905, Theobald Smith, after giving further cases fully worked out, states that Vagades (*Zeitschr. für Hygiene*, 1898, xxviii. p. 276) found " one culture among 28 isolated from man, which, it seems to me, was a bovine bacillus." He also quotes Lartigau (*Journal of Medical*

Research, 1901, vi. p. 156) as finding at least one bovine culture of maximum virulence among nineteen cultures of human source ; and he quotes Ravenel as having, like himself, isolated from mesenteric glands two cultures, of which one was of the human and the other of the bovine type.   He emphasises (1905, p. 296) the fact that

but few experimenters have taken the time necessary to isolate and carefully compare cultures. The literature does not therefore offer that precise basal information upon which far-reaching conclusions may be built.

Since the above quotation was written, the Imperial Board of Health in Berlin and the English Royal Commission have both issued reports, the latter of which is quoted on p. 126.   In the former Kossel (1905, p. 1448) states :

The result of the far-reaching experiments conducted under my direc-tion in the Gesundheitsamt at Berlin has been to show that in human tuberculosis tubercle bacilli may exist that correspond in every respect in their morphological, biological, and pathogenic qualities to bacilli of cattle tuberculosis—that is, such as belong to the *Typus bovinus*.

Among 56 cases of human tuberculosis we found these germs 6 times—that is, in 10 per cent. of the cases. It would, however, be erroneous to conclude from these figures alone that 10 per cent. of all cases of human tuberculosis in Berlin were caused by infection with tubercle bacilli of the *Typus bovinus*, and that for the following reason : We included in the number of our experiments chiefly cases in which we could assume that the tuberculosis owed its origin to an intestinal infection, and possibly, therefore, to food containing tubercle bacilli.

Tubercle bacilli of the *Typus bovinus* appear chiefly in tuberculous lesions in children, and among our cases we found that, with one excep-tion, it was the mesenteric glands or intestinal ulcers that contained the bovine germs. When, on the other hand, the sputum of adults suffering from pulmonary phthisis was examined, only bacilli of the *Typus humanus* were found. That tubercle bacilli of the *Typus bovinus* can, however, also enter the adult body was ascertained by our finding them, together with those of the *Typus humanus*, in a case of extensive tuberculous ulcers of the intestines in a woman.

RESULTS OF THE ENGLISH ROYAL COMMISSION.—As already indicated, the bacilli obtained from sixty cases of human tuber-culosis were exhaustively examined by every known method, with the results as to type of bacillus set out on p. 126.   These results are so important from other points of view that I have set them out in tabular form below, in a table modified from the table on p. 72 of the report of the above Commission.

TABLE XXIII

Summary of Results of Examination of Different Strains of Human Tubercle Bacilli

Nature of Case.	Part used for Experiment.	Viruses Virulent for Bovines and Rabbits.	Viruses slightly Virulent for Bovines and Rabbits.	Virus of Irregular Virulence for Bovines and Rabbits.	Viruses slightly Virulent at first for Bovines and Rabbits; becoming Virulent afterwards.
1. Sputum (4 cases) . .	Sputum . . .	1	2	...	1
2. Primary Pulmonary Tuberculosis (10 cases) .	Lung . . .	...	9	...	...
	Lung and cervical gland . . .	...	1	...	...
3. General Tuberculosis (1 case) . . .	Bronchial glands .	...	1	...	...
4. Bronchial Gland Tuberculosis (4 cases) . .	Bronchial glands .	...	2	...	2
5. Cervical Gland Tuberculosis (9 cases) . .	Cervical glands .	3	6	...	...
6. Primary Abdominal Tuberculosis (19 cases) .	Mesenteric glands .	6	7	1	...
	Mesenteric gland, cervical gland, meninges . .	...	1	...	...
	Mesenteric gland, bronchial gland .	1	...	...	...
	Mesenteric gland, lung, cervical gland, meninges .	1	...	...	...
	Mesenteric gland, meninges . .	1	...	...	..
	Mesenteric gland, lung, meninges .	1	...	...	...
7. Joint Tuberculosis (10 cases) . . .	Scrapings from joints	...	6	...	1
	Pus from lumbar abscess . . .	...	3	...	...
8. Tuberculosis of Testis (1 case)	Testis . . .	...	1	...	...
Tuberculosis of Kidney (1 case) . . .	Kidney . . .	...	1	...	...
9. Lupus (1 case) . .	Scrapings of the lesions . .	...	...	1	...
Total . . .	. . . .	14	40	2	4

It will be noted that 14 out of the total number of strains obtained from human sources conformed to the bovine type. Out of 19 cases of primary abdominal disease, in which infection might be through ingestion, 10 were of bovine type; out of 8 cases of tuberculous cervical glands, in which similar infection during swallowing might occur, 3 were of bovine type; whereas only 1 strain of the bovine type was obtained from sputum out of 4 examined, and none from diseased lungs out of 10 examined. Of 4 cases of bronchial gland disease 2 were of the human type and 2 doubtful. Of 10 cases of joint tuberculosis, all were of the human type.

It would be unjustifiable to infer from the above figures that probably 14 out of 60, or about 23 per cent., of all cases of human tuberculosis are derived from tuberculous cattle. If the single sputum case be omitted, the parts affected in the above cases of tuberculosis of bovine type are the mesenteric and cervical glands. But primary tuberculosis of these parts causes less than 10 per cent. of the total mortality officially recorded as due to all forms of tuberculosis in this country. If the 28 cases of cervical and primary abdominal tuberculosis are assumed to be typical of what similar examination on a larger scale would show, it is noteworthy that 13 of these, i.e. about half, were of the bovine type. This would reduce the 10 per cent. above mentioned to 5 per cent.; and until further evidence accumulates it may be convenient to assume that from 5 to 10 per cent. of the total human mortality from tuberculosis is due to infection from bovine sources.

This assumption will be subject to modification if future investigations show that the bovine bacillus can be transformed into the bacillus of the human type. We may next consider with advantage the evidence at present available on this point.

What Evidence is there that Tubercle Bacilli of one Type can be transformed into Tubercle Bacilli of another Type ?—Many investigators hold that the characteristics given on p. 124 as distinguishing races of mammalian tubercle bacilli are variable elements, and can be modified by growing the bacilli in different culture media. Theobald Smith (1905, p. 297), however, observes :—

This view, I think, would be rejected by all who have studied continuously bacilli from different species. Virulence necessarily declines with prolonged cultivation, and bacilli may assume slightly different forms on different culture media.   These do not overthrow, but simply mask, racial characters.

On the other hand, Ravenel (1902, p. 45) says :—

With these facts before us I do not think we are forcing a point in believing that it is at least possible for the bovine bacillus to become rapidly so changed in the body of man that it will show the cultural and pathogenic peculiarities which we find usually in cultures of human origin.

In support of this view he quotes Nocard, who by introducing bovine and human bacilli into the peritoneal cavity in collodion sacs showed that in five to eight months both bovine and human bacilli acquired the cultural characteristics of the avian tubercle bacillus, and to a certain extent also its pathogenic action. Möller thought that he had so changed the human tubercle bacillus by passage through the blind worm for a year, that it grew best at 20° C. like the bacillus of fish tuberculosis.

According to von Behring and De Jong passage through goats is able to change the bacillus of the *Typus humanus* into the *Typus bovinus*.   Kossel is incredulous as to the transformations enumerated above, believing the results obtained to be due to inaccurate methods.   He quotes as an analogous case the fact that before Koch discovered a method of separating bacteria and growing them in pure culture on solid media, examples of transformation of one species of bacteria into another were described, to be rejected on more accurate investigation.   The experiments of Weber and Taute indicate the need of great caution.   They have shown that the tubercle bacilli of fishes, mentioned above, are really acid-fast saprophytes derived from mud.   Similarly in De Jong's experiment a goat was left for 3½ years after inoculation with tubercle bacilli of the human type before cultures were taken from it.   The possibility under these circumstances of extraneous infection by bovine tuberculosis is considerable. Kossel, Weber, and Heuss passed bacilli of the human type through goats and cattle, and found that after five passages they still remained of the same type, although they had been in the goats up to 202 days and in the cattle up to 381 days.

So far the evidence favours the view of a racial difference between tubercle bacilli of the bovine and those of the human types.   Against this view is urged the fact that it is possible—in the words of Kossel (p. 1448)—to

immunise cattle with the aid of tubercle bacilli of the *Typus humanus* against the bacilli of the *Typus bovinus*.   This fact is adduced as proving that one is dealing with one and the same germ, on the ground that immunity against a bacterium can only be produced by an identical microorganism.   Especially von Behring and Lorenz have emphasised this fact as conclusive.

But Kossel then remarks :—

On the other hand, it must be remembered that immunity in this direction is not equally specific in all species of bacteria.   The fact that efficient tuberculin can be prepared from avian tubercle bacilli as well as from mammalian by itself suggests caution in applying to tuberculosis such experiences as have been gained with regard to immunity in other groups of bacteria.   Furthermore, Beck observed that animals injected with acid-fast bacilli had become hypersensitive to tuberculin ; and Koch stated that by injection of tubercle bacilli into animals a serum could be produced which possessed agglutinating power, not only on tubercle bacilli, but also on saprophytic acid-fast bacilli.

Finally, opinions are not wanting that the treatment of experimental animals with saprophytic acid-fast bacilli—that is, by micro-organisms in no way identical with tubercle bacilli—has a protective influence against the infection by tubercle bacilli (Moeller, Friedmann).   I do not deny that the tubercle bacilli of the *Typus humanus* are nearly related to those of the *Typus bovinus*, and that their origin may be traced to a common stock ; but these are considerations for which sufficient foundation is wanting.   To-day we are dealing with two types that do not play the same part in the distribution of tuberculosis in animals and man, and therefore must not be confounded.   It is not essential whether these types are defined as different species, or races, or varieties, for in any case they are not identical.

The position of the problem is well summarised in the above extract from Kossel's report ; but on the same question the very elaborate and important experiments made on behalf of the English Royal Commission should also be consulted.

We are now in a position to consider

VON BEHRING'S VIEWS AS TO HUMAN TUBERCULOSIS.—These are given in short in the extracts on p. 129.   He holds that bovine tubercle bacilli, after long residence in human tissues from infancy onwards, become the source of adult phthisis, the chief cause of mortality from tuberculosis.   Dr. Römer showed that true albumins penetrate unchanged the intestinal mucous membrane of new-born foals, calves, and small laboratory animals, without being converted into peptones as in adult animals. Following up this observation, von Behring found that similarly bacteria passed much more easily through the alimentary mucous membrane of new-born than of adult guinea-pigs. He concluded that the penetrability of infantile mucous membrane in artificially fed infants is the important cause of tuberculosis. He says :—

> The tubercle bacilli which gain access to the system through the alimentary tract in infancy constitute the important etiological factor in the production of the tuberculous infection which leads to consumption. . . .
> The virus of tuberculosis . . . creeps in most insidiously, all unnoticed, being in this respect analogous only to the virus of leprosy, of syphilis, or possibly of malaria in tropical countries. It may be months, years, or decades before the infection leads to manifest disease. This depends on the virulence of the virus . . . and on the number of bacilli introduced.

Although von Behring states very lucidly the important fact of prolonged latency, his view that nearly all or all tuberculosis in man is due to a primary infection by the bovine bacillus cannot be accepted, for the following reasons :—

(*a*) As inferred on p. 134, the results of the Royal Commission can be regarded only as proving that a relatively small proportion of human tuberculosis is of bovine type.

(*b*) The evidence given above points against the conclusion that transformation of *Typus bovinus* into *Typus humanus* occurs ; so that, until further investigations have been made, von Behring cannot justifiably explain the relatively small proportion of the bovine type as being due to transformation in the body into the human type.

(*c*) Doubtless other observers have, like myself, collected a number of cases of fatal infantile tuberculosis where human milk alone had been given. The element of doubt attaching to tubercle bacilli of uncertain or variable type (Group III. p. 127) mentioned in the report of the Royal Commission (1907) is summarised in the following extract (par. 63) from that report :—

> Should it be proved that the cases in question were due to an admixture with the bacilli of human source of a few bacilli of bovine source, the two kinds always remaining distinct the one from the other and never becoming changed the one into the other, we should have no need to enlarge appreciably our conception of the extent to which the human body is subject to bovine tuberculosis. Such cases of admixture must be few and their effect slight ; bovine tuberculosis in the human body

would practically be limited to cases such as those which furnish Group I. (p. 126).

Should, however, it be conclusively proved that a eugonic [1] bacillus of low virulence may be modified under certain conditions into a dysgonic bacillus of high virulence and *vice versâ*, our views as to the relation of human to bovine tuberculosis must be very different. Such a conclusion would lead to the following view. Bacilli from a bovine source entering a human body in scanty numbers may become lodged there without immediately provoking a generalised progressive tuberculosis. During their sojourn there they may become modified into eugonic bacilli of low virulence ; and they may then give rise either to a limited tuberculosis only or, under the influence of certain conditions, to a generalised progressive tuberculosis. For some time after the change they may remain unstable and capable of reverting to their bovine character under changed conditions, when subjected for instance to the influence of bovine tissues as in the passage experiments. Or after a long stay in the human body their character may become so fixed that they cannot be distinguished from bacilli conveyed directly from man to man.

It is on account of the far-reaching bearings of the conclusion that we are unwilling to make any statement at all premature.

We may take this opportunity of pointing out that time is an essential factor in dealing with a disease of so chronic a nature as tuberculosis. Some of its problems, such for instance as the possible change in virulence and other characters of the virus obtained from one kind of animal by repeated passage from animal to animal of another species, can only be settled after constant observations extending over a long period of time.

From a survey of the evidence we must conclude that the conversion of *Typus bovinus* into *Typus humanus* during the lifetime of a single person and in his tissues is unproved. The third of the three alternatives given in Chapter XVI., pp. 128–129 fits in best with all the facts at present known ; and we are justified, in view of the balance of evidence, in concluding that (1) both *Typus bovinus* and *Typus humanus* are competent to produce tuberculosis in the human being ; (2) both forms of the disease have been identified in man (p. 126) ; (3) the bovine type is more common in children than in adults ; (4) the bovine type retains its special characters even in the human subject ; and (5) tuberculosis of bovine origin is much less frequent in the human subject than tuberculosis of human origin.

Conclusions (1), (2), and (3) are established with certainty ; (4) and (5) are probable.

---

[1] A *eugonic* bacillus is one which grows readily, a *dysgonic* bacillus one which grows with difficulty on artificial media.

CHAPTER XVIII

TUBERCULOSIS FROM MEAT AND FROM MILK AND OTHER DAIRY PRODUCTS

IN this chapter it is assumed that a certain — probably a relatively small — proportion of human tuberculosis is caused by tubercle bacilli of the bovine type ; and it is proposed to consider the extent of the disease in cattle and the frequency with which tubercle bacilli are found in milk and other dairy products.

AMOUNT OF TUBERCULOSIS IN CATTLE.—According to the evidence of Mr. (now Sir) T. H. Elliott, Secretary to the Board of Agriculture, before the Royal Commission on Tuberculosis, 1898, at least 20 per cent. of the cows in this country are tuberculous. Delépine (1899) found that in farms which had careful sanitation the proportion varied according to age from 20 to 31 per cent. in milch cows, and that on some farms from three-fourths to all of the cows were affected. MacFadyean (1901) states : " We know that about 30 per cent. of all the cows giving milk in this country are tuberculous in some degree." This undoubtedly implies a most unsatisfactory state of things ; and if tuberculosis is easily communicable to man from tuberculous cattle, the wonder is not that the disease is common in man, but that it is not much more common.

Tuberculous cattle might be a source of human tuberculosis (1) by dust or spray infection from cattle suffering from lung disease ; (2) by the eating or handling of the flesh of tuberculous cattle ; or (3) by consuming milk or some milk-product derived from tuberculous cows.

There is no evidence on the first point, and it may be ignored, as an unlikely or at least an uncommon source of infection.

TUBERCULOUS FLESH.—Butchers and others dressing tuberculous animals may receive accidental inoculations through wounds ; but the development of fatal tuberculosis after such accidents is excessively rare.

The flesh from tuberculous cattle is undoubtedly sometimes infective.   Much evidence on this point was collected by the English Royal Commission of 1895.   It was shown that uncooked tuberculous material given as food to guinea-pigs, calves, pigs, and cats produced tuberculosis.   In " joints " of meat it is exceptional to find tuberculous nodules or other evidence of disease, though to a practised eye the " stripping " of the pleura lining the ribs gives rise to suspicion of tuberculous " grapes " removed in the dressing of the animal.   S. Martin in his experiments for the above Commission frequently produced tuberculosis by inoculating or feeding animals with flesh from tuberculous cattle, " in which no tubercle could be detected by his ocular tests." This led him to consider the " real and considerable danger " of the meat becoming contaminated by the butcher's hands, knives, and cloths, which had been previously in contact with tuberculous lesions in the animal.   " The greater the amount of tubercle there is in the cow " the more likely " is the sticky caseous matter to get smeared over the carcass."   Thus he failed to produce tuberculous disease by feeding animals on meat from cows with mild or moderate tuberculosis, though inoculation of test animals might be successful ; while feeding with meat from cows with advanced or generalised tuberculosis succeeded in producing tuberculosis.

The main tuberculous lesions in cattle are found in the organs, membranes, and glands; but seldom in the flesh or meat substance.   Naked-eye evidence of disease - has therefore usually been removed from the dressed carcass, with the possible exception of a few pea-like tubercles internal to the ribs or about the diaphragm, or a few small glands in certain " joints."   As will be seen subsequently, cooking processes may with certain exceptions protect the adult (p. 404) ; but meat juice made from tuberculous flesh is distinctly dangerous.

The fact that during a period in which the consumption of meat has greatly increased, human tuberculosis has greatly declined does not favour the view that tuberculous meat has played a large part in its causation.   I am not aware of any evidence that the proportion of tuberculous cattle is markedly less than formerly.

TUBERCULOUS MILK.—The evidence of the pathogenicity of cows' milk to a dangerous extent is much clearer than that of cows' flesh. Thus S. Martin reporting to the same Commission (p. 16) found that out of 15 tuberculous cows 8 had healthy udders ; 2 had udder disease, which was proved after slaughter not to be tuberculous ; and the remaining 5 had tuberculous udder disease. With the milk from these cows, tests were made with the following results (Report, p. 16) :—

(*a*) The 8 tuberculous cows which had healthy udders showed him no tubercle bacilli whatever in the milk of any one of them ; 41 test animals fed with their milk remained perfectly free from tuberculous disease ; 28 test animals inoculated with their milk also remained quite free from tuberculous disease.

(*b*) The 2 tuberculous cows which had udder disease, found post-mortem not to be tuberculous in nature, showed him no tubercle bacilli in their milk. Three test animals, fed with their milk and 14 other test animals inoculated with their milk, remained, all of them, perfectly free from tuberculous disease.

(*c*) Of the 5 tuberculous cows which had udder disease, found post-mortem to be of tuberculous nature, 3 showed him tubercle bacilli in their milk. He could not find tubercle bacilli in the milk of the other 2. With milk from the 3 cows, 15 test animals were fed, with the result of producing tuberculosis in every one of them. With milk from one or other of the same 3 cows, 13 test animals were inoculated, with the result of all 13 acquiring tuberculous disease. The milk of the fourth cow (one of those which had not shown tubercle bacilli) was used to feed 10 test animals, and produced tuberculosis in 4 of them. Inoculated into 6 test animals, all of them became tuberculous. The milk of the fifth cow (in which also no tubercle bacilli had been seen) was used to feed 2 animals, but without result. Yet when it was used to inoculate 2 other animals, both of them acquired tuberculous disease.

(*d*) It remains to note these tests as applied to the milk of the two cows found after slaughter to be suffering under another disease, but not tubercle. The results were : no tubercle bacilli found in the milk of these cows ; inoculated into 17 test animals, it did not produce tuberculosis in any one of them ; milk from one of the cows, however, in some test animals gave rise to various abscesses.

The Report of this Commission goes on to say (p. 17) that

according to our experience, then, the condition required for ensuring to the milk of tuberculous cows the ability to produce tuberculosis in the consumers of their milk, is *tuberculous disease of the cow affecting the udder*. It should be noted that this affection of the udder is not peculiar to tuberculosis in an advanced stage, but may be found also in mild cases.

All are agreed that when there is tuberculosis of the udder the milk is found to be dangerously infectious, and so likewise are all products of such milk, as butter, skimmed milk, buttermilk, cheese. Thus the report of the same Royal Commission states : " The milk of cows with tuberculosis of the udder possesses a virulence which can only be described as extraordinary " (par. 61). It is also ominous that " the spread of tubercle in the udder goes on with most alarming rapidity." Sims Woodhead remarks (par. 62), " I have noticed on several occasions, during the interval between fortnightly inspections carried on along with a veterinary surgeon, that the disease had become distinctly developed. It may be, of course, that the early evidence has been overlooked at the previous inspection, but whether this is the case or not, the spread of the disease was so rapid as to afford very good ground for alarm. The very absence of any definite sign in the earlier stage is one of the greatest dangers of this condition."

Professor (now Sir) J. MacFadyean (1901, p. 84) points out in the following remarks,

not every cow that is tuberculous gives milk containing tubercle bacilli. It is true that opinions with regard to this point are not absolutely unanimous, but there is ample evidence to justify the assertion that, as a rule, the milk is not dangerous until the udder itself becomes diseased. The experiments pointing to an opposite conclusion form only a small minority, and the results obtained in most of them were probably due to carelessness on the part of the experimenter. In a few of the cases in which the milk of an apparently healthy udder was found to be infective it is probable that the gland tissue was in reality diseased, though not to an extent discoverable without microscopic examination. The important question, therefore, is not what proportion of milch cows are tuberculous, but what proportion of them have tuberculous udders. Some authorities have estimated this to be as high as 10 per cent., but the proportion is certainly much less than that in Great Britain. My own experience leads me to think that about 2 per cent. of the cows in the milking herds in this country are thus affected. Now, the milk secreted by a tuberculous udder always contains tubercle bacilli, and it sometimes contains enormous numbers of them, and when these facts are apprehended one begins to realise the seriousness of the danger to which, in the present state of affairs, those who drink uncooked milk are exposed. But there are one or two considerations that make the danger greater than the mere statement of the number of cows affected would at first sight indicate. In the first place, the udder disease is not attended by any pain or tenderness in milking, and the milk for a considerable time after the udder has become manifestly diseased may appear quite wholesome, though in reality it is charged with the germs of tuberculosis. It there-fore often happens that the gravity of the condition is not realised by the milker or the owner of the cow, and the milk continues to be sold for human consumption. There is scarcely any room for doubt that if it were sold and consumed unmixed with other milk some of the persons partaking of it would become infected. In practice it is usually mixed with the milk from other cows that have healthy udders, and thus the germs are distributed among a large number of persons. Even tuber-culous milk that has been thus much diluted may prove infective, but the danger to the individual consumer is in inverse proportion to the degree of dilution. Since about one cow in 50 is the subject of tuberculosis of the udder, and the average number of cows in the milking herds of this country is less than 50, it follows that the majority of dairies and farms supply milk that is free from tubercle bacilli, or at least does not contain any derived from this source. On the other hand, when the infected material is present, it operates with the greatest intensity in the milk of single cows and in the mixed milk from small herds.

By other observers the percentage of milch cows with tuber-culous udders is put somewhat higher. Thus Professor Delépine puts it at 3·7 per cent. (1899, p. 19).

Müller (1905) found that the udder was tuberculous in from 1·1 to 3·7 per cent. of the tuberculous cows slaughtered in Saxony during the years 1888–97, and in 1·6 per cent. of the tuberculous cows in the whole of Germany. In Denmark in 1901–02 the number of cases in which tuberculosis of the udder was detected and the cows subsequently slaughtered was 584, or 0·55 per 1000 of the total stock. In the experience of the East Prussian Herd-book Society, a half-yearly examination of the herds and a quarterly examination of the milk, implying a very thorough control, only showed 62 cases of tuberculous udder in 15,000 cattle, or 0·4 per cent.

ARE TUBERCLE BACILLI FOUND IN COWS' MILK IN THE ABSENCE OF TUBERCULOUS UDDER DISEASE ?—From the experi-ments of the English Royal Commission already quoted, it would be inferred that this question must be answered in the negative, or that tubercle bacilli when found are too few to be dangerous. Other experimenters have published results con-tradictory to these, tubercle bacilli being found in milk when udder disease was absent in cows suffering from clinical tuber-culosis, or even when cows had no obvious evidence of tuber-culosis but reacted to the tuberculin test. These results have failed to be substantiated. Thus Ostertag examined 77 such cows without finding tubercle bacilli in the milk after testing it microscopically, by inoculation, and by prolonged feeding experiments. Ascher, M'Weeney, and Strenström obtained like results. The latter concluded that tubercle bacilli found in the milk by observers obtaining different results must have gained access to it during milking. This may have been derived from tuberculous milkers ; but Ebers regards the very common fouling of the milk with particles of cow-dung as the source of tubercle bacilli. Tuberculous cows after coughing commonly swallow their expectoration, which would subsequently appear in the fæces. This evidence has been more recently confirmed.

The detailed results of the East Prussian Herdbook Society are interesting in this connection. Samples of milk were taken from the total milk of 1596 herds, and tubercle bacilli were found in 97 samples. In 59 of these tuberculous udders were discovered, and in the other instances there was reason to believe that contamination of the milk after leaving the animal had occurred. The above experiment represented the milk of about 20,000 cows, and it may be assumed in accordance with average experience that 6000 to 7000 of these were tuberculous ; and yet in 1499 out of 1596 herds no tubercle bacilli were found in the milk. The evidence that contamination of the milk is most often due to udder disease is very strong, though contamination by cows' dung or from milkers also occurs, and cannot be left out of count.

PROPORTION OF INFECTIVE MILK IN MIXED SUPPLIES TO THE PUBLIC.—The preceding experience of the Herdbook Society must be regarded as exceptional, in the fewness of the herds containing infective milk. English experience shows that a very large percentage of ordinary mixed milk contains tubercle bacilli. Thus Delépine (1898) found tubercle bacilli in 22 out of 125, or 17·6 per cent., of samples of milk from country dairy-farms collected at railway stations in Liverpool and Manchester. Kanthack and Sladen found that specimens of 9 dairies were infected out of 16 examined. Woodhead and Wood found virulent tubercle bacilli in 5 out of 50 specimens, and Rabinowitsch and Kempner in 7 out of 25 samples in Berlin. Taking these as fair samples of a much larger number of examinations, it would appear that about 20 per cent. of the mixed milk supplied to towns contains living tubercle bacilli.

Tubercle Bacilli in other Dairy Products.—Many observations have been made and tubercle bacilli have been found. It is not unlikely that the earlier observations over-stated the facts, acid-fast bacilli simulating the tubercle bacillus having been confused with it.   There can be no doubt, however, that when milk contains tubercle bacilli, cream, butter, cheese, skimmed milk, and buttermilk are likewise infective.   Margarine may also contain tubercle bacilli, introduced with the milk which is blended with it.   Cream is likely to be particularly dangerous, as the cream in rising is found to carry an excessive proportion of the bacilli with it.   The feeding of calves and pigs on skimmed milk, buttermilk, whey, and the refuse collected on centrifuges is a common source of tuberculosis in them.   The horse has also been shown, especially in Denmark, to be very liable to tuberculosis when fed on milk or its products.   Pigs are rarely infected from one another, but mainly by their food. Tuberculosis is very prevalent in pigs only when a large dairy industry is carried on.   The slaughter-house reports of Copen-hagen for 1897 show that the proportion of tuberculous pigs varied from 3 to 14 per cent. ; while in Bavaria, in which there is only a small dairy industry, only 0·2 to 0·4 per cent. of the pigs slaughtered in 1896–1900 were tuberculous.   In Denmark pig tuberculosis has become much less frequent since it has been made compulsory to heat separated milk before it is returned from the creameries.

CHAPTER XIX

DOMESTIC INFECTION

TUBERCULOSIS is undoubtedly caused most often by domestic infection. Koch (1906, p. 1449) says that tuberculosis " has been frankly and justly called a dwelling disease " ; while Biermer goes further and describes it as essentially a bedroom disease. There is little doubt that its infection is chiefly acquired in bedrooms. Industrial conditions, although an important source of infection, probably act to an even greater extent by removing or paralysing influences inhibitory to infection, thus opening the door to infection or stirring into activity infective material latent in the tissues.

In treating of domestic infection it is necessary to distinguish between indirect or mediate and direct or immediate infection. The influence of overcrowding is complex, and is concerned partly with infection and partly with the conditions of imperfect sanitation usually associated with overcrowding.

INFECTION DUE TO THE DWELLING PROPER.—The experimental results of Cornet and others (p. 98) show that tubercle bacilli are present, but only in the immediate environment of consumptives. Given that a house has become infected through the uncleanly habits of a consumptive who has recently lived and possibly died in it, there are the great limitations to infection already enumerated on pp. 101–105. Although it is in the highest degree desirable that such a house should be efficiently cleansed and disinfected, it is unlikely to form a large element in the production of phthisis by domestic infection. It may be, however, that apart from this additional source of infection, evil conditions of housing lower vitality, diminish the resistance to infection, and thus increase the amount of tuberculosis among the poor. This point is further discussed on p. 192. Such influences undoubtedly favour tuberculosis by hastening the occurrence of infection, and no preventive measures can be regarded as efficient and complete which do not vigorously attack and re-move housing defects. It is possible, however, to obtain some indications of the chief agency which causes the dissemination of tuberculosis in overcrowded quarters.

OVERCROWDING.—There is abundant statistical evidence of the close association between overcrowding and excessive mortality from phthisis. Thus Sir Shirley Murphy has shown that in London the death-rate from phthisis steadily increases with the proportion of the total population living more than two in a room, in tenements comprising less than five rooms. This experience is summarised in the following table :—

TABLE XXIV

London.—Proportion of Population living more than Two in a Room (in Tenements of less than Five Rooms).	London.—Average Annual Death-rate from Phthisis per 100,000 of Population, 1894–98.
Districts with under 10 per cent. . .	111
,, ,, 10–15 ,, . .	144
,, ,, 15–20 ,, . .	161
,, ,, 20–25 ,, . .	177
,, ,, 25–30 ,, . .	209
,, ,, 30–35 ,, . .	231
,, ,, over 35 ,, . .	259

When the same facts are subdivided according to ages of the patients dying from phthisis, it is found that the excess of the death-rate from this disease in the most overcrowded districts is greatest at the ages at which the mortality from it is heaviest. Sir Shirley Murphy in commenting on the table summarised above says (Ann. Rep. 1898, p. 46) :—

There is obviously a relation between the amount of overcrowding and the phthisis death-rate. The figures do not, however, suffice to show whether the overcrowding caused phthisis, or whether the disease, by adding to family expenditure or by diminishing the wage-earning power, left less money available for rent and thus brought about the over-crowding, or whether again overcrowding is associated with some other condition or conditions which are favourable to disease. In all probability all these circumstances have tended to produce the results shown in the table.

There is a further difficulty in accepting the above figures as completely satisfactory evidence that crowding is a main influence in causing tuberculosis. The house where a person dies of this disease is not necessarily the house in which he acquired it. In view of the frequent changes of house among the poor, and of the protracted duration of phthisis, the coincidence between the two is probably exceptional. The usual course of events is for a person who becomes consumptive to drift, owing to his impaired working powers, from the class of skilled to that of unskilled and casual labour ; and with each step downwards his housing conditions deteriorate to a corresponding degree.

In Part II. pp. 220 to 229 a comparison of different countries shows that the death-rate from phthisis does not vary in accordance with their relative position as to sanitation and housing, whether the different countries are compared with each other, or whether the death-rate and housing conditions of the same country are compared at different times.

The following additional evidence, quoted from a recent address by the writer (1907), bears on the same point. The figures as to housing are taken from a paper by Sir W. Matheson, Registrar-General of Ireland :—

TABLE XXIVA

	Number of One-roomed Tenements Per Cent. of Total Dwellings or Tenements.	Number of One-roomed Tenements having Five or more Occupants each in every 100 Tenements of all Classes.	Number of Persons in One-roomed Tenements, with Five or more Occupants in every 100 of the Total Population.	Average Death-rate from Phthisis, per 100,000 living, in the Three Years 1900–1–2.
Dublin . . .	36·70	8·69	10·61	329
Belfast . . .	1·00	0·09	0·10	313
London . . .	14·66	0·57	0·70	171
Liverpool . . .	6·14	0·22	0·24	190
Manchester . . .	1·90	0·04	0·05	208
Edinburgh . . .	16·98	1·80	2·33	164
Glasgow . . .	26·11	4·28	5·24	177

Thus in Glasgow, which has 26 times as large a proportion of one-roomed tenement dwellings as Belfast, and 52 times as many persons in its one-roomed tenements with 5 or more occupants, the death-rate from phthisis instead of being higher is 43 per cent. lower than that of Belfast. This does not imply that in a given town the death-rate from phthisis is not higher in the smaller and more overcrowded tenements. Abundant statistics show this to be the case. But it is clear from the above table that size of dwelling or even degree of overcrowding may be overshadowed by the effect of other influences.

It may be taken as an axiom that overcrowding favours tuberculosis. Doubtless there is more than one *modus operandi* in bringing about this result. Two things, however, are certain :—

(*a*) Tuberculosis cannot be produced, however strong may be the favouring circumstances, unless its infection is received ; and (*b*) although, as seen above, the death-rate from phthisis in a given community is always greater in proportion to the amount of overcrowding, there is, when different countries or different cities are compared with each other, no direct relation between the amount of overcrowding and the amount of phthisis.

It will be subsequently seen that a given amount of over-crowding with a large amount of institutional segregation of consumptives is associated with less phthisis than when over-crowding is less but accompanied by only a small amount of institutional segregation of consumptives (pp. 224 to 295). We are justified in concluding therefore, that *the quickest way to diminish the risks of overcrowding is to favour by every means of persuasion the removal of the sick from among the healthy.* This should, of course, be accompanied by strenuous endeavour to diminish over-crowding, apart from the question of such removal.

FAMILY INFECTION.—The facts already given indicate almost sufficiently the risks of family life when one member is a con-sumptive, though they also happily indicate with what ease and how simply these dangers may be avoided. The histories of family infection given on pp. 64–68 are examples of the conditions under which tuberculosis spreads.

It is sufficiently clear that young children are particularly prone to be infected, partly because they are more caressed, and possibly also because they are more susceptible than their elders. Girls are more exposed to infection than boys (see p. 171). The most intimate relationship in family life is that of husband and wife, and the evidence as to infection between these may therefore be examined.

INFECTION IN MARRIED LIFE.—When a married man or woman is consumptive, is the proportion of instances in which the partner is also consumptive greater than the average for persons of the same age and sex apart from married life? There cannot be said to be sufficiently full evidence to settle this point. The following table is given to show the varying percentages stated by different collectors of statistics:—

TABLE XXV

Number of Married Couples with One or Both Consumptive

Authority.	No. of Couples with one or both Consumptive.	No. of Couples with both Consumptive.	Percentage in which both were Consumptive.	Quoted from—
Brehmer . .	159	19	11·9	Cornet *On Tuberculosis* (Nothnagel), p. 265.
Haupt . . .	260	30	11·5	,,
Cornet . . .	594	135	22·7	,,
Schuyder . .	844	32	3·8	*Lancet*, Sept. 19, 1891.
Rivers . . .	84	6	7·1	K. Pearson, 1907.
Weber . . .	80	19	23·7	Weber, 1874.

Clearly figures giving such discrepant percentages cannot be comparable. Observations of supposed infection between married couples or its absence are trustworthy only if they accurately state the length of the married life of the couples under observation, and the subsequent history through life of the surviving partner. In other words, to arrive at the truth one must have the complete life-experience of the married couples, and a sufficient number of these to avoid accidental errors. I do not think that most of the observations tabulated above will bear this test. Even when these tests are satisfied, it has to be remembered that frequently patients having had phthisis die as the result of other diseases. The long latency of phthisis in a considerable proportion of the total cases is one of the most serious difficulties in the more detailed and elaborate investigation on this point that is needed.

Even when allowance is made for coincidence, the following instance of apparent communication of pulmonary tuberculosis by a husband to successive wives, given by Sir Hermann Weber (1874, p. 144), is sufficiently striking to deserve reproduction:—

A. B. lost his mother, two brothers, and a sister from pulmonary tuberculosis. He had hæmoptysis at the age of 20. He then became a sailor. He married when 27 years old, and was then quite well.

His first wife came of a healthy family, and had good health till towards the end of her third pregnancy, and she died after her confinement.

After a year he married again, his wife being apparently healthy. She developed a cough after a year of married life, and died of pulmonary tuberculosis.

His third wife was 25 years old when he married her. She came of an exceptionally healthy family. In her second pregnancy she began to cough, and died after the second confinement.

His fourth wife, who was 23 years old when he married her, and who had come of a healthy family, began 13 months later, *i.e.* 3 months after her first confinement, with a cough, and died later of phthisis.

A. B. did not marry again. When examined in 1854 after the death of his third wife he showed evidence of old pulmonary tuberculosis. He died in 1871 of this disease, and an autopsy showed old cicatrised disease, and recent tuberculosis.

Dr. Weber states that in 29 marriages between consumptive wives and healthy husbands only one husband became consumptive ; while in 51 marriages between consumptive husbands and healthy wives 18 wives became consumptive.

There is, I think, in view of our general knowledge of tuberculosis, no reasonable doubt that the close intimacy of married life has, in the absence of intelligent precautions, been a not infrequent cause of phthisis when one partner is already affected. The wife is more likely to suffer from her diseased husband, than the husband from his wife; as the wife has more protracted opportunities of receiving infection, especially in the later stages of the disease.

CHAPTER XX

INFECTION IN ATTENDANCE ON THE SICK

THE majority of consumptives, when ill enough to require nursing, are nursed by their own relatives. The degree to which infection occurs among them has already been discussed (p. 149). In view of the evidence already given, and that cited in Part II., there can, I think, be little difficulty in agreeing that the home-treatment of advanced consumptives in crowded dwellings, in which the necessary precautions cannot be taken, is a predominant cause of the continued spread of tuberculosis. It still remains to discuss the possibilities of infection of nurses and other attendants in the institutional treatment of phthisis, and the possibilities of infection of doctors who attend consumptive patients at their homes or in institutions.

The most carefully investigated experiences are those of the Brompton Hospital and of the Victoria Park Hospital for Diseases of the Chest, the former investigated by Drs. Cotton and Theodore Williams, the latter by Dr. Andrew. Wilson Fox (1891, p. 563) summarises these experiences in the table on the following page.

In the Brompton returns the number of nurses and servants is given only for 20 years, the deaths for 36 years. It appears that, so far as could be ascertained, during 36 years only one death from phthisis occurred among the physicians, and only five cases among the nurses during or subsequent to their work in the hospital. The results for the Victoria Park Hospital are somewhat similar. It is very difficult to analyse this evidence. It is very scanty. It is not certain how thoroughly the subsequent history of workers in these hospitals was traced. It is likely that such workers as had died were less completely traced than those still alive. Again, we do not know the total duration of hospital work of the above persons. If we assume that, including servants, it averaged two years, then among the 377

workers in the Brompton Hospital the annual number of cases
of phthisis among the staff while still at the hospital (excluding deaths) was about 1 in 94, or including cases developing
later was 1 in 37, which is much higher than the estimated
number in the general population (p. 63).   I do not think,
however, that the evidence as collected is sufficiently accurate
to bear such a comparison as this, and it is made only to in-

TABLE XXVI

| | Brompton. | | | | | Victoria Park. | | |
| | Number of Staff. | Number of Cases of Phthisis. | | | Total Deaths from Phthisis. | Number of Staff. | Number of Cases of Phthisis. | Total Deaths from Phthisis. |
		Before Admission.	During Stay.	Subsequently.				
Resident Medical Officer .	4	...	...	...	...	12	1	1
Clinical Assistants . .	150	1	1	6	5	51	3	3
Matron	6	...	...	...	...	4	...	...
Nurses	101(?)	...	1(?)	4	5(?)	}255	1(?)	1(?)
Servants	32(?)	...	...	...	...			
Porters	20	...	...	...	...	34	1	1
Secretary and Clerks .	9	...	3(?)	...	...	3	1	1
Dispensers . . .	22	...	3	2	3	7	...	...
Chaplain	4	...	...	...	...	5	...	...
Physicians and Assistant Physicians . . .	29	...	...	...	1	31	1	1(?)
Total . .	377	1	8	12	14	402	8 (7?)	8 (7?)

dicate that the data, if completely accurate, do not contra-
indicate a considerable possibility of infection among the staff
of these hospitals, and do not, as commonly supposed, offer
any presumption of freedom from infection.

A similar remark applies to Dr. Robertson's figures for the
Ventnor Hospital for Consumption (Bulstrode, 1903, p. 76).
During the 22 years 1881–1902, 15,500 phthisical patients were
treated in this hospital, and during the same period 62 officers,
208 nurses, 407 housemaids, and 1 charwoman — total, 678
—were engaged in the institution.   None of the officers have
contracted tuberculosis.   Six nurses, of whom two died, have

had phthisis, but apparently three had the disease on admission. The records for housemaids are not very definite. Here, again, one would wish for exact information as to the length of service and of the subsequent period over which each member of the staff could be traced. In view of what has been said about prolonged latency of tuberculosis (p. 73), this is an essential condition of an accurate investigation.

The above experiences are usually quoted as instances of non-infection in hospitals. They should rather be described as examples of investigations, in which the data are, possibly owing to insuperable difficulties, incomplete and insufficient to justify any dogmatic statement.

In attempting to ascertain the true inwardness of the statistics of hospital staffs relating to phthisis, generally quoted, it is not suggested that the nursing of consumptives under the hospital conditions of to-day, including the adoption of the best precautionary measures, involves considerable risk.

All that is suggested is that the danger is to a definite extent greater than that for the general population, though much less so than formerly. In all well-regulated workhouse infirmaries, hospitals, and sanatoria, absolute cleanliness is maintained ; and soiled handkerchiefs and the contents of spittoons are prevented from becoming sources of infection. The chief remaining source of danger is direct infection, which the careful nurse avoids. The conditions are altogether different from those of the wife who attends on the consumptive breadwinner. She is in intimate personal contact with the patient day and night ; may have insufficient rest ; is overfatigued, and often underfed. Mental anxiety still further lowers her powers of resistance to infection. It is not strange, therefore, if she falls a victim, while the hospital nurse escapes. There is little difficulty in agreeing with Koch's summing up of this subject (1906, p. 1449) :—

In hospitals for pulmonary phthisis it is in certain circumstances possible that no cases of infection occur among the attendants, or at any rate so few that in former times it was thought necessary to regard this as a proof of the non-contagiousness of tuberculosis. But if one examines such cases more carefully there are good reasons for the apparent non-contagiousness. It then appears that the patients in question are people who are very cautious about their sputum, see to the cleanliness of their dwellings and clothing, and live in copiously aired and lighted rooms, so that the germs that get into the air can be swiftly swept away by the current or killed by the light.   If these conditions are not fulfilled, there is no lack of infection even in hospitals and the dwellings of the well-to-do, as experience teaches daily.   And it becomes the more frequent the more uncleanly the patients are as regards their sputum, the more lack there is of light and air, and the more closely crowded together the sick live with the hale.   The danger of infection becomes especially great when healthy people have to sleep in the same rooms with sick people, and even, as unfortunately still frequently happens among the poor, in the same bed.   This kind of infection has struck attentive observers as so important that tuberculosis has been frankly and justly called a dwelling disease.

Doctors are not exposed to infection so often, or for such long periods, as nurses.   They have no difficulty in their work in escaping direct infection from coughing, and one would not expect to have among them any definite evidence of risks markedly greater than those of the general community, of acquiring tuberculosis.   The data in Table XXVI. are too scanty to form the basis of a sound conclusion.   The official occupational figures given by Dr. Tatham in the Decennial Supplement of the Registrar-General's Report (1881-90) offer a much wider basis of induction.   In these figures the death-rate from all causes and from certain specified causes among males, aged 25-65, are compared in groups, whose composition as to age is identical.   In these groups the number of the general population that would furnish 1000 total deaths from all causes (*comparative mortality figure*) is found to furnish 966 deaths among doctors, 821 among lawyers, and 533 among the clergy. Ogle in 1871-80 found that the death-rate from phthisis and from respiratory diseases was lower among doctors than among the general male population.   The figures for 1881-90 confirm this result, as shown in the following table :—

TABLE XXVII

Comparative Mortality Figures of Males aged 25-65, during 1881-90, in Different Occupations, from

	All Causes.	Phthisis.	Bronchitis.	Pneumonia.	Influenza.
All Males .	1000	192	88	107	33
All occupied					
Males .	953	185	88	105	34
Clergy . .	533	67	11	45	36
Doctors. .	966	105	12	93	51

Doctors have a much lower death-rate from phthisis than the average male population. It will be observed that their death-rate from influenza is excessive, and the comparison is interesting, illustrating as it does the much more rapid and more intense infectivity of the latter disease.

CHAPTER XXI

INDUSTRIAL INFECTION

IN considering the possibilities of infection in various industries, the general considerations already emphasised must be borne in mind. (1) Prolonged exposure to infective material is more likely to be successful than intermittent and occasional exposure. (2) Intimate contact, as between husband and wife, and still more—because of the possibilities associated with long latency — between parent and child, is more likely to cause infection than the less intimate contact which characterises the usual conditions of work.

It has to be remembered, however, that the dust inhaled in many occupations may not only serve as a vehicle for the tubercle bacillus; but if, as frequently happens, it is angular or rough, may serve as an inoculating needle for the bacillus; and by this means it is conceivable and in fact likely that smaller doses of infective material than in domestic life may be made almost equally efficient.

TABLE XXVIII.—PHTHISIS

Comparative Mortality Figures of Males aged 25-65, the total Deaths of all Males at these Ages being taken as 1000

Among	1890–91–92.	1900–01–02.	Percentage Decline or Increase in Ten Years.
Occupied Males—			
(a) in England and Wales as a whole	214	175	– 18
(b) in London	321	262	– 18
(c) in industrial districts . . .	258	202	– 22
(d) in agricultural districts . .	157	125	– 20
Unoccupied Males	521	583	+ 12

The chief available and approximately accurate statistics of phthisis in relation to industrial occupations are those supplied in the Decennial Supplements to the reports of the Registrar-General of Births and Deaths. The results of the last two of these reports, which are by Dr. Tatham, are given in Table XXVIII. on previous page. The meaning of the words *comparative mortality figure* has already been explained on p. 155.

Unoccupied males represent a large proportion of invalids, and we may leave them out of consideration. The excess of phthisis in industrial over agricultural districts will be noted,

TABLE XXIX.—PHTHISIS

Comparative Mortality Figures of Males aged 25–65, the total Deaths of all Males at these Ages being taken as 1000

Occupation.	Comparative Mortality Figure.		Percentage Decline or Increase in Ten Years.
	1890–91–92.	1900–01–02.[1]	
Occupied males	214	175	− 18
General shopkeeper . . .	272	344	+ 26
Lead miner	440	317	− 28
Tool, scissors, file-maker . .	390	353	− 9
File-maker	467	375	− 20
Copper miner	384	501	+ 30
Cutler, scissors-maker . . .	442	516	+ 17
Tin miner	586	838	+ 43
Messenger, porter	376	368	− 2
General labourer (England and Wales)	295	450	+ 53
Costermonger, hawker . . .	514	516	+ 0
General labourer (London) . .	445	531	+ 19
General labourer (industrial districts)	363	567	+ 56
Inn, hotel servant (agricultural districts)	412	410	− 0
Inn, hotel servant (industrial districts)	415	426	+ 3
Innkeeper, servant, etc. (London) .	519	443	− 15
Inn, hotel servant (England and Wales)	552	533	− 3
Inn, hotel servant (London) . .	705	669	− 10

[1] The above corrected figures are supplied through Dr. Tatham's kindness, before the publication of Part II. of the Decennial Supplement for 1891–1900.

and the still greater excess in London. It is also noteworthy that the decline of phthisis among occupied males is about equal in industrial and agricultural districts.

In Table XXIX. is shown the relative position of the chief occupations in association with which fatal phthisis is particularly prevalent.

Among all occupied males there has been in ten years a decline of 18 per cent. in phthisis, as compared with a decline of 22 per cent. in the general population. The great excess of phthisis among males in towns and the special figures in the preceding table indicate that a most fertile line of work is open in the prevention of industrial phthisis. The class of occupations in which the excess of phthisis is greatest, and in which this excess is increasing, throw much light on the lines of preventive work which are indicated. The occupations in Table XXIX. can be classified under three heads: (1) Those in which the workers are exposed to irritating and injurious dust, as scissors-makers, file-makers, tin miners; (2) those who are particularly prone to alcoholic excess, and are particularly exposed to infection from indiscriminate expectoration, as innkeepers and inn servants; and (3) those whose work is casual in character, and who likewise are addicted to frequenting public-houses, as general labourers, messengers, costermongers. The occupation of a "general labourer" includes many loafers, as well as many who have fallen from skilled occupations owing to illness; and it is difficult to distinguish between the public-house and the industrial factors, or to state in the case of how many the ill-health prevented the patient securing a more stable occupation. It will be noted that general labourers showed a marked increase, while hawkers and messengers showed little or no decrease, of phthisis. Innkeepers and inn servants have in some districts made their previous bad record worse. Lead miners and file-makers show considerable improvement, while tin miners, copper miners, and cutlers have become worse.

The obvious indications for prevention are the diminution or removal of dust, the substitution of wet cleansing for sweeping, the use of fans to divert dust from the workshop. The operation of the Workshops and Factories Acts is gradually improving the condition of workshops and factories; but evidence of improvement has not yet shown itself to a marked extent in the death-returns for phthisis among miners and among general shopkeepers, as is indicated in Table XXIX. Another decade will doubtless see great advance in the directions indicated above, and will bring nearer the realisation of the benefit from preventive work already being done.

CHAPTER XXII

SUSCEPTIBILITY TO INFECTION

A SPECIAL susceptibility to infection, hereditary or acquired, is generally regarded as appertaining to those who become tuberculous, and as being indeed necessary for the development of tuberculosis when infection is received. In those showing this special susceptibility vital resistance to invasion by disease is supposed to be deficient, or the patient is said to be abnormally vulnerable to disease. The resulting amount of disease which will follow infection by the tubercle bacillus will vary on the one hand according to the number and virulence of the particular bacilli introduced into the system, and on the other hand according to the resistance of the patient to invasion.

It is extremely difficult to resolve resistance into its constituent factors, and in fact it cannot be done with exactitude. In part it consists of innate, and in part of acquired powers, and the resistance may prove its power after as well as at the time of the invasion by bacilli. The difficulties of estimating resistance are particularly great in a disease which is so prevalent as tuberculosis. Nearly one-ninth of the deaths in the total population result from invasion by the tubercle bacillus, and, judging by hospital experience, as many as half of the adults of the working classes dying of other diseases show indication post-mortem of some degree of past tuberculous invasion, either in the lungs or elsewhere. The latter evidence may be regarded as indicating either almost universal proclivity to a certain extent, or some measure of immunity on the part of a very high proportion of the total population. The former view appears to me to be nearer the truth, as all degrees of lesions are found in the above cases, and a very high proportion of the total number of those who have suffered severely from tuberculosis recover completely and die from other diseases. In view of the two aspects of the case it is not surprising that the clinician

G. Sée (quoted by Cornet, p. 328) should say that " la prédisposi-
tion est un mot pour masquer notre ignorance"; or that, on the
other hand, J. Kingston Fowler (1898, p. 305) should say :—

Although infection must be regarded as the *causa sine quâ non*, it is
not necessarily of most importance from a practical point of view.   If
of a large number of persons exposed to infection only a few acquire
a disease, the susceptibility of the individual becomes a factor in causation of greater moment than exposure to infection.

The underlying assumption in the position taken up by those
holding the view expressed in the above quotation appears to be
that everybody " exposed " to infection necessarily receives an
efficient dose of infection.   The error of this assumption can be
seen by ascertaining what happens when a given number of
persons are exposed to the infection of acute infectious diseases
like scarlet fever, diphtheria, and enteric fever.   The instances
best lending themselves to such an inquiry are milk outbreaks
of these diseases, as in these the element of chance appears to
be largely eliminated, and it is reasonable to believe that the
infective material is distributed throughout the milk.   In such
outbreaks the families invaded by the disease in question may
be as low as 6 per cent. of those supplied with the infected milk in
scarlet fever, 11 per cent. in typhoid fever, and 7 per cent. in
enteric fever (Newman and Swithinbank, 1903, p. 268).   I have
known two milk outbreaks of scarlet fever in which the percentage
of families affected was considerably lower than 6 per cent.
It has to be noted, furthermore, that the percentage *of persons*
affected in the families supplied with milk from the infected
source would be much less than the above.   The fact is that
in all these diseases a very large proportion of the persons exposed either escape because they do not receive any infection,
just as in battle the majority of soldiers are not shot, or else
receive an inefficient dose of infection, like soldiers who are
touched by spent bullets.   The circumstances which limit infection among those " exposed " to tuberculosis have been already
fully discussed (p. 101).

It should be noted further that in comparing tuberculosis
with the three acute infectious diseases just named, we are in
tuberculosis, with a few imperfect exceptions, restricted to
mortality statistics, while we have complete records of total cases
in the other diseases.   The fact that old localised and cured

tuberculous lesions are so often found at autopsies does not appear to me to indicate that the majority of the population are naturally immune to tuberculosis ; any more than it would be justifiable to state that the majority of the population are naturally immune against the three following infectious diseases, because in scarlet fever about 95 out of every 100 attacked, in enteric fever about 85, and in diphtheria 80 to 90 out of every 100 attacked, recover.

When, therefore, we use Allbutt's (1899, p. 1149) phrase of " openness to consumption," it must be remembered that the presence of a constant and inherent " openness " in certain individuals or in certain families is not demonstrated, however likely it is. It is useful to assume its existence, as a reason for additional precautions in the cases in which the family or personal history points to such " openness " ; but in experience it is difficult if not impossible to obtain exact evidence of such " openness," in which the disturbing factor of excessive exposure to or excessive dosage of infection can be entirely eliminated.

In Chapter XXIV. we shall deal with those personal conditions, often temporary in character, which appear to diminish the resistance to infection ; such as the state of nutrition, alcoholism, overfatigue, and injuries. Age and sex as bearing on the same problem are discussed in Chapter XXIII., while in Chapter XXV. the possible influence of heredity in producing a congenital susceptibility will be discussed.

CHAPTER XXIII

AGE AND SEX

ALL investigators agree that tuberculosis is rare in infancy, when stated in proportion to the infantile population. This is true, notwithstanding the national statistics as to the number of deaths caused during infancy by tuberculous meningitis and tabes mesenterica. Even when stated in proportion to the total infantile deaths from all causes, the number verified by autopsies is small. Thus Hervieux at the Paris Foundling Hospital found on careful post-mortem examination only ten cases of tuberculosis, or about 1 per cent. in 996 infants who had died in the first year of life. Frebelius in ten years had 16,581 autopsies on infants aged one to four months at the St. Petersburg Crèche, and found tuberculosis in 416, or 0·4 per cent. Schwer, in 690 infants dying under one year of age, found 44 tuberculous, or 6·3 per cent. These were distributed as follows :—

263 infants aged	1 day to 4 weeks—	0 tuberculous	= 0	per. cent.
123 ,, ,,	5 to 9 weeks—	1 ,,	= 0·8	,,
144 ,, ,,	9 weeks to 5 months—	15 ,,	= 10·4	,,
160 ,, ,,	6 months to 1 year—	28 ·,,	= 17·5	,,

The number of deaths from tuberculosis rapidly became more numerous in the second year of life; and, according to Papassine, Rilliet, and Barthez, towards the age of five, half the deaths of children which occur are due to tuberculosis. This figure does not correspond with the figures for England and Wales in 1901. If reference be made to Tables XIV. and XV. it will be seen that the highest recorded death-rates from tuberculous meningitis (109) and from tabes mesenterica (125 per 100,000) are at ages 0–5, while that from phthisis (315 per 100,000 for males) is at the age-period 45–55. Without accepting the complete accuracy of the rates for the two first, it is at least evident that as fatal diseases they are chiefly children's diseases, while fatal phthisis is chiefly a disease of adults. Tatham has drawn attention to the fact that the age of maximum mortality from phthisis has been postponed in both sexes as shown below :—

TABLE XXX.—AGES OF MAXIMUM MORTALITY FROM PHTHISIS
(*The age-periods in heavy type have the maximum rates, the others being approximate*)

Periods.	Males.	Females.
1851–60	**20–25**, 25–35, 35–45	**25–35**
1861–70	**25–35**, 35–45	**25–35**
1871–80	**35–45**	**25–35**
1881–85	**35–45**	**25–35**
1886–90	**35–45**, 45–55	25–35, **35–45**
1891–95	**35–45**, 45–55	**35–45**

This postponement may be ascribed to a greater saving of life at those ages formerly most liable to death from this disease, or to a postponement of death in those who are attacked by it. Probably both causes are at work. In the following diagram, taken from Dr. Robertson's annual report for Birmingham (1905), the age distribution of the death-rate from phthisis is shown for both males and females, in Birmingham, Sheffield, and England and Wales as a whole.

The diagram on the next page enables us also to compare the death-rate from phthisis in the two sexes, and to see the general excess of the male rate. It will also be observed that the difference between the adult death-rate of males and females respectively is much greater in the two great urban centres than in England and Wales as a whole, which coincides with the difference noted on p. 221, where it is pointed out that urban life is not in England materially less favourable to women than rural life, in respect of phthisis. In this diagram the female death-rate from phthisis is seen to be higher in England and Wales as a whole during a large part of adult life than in Sheffield and Birmingham, again illustrating the point emphasised on p. 221 as to the failure of urban conditions of life to raise the female phthisis death-rate. The contrast with the male death-rates from phthisis in adult life is very striking.

In Table XII. and Fig. 6 the death-rates from phthisis among

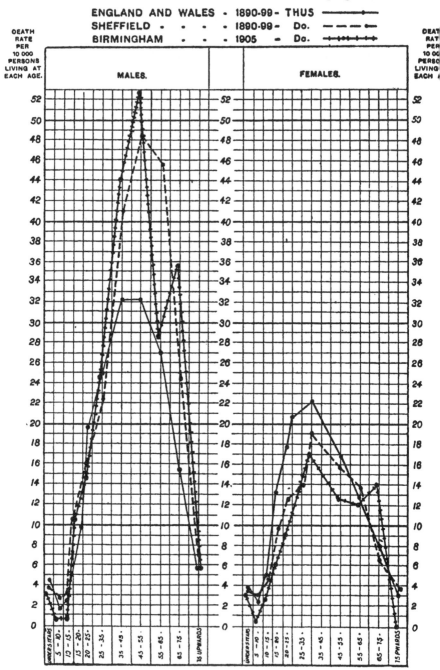

FIG. 13.—Death-rates from Phthisis for Males and Females at different Age-periods in England and Wales, Sheffield, and Birmingham (Robertson)

males at each age - period in 1861–70 and 1901 respectively are compared.

For 1901, the death-rates for children under five have been calculated in Dr. Tatham's reports for each year of life, and these have been compared with the official figures for 1871–80 in the following table :—

TABLE XXXI.—PHTHISIS

Death-rates per 100,000 of Population living at each of the First Five Years of Life

Period.	0–1.	1–2.	2–3.	3–4.	4–5.	All Ages under 5.
1871–80 . . .	141	117	54	34	30	77
1901	49	44	26	18	15	31

It has not been thought necessary to subdivide these according to sex.

˥ In the following table the male and female death-rates from phthisis in four successive decennia are given for the first twenty years of life :—

TABLE XXXII.—ENGLAND AND WALES

Pulmonary Tuberculosis

Period.	Death-rates per 100,000 of Population living at Ages								Relative Death-rate of Females, that of Males being stated as 100.			
	0–5.		5–10.		10–15.		15–20.		0–5.	5–10.	10–15.	15–20.
	M.	F.	M.	F.	M.	F.	M.	F.				
1861–70 . .	99	95	43	48	61	105	219	311	96	111	173	142
1871–80 . .	78	75	34	38	48	85	168	240	96	110	176	143
1881–90 . .	55	52	25	33	34	70	129	180	94	129	204	140
1891–1900 .	44	39	17	24	23	50	100	129	87	137	215	130

Taking the first five years of life together, it will be noted that in 1891–1900 the female is 13 per cent. lower than the male death-rate, a difference which has not hitherto been explained. The sex difference at ages 0–5 in the three previous decades varied from 6 to 4 per cent. At ages 5–10 there has been throughout the forty years a greater female than male rate. At first the excess of the male rate was 10 to 11 per cent., it then increased to 29 per cent., and in the last decade became 37 per cent. In the next age-period 10–15, the excess of the female rate is even more striking: in 1861–80 it was 73 to 76 per cent. higher than the male rate, in the last twenty years the female has been more than double the male rate, and the sex difference has increased in the last decade. At ages 15–20 an inverse process on a smaller scale is visible. The female rate was 42 to 43 per cent. higher than the male in the first twenty years, in the third decade it was 40, and in the last decade it was 30 per cent. higher. It is most difficult to explain these differences and the changes in the differences, assuming that they represent actual facts. Sir Hugh Beevor (1899) thinks that there is a true sex difference as regards this disease at the ages of rapid growth. The growing lung "is able to resist infection; resistance of the growing lung effectively accounts also for the very regular difference in the sex incidence of phthisis up to the age of 20." He draws attention to the

TABLE XXXIII.—PHTHISIS

Death-rates per 100,000

	Males.		Females.		Relative Death-rates in 1891–1900, the Death-rate for 1861–70 being stated as 100.	
Ages.	1861–70.	1891–1900.	1861–70.	1891–1900.	Males.	Females.
0–	99	44	95	39	45	41
5–	43	17	48	24	40	50
10–	61	23	105	50	39	48
15–	220	100	312	129	46	41
20–	389	189	397	159	49	40
25–	411	237	440	192	58	44
35–	417	310	391	212	74	55
45–	388	314	287	164	81	58
55–	331	262	208	124	79	60
65–	204	158	125	81	78	66
75 and upwards	66	56	45	35	84	79
All Ages	254	158	255	121	62	48

earlier and more rapid general development, and particularly of the lungs in girls. Thus growth in height in girls is completed at the age of 15 years, while boys go on growing two or three years later, and he connects this fact with the higher female phthisis rate at ages 10–15. However applicable this explanation may be for the ages 10–15, it can scarcely be applicable to the ages 5–10, in which the female rate is to a less extent excessive. It is likely that the excess at all ages 5–20 among girls is partially explicable on the ground that they live a much less outdoor life than boys, and are much more constantly exposed to domestic infection.

In the table on the preceding page the death-rates at different ages from phthisis are given separately for the two sexes at intervals of thirty years.

It will be seen that at ages 0–5 the decline in the male death-rate from phthisis has been 4 per cent. less than that in the female rate ; that at ages 5–15, the decline has been 10 per cent. greater in the male than in the female rate. At ages 15–20, the difference is only 5 per cent. At all subsequent ages the decline has been less among men than among women, this being most markedly so at ages 45–65.

The relation between the death-rates from phthisis in the two sexes can be further studied in the following table :—

TABLE XXXIV.—PHTHISIS

Relation of Female to Male Mortality at each Age and in each Period, that of Males for the same Age and Period being stated as 100

Period.	0–	5–	10–	15–	20–	25–	35–	45–	55–	65–	75 and upwards.
1861–70 .	96	111	173	142	103	107	94	74	63	61	68
1891–1900 .	87	137	215	130	84	81	69	52	47	51	63

The relations shown in this table are set out graphically in Fig. 14.

It will be observed (*a*) that at the two extremes of age there is little change in the relation which the male and female death-rates bore to each other in 1861–70 and in 1891–1900 ; (*b*) that in adult life women have gained considerably more than men ; and (*c*) that they have lost as compared with boys at ages 5–15.

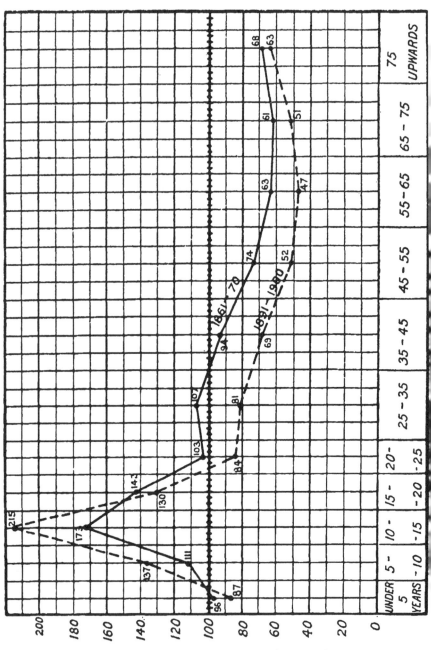

Fig. 14.—Female Death-rate from Phthisis at each Age-period, that of Males at the same Age-period being stated as 100

1861–70 . . ●━━●━━●━━●

1891–1900 . . ●----●----●----●

It is necessary to bear in mind that all the preceding figures deal with deaths. The date at which infection was received may have been less than a year, or may have been very many years before death (Chap. X.). Thus the excessive death-rate of girls aged 10-15 may be in part due to the strain of the changes undergone at puberty,—a strain greater than in boys,—calling latent infection into activity, as well as to recent infection caused by their indoor habits, as suggested on p. 169.

CHANGES IN THE SEX INCIDENCE OF PHTHISIS.—This subject deserves further study from the historical standpoint. In England and Wales the female death-rate from phthisis has been lower than the male rate from 1866 onwards, in Massachusetts it was as high as or higher than the male rate until 1896. In Prussia since 1876, when statistics first became available, the male has always been higher than the female rate. In Scotland the female was higher than the male rate until 1885, when the rates for the two sexes were nearly equal. In more recent years the position of the two has changed without consistency, but from 1898 onwards the female has always been lower than the male

TABLE XXXV

The Relative Male and Female Death-rates from Phthisis, that of Males being stated as 100 [1]

	England and Wales.		Massa-chusetts.		Providence, U.S.A.		Prussia.	
	Male.	Female.	Male.	Female.	Male.	Female.	Male.	Female.
1851–55 . .	100	107	100	137	...	...	...	...
1856–60 . .	100	108	100	123	100	131	...	...
1861–65 . .	100	104	100	109	100	91 ?	...	...
1866–70 . .	100	103	100	112	100	101	...	...
1871–75 . .	100	93	100	113	100	109	...	...
1876–80 . .	100	91	100	119	100	112	100	80 in 1876
1881–85 . .	100	84	100	114	100	101	100	84 ,, 1881
1886–90 . .	100	84	100	106	100	93	100	83 ,, 1886
1891–95 . .	100	80	100	104	100	92	100	85 ,, 1891
1896–1900 . .	100	74	100	95	100	86	100	83 ,, 1896 and 1901

[1] The correction of the death-rates for males and females respectively for differences due to age distribution of population in the two sexes was not practicable. It is unlikely that such correction would seriously alter the comparisons in the above table.

rate. In Ireland from 1864 to 1873 the male and female rates were close together ; afterwards the female became increasingly higher than the male rate. In the last few years the two rates have approached again ; in 1903 the female death-rate was 2·2 as against 2·1 per 1000 for males. In the table on preceding page the relative sex incidence of the death-rate in Massachusetts and England is given for a series of years.

MORTALITY IN THE TWO SEXES IN URBAN AND RURAL LIFE.— The influence of urban or rural conditions of life on the relation of the male to the female phthisis rate is also of interest. For Prussia this is seen in the following table :—

TABLE XXXVI.—PRUSSIA

The Relative Male and Female Death-rates from Phthisis,
that of Males being stated as 100

Year.	Towns.		Rural Communes.	
	Male.	Female.	Male.	Female.
1876	100	74	100	88
1881	100	76	100	89
1886	100	73	100	90
1891	100	74	100	95
1896	100	72	100	93
1901	100	73	100	95

This table fits in with the facts set forth on pp. 220 to 224, which showed that the female death-rates from phthisis are nearly equal in rural and urban counties of England, while the male death-rates are much higher in urban than in rural counties. The comparison in the case of England and Wales can be pursued into the different age-periods. The result is shown in Figs. 15 to 18, the data from which are taken from p. xcvi of Dr. Tatham's Letter to the Registrar-General (1905).

(a) *Comparison of urban and rural life for males.* In Fig. 15 it will be observed that throughout the early part of life up to the age-period 25–35 the male phthisis rate is higher in rural than in urban counties. After that age the rural rate ceases to rise and falls slowly, while the urban rate rises, being highest at the age-period 45–55. The evil effects of urban conditions of life

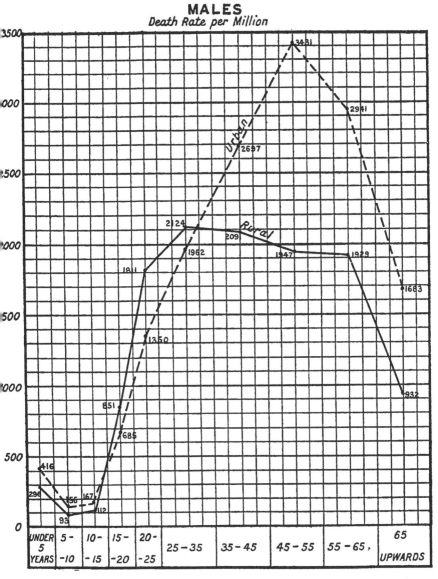

FIG. 15.—1905. Death-rate from Phthisis per million of Males living at each Age-period, in Urban and Rural Counties

and work in increasing the male phthisis rate at the higher ages are well shown.

(b) *Comparison of urban and rural life for females.* In Fig. 16

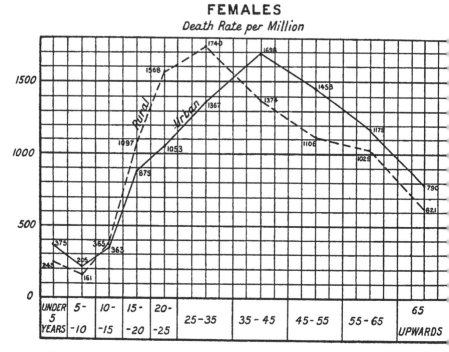

FIG. 16.—1905. Death-rate from Phthisis per million of Females living at each Age-period, in Urban and Rural Counties

the contrast to the male experience is very evident. At the ages 5–15 urban and rural experiences are almost identical. From 15–20 to 25–35 the rural phthisis rate among females is much higher than the urban. From that age-period onwards the rural is lower than the urban rate.

(c) *Comparison of males and females in urban districts.* The failure of the female rate to rise to the same extent as the male rate at ages after 20 is well seen in Fig. 17.

In Fig. 18 is given a similar comparison for rural counties.

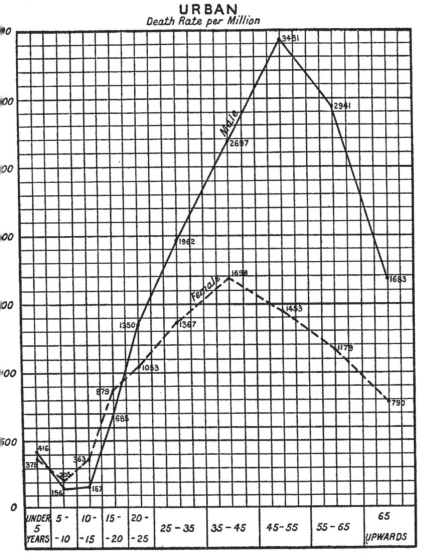

Fig. 17.—1905. Death-rate from Phthisis per million of Males and Females living at each Age-period in Urban Counties

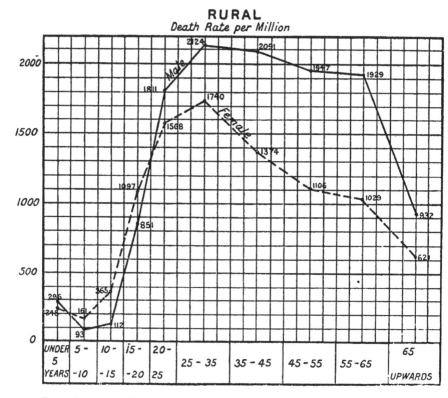

Fig. 18.—1905. Death-rate from Phthisis per million of Males and Females living at each Age-period in Rural Counties

CHAPTER XXIV

PERSONAL CONDITIONS LOWERING RESISTANCE TO INFECTION

IT has already been stated, that not only differences in age and sex, but also more or less temporary individual conditions, affect the proclivity to tuberculosis. Of these fatigue, injuries, and attacks of diseases other than tuberculosis are important ; and the state of nutrition, with particular reference to alcoholism, also needs discussion.

FATIGUE.—Over-exertion is well known to predispose to infection. The common method of origin of an ordinary catarrh is an illustration of this, and there are numerous instances in experimental bacteriology. Thus Charrin and Roger showed that normal rats, which are but slightly susceptible to anthrax, become highly susceptible when fatigued by working at a tread-mill.

Clinically a history of bodily or mental over-exertion, of protracted emotional excitement or anxiety, as after a competitive examination or the prolonged nursing of a sick relative, is a frequent prelude of acute phthisis. On this point Dr. Burton-Fanning (p. 24), says :—

To my mind there are few causes more powerful to determine the outbreak of pulmonary tuberculosis than physical over-exertion. In at least 10 per cent. of my patients the disease seemed directly attributable to their having overdone themselves. A feat of endurance is apt to overstrain the constitution, and break down the defences of an apparently healthy man against the tubercle bacillus. It had already gained, we assume, a footing in his system, and only waited an opportunity to manifest its activity. I have been struck by the frequency with which consumption attacks men who have distinguished themselves in various athletic pursuits. This remark particularly applies to such sports as tax the powers of endurance, such as long-distance bicycle riding or running, rowing, or, in fact, any exhausting exercise. It is important to recognise that, although such exercise be taken in the open air, it is conducive to the development of consumption if it entails exhaustion or fatigue.

12

INJURY.—The apparent influence of local injury in determining the site of tuberculous disease of bones and joints is well recognised. Injury to the chest wall has sometimes appeared to light up active phthisis. There is no reason to doubt that injury may, by lowering the local phagocytal influence, enable latent tubercle bacilli to assume active life.

DISEASES OTHER THAN TUBERCULOSIS. — Tuberculosis is commonly associated with certain diseases, especially with chronic insanity. The death-rate from phthisis is very excessive in the insane in asylums. From the pathological evidence collected by Dr. Mott it is clear that a very large part of this tuberculosis was present in a latent condition when the patients were admitted to the asylums ; and that the tuberculosis must be regarded as acting in insanity as it does in diabetes by hastening death, the devitalised condition of these patients enabling the tubercle bacillus to proceed with its ravages unmolested. The annual death-rate from tuberculosis in borough and county asylums is about 16 per 1000 occupants, which is more than seven times as high as that in the total adult population of England and Wales.

Certain acute infectious diseases, especially influenza, whooping-cough, measles, and to a less extent scarlet fever and enteric fever, undoubtedly favour the occurrence of tuberculosis. Probably they act in two ways : (a) in all these diseases irritation of mucous membranes and denudation of their epithelium is caused, and the way is opened for the entrance of the tubercle bacillus ; (b) probably these diseases act more commonly by

TABLE XXXVII.—ENGLAND AND WALES

Annual Death-rate per million of Population

	1888.	1889.	1890.	1891.	1892.	1893.
Influenza . . .	3	2	157	574	533	325
Phthisis . . .	1568	1573	1682	1599	1468	1466

Note.—In 1890, although probably doctors had not yet begun to record deaths as due to influenza to the full extent which the facts justified, it was already widely prevalent, and the sudden excess of deaths ascribed to phthisis occurred in this year. Probably many phthisical patients with an unstable tenure of life died as the result of intercurrent influenza.

causing swelling and infiltration of lymphatic glands, often already containing tuberculous foci, the migration from which of tubercle bacilli to internal organs is thus greatly favoured. The influence of influenza in increasing the death-rate from phthisis is shown in our national death returns. As a rule, the annual death-rate from phthisis shows no epidemic peaks, but declines smoothly by a small percentage year by year. This course was interrupted in the years 1890–91 in which influenza after a long interval again became epidemic, as shown in the table on the preceding page.

Common catarrhs are credited with an important influence in causing phthisis, especially when neglected. Possibly they act like acute specific fevers by denuding epithelium and by causing glandular enlargements, thus setting free encysted tubercle bacilli. More often the real connection is one of identity. What is regarded as a " severe cold," a slight " attack of influenza," or a " touch of bronchitis," is in fact an attack of pulmonary tuberculosis, from which the patient temporarily recovers, with frequent relapses. Whether there be any connection between neglected catarrhs and phthisis or not, it is certain, as pointed out by Clifford Allbutt, that the belief in it has had a lamentable effect on the treatment of the latter disease. Indoor confinement and stuffy rooms have been prescribed, when abundant fresh air was indicated. The common indication for treatment both in catarrh and in febrile phthisis is absolute rest with as close an approximation to open-air conditions as possible.

The association between bronchitis and phthisis has been much discussed. Many cases of senile phthisis are overlooked on account of the presence of emphysema. It is likely that many cases starting as true bronchitis have phthisis engrafted on this disease. This is especially so in many occupational diseases.

MALNUTRITION.—As shown on p. 230, good nutrition is considered by some authorities to play a very important part in the prevention of tuberculosis, although the evidence given on pp. 230 to 243 does not justify the conclusion that on a national scale any marked inverse relationship between phthisis and nutrition holds good. The same remark applies to exposure to weather, cold, and hardship, which may be regarded as representing so much excessive loss of benefit derivable from a given amount of food. Thus Ransome (1890, p. 50) says :—

> The Highlanders, who inhabit well-built houses on the mainland of Scotland, are subject to the same fate as the other inhabitants, whilst the ill-fed, ill-clothed fishermen of St. Kilda and the Hebrides, who are of the same race, hardly ever contract the disease.

In another paragraph on the same page Ransome gives a second illustration, which may also be quoted :—

> The terrible mortality from phthisis that prevailed at one time amongst the finest soldiers of the British Army was certainly not brought on by starvation or misery. It occurred for the most part when they were not on active service, but in a time of peace, when they were well fed and well cared for so far as their bodily comfort was concerned—far better, in fact, than the half-starved workpeople and labourers, who only died of the disease at one-third the rate they did.

The experience of Ireland, given more fully on pp. 217 and 233, tells the same story. Between 1870 and 1903 the wages of its agricultural labourers have increased 42 per cent., while the cost of food has greatly diminished and its death-rate from phthisis has increased.

Dr. Stafford of the Irish Local Government Board has recently given the death-rates from phthisis in the years 1900–02 in the two Dublin Poor Law Unions and in the county of Mayo respectively. In Dublin the phthisis death-rate is 3·4 and in Mayo 1·4 per 1000. He adds that

> for scantiness of the means of subsistence the general condition of the inhabitants of County Mayo could scarcely be surpassed. It is clear, therefore, that poverty alone may be present in an acute form and on a large scale without producing an excessive mortality from tuberculosis, and that some other factor or factors as well as poverty exercise a determining influence in producing the excessive death-rate from tuberculosis.

It is important to bear in mind these illustrations following from the fact that circumstances other than differences of nutrition affect the proclivity to tuberculosis. They show that no general measures of improvement in well-being by themselves suffice to control the disease. But beyond question malnutrition favours tuberculosis, and while the evidence in Part II. amply shows that other factors are more important, no system of measures for controlling tuberculosis can be regarded as final which omits to do what is practicable for preventing malnutrition.

ALCOHOL.—That alcoholic indulgence favours the occurrence of phthisis is shown by abundant evidence, and is well recognised. Thus the late Professor Brouardel (1901) of Paris said :—

Alcoholism is in fact the most powerful factor in the propagation of tuberculosis. The most vigorous man, who becomes alcoholic, is without resistance before it.

Although some have obtained opposite results, there are many experiments on record tending to show that infections in general are more rapid and more grave in alcoholised animals. Drs. Achard and Gaillard found in experimenting on rabbits that giving alcohol hastened the progress of experimental tuberculosis. For the human being Landouzy has expressed the influence of alcoholism as follows : " l'alcoölisme fait le lit de la tuberculose."

Alcohol and phthisis are related as indicated above, through the diminished resistance to the disease caused by alcohol, and with that we are chiefly concerned in this chapter. Alcoholic indulgence, and still more the occupation of selling alcoholic drinks, commonly expose persons to more frequent infection ; and this is a prominent factor in causing the excessive death-rate from phthisis in certain occupations (p. 159).

CHAPTER XXV

HEREDITARY DISPOSITION TO PHTHISIS

SO far we have been chiefly concerned with factors of causation which are all more or less ascertained and defined.

The influence of heredity differs from these in being still more or less *sub judice*.

It is considered as acting in two ways : by direct transmission before birth from parent to infant of the germs of disease ; or by the transmission from parent to offspring of a special weakness or openness rendering certain persons more liable to infection than others.

THE DIRECT TRANSMISSION OF TUBERCULOSIS from parent to child may occur before birth, either germinally—a very rare phenomenon—or during intra-uterine life, a more common, but still rare, event.

The passage of the tubercle bacillus through the placental tissues to the fœtus has been proved by a number of pathologists. Thus Johne found tubercles in the lungs and bronchial glands of the eight months' fœtus of a tuberculous cow. MacFadyean found cheesy foci in the liver and portal glands of a five days' old calf. Similar cases have been described in the human fœtus. Fränkel (1906) thinks that the danger of hæmatogenous infection through the placenta is commonly understated. He quotes Schmorl, who found tuberculous nodules in 9 out of 20 or 45 per cent. of the placentas of tuberculous women examined by him ; and these were found not only in cases of miliary tuberculosis or advanced phthisis, but also in a case of incipient phthisis. It is possible, furthermore, that the instances in which obvious tuberculous lesions are found in the new-born child do not cover the entire ground. Other infants may have latent tuberculosis, which develops into obvious disease later in life.

This view is commonly associated with the name of Baumgarten, though it was held before his day. He believes that either germinal or intra-uterine transmission of infection is the most common cause of tuberculosis, and that long latency of the infection is the rule rather than the exception. He goes further, believing even that a person may have been infected by transmission through two generations from a tuberculous grandparent.

The views of Baumgarten, apart from the last-named point, are supported by the fact that microscopic examination of the liver and inoculation experiments with fœtal tissues showing no naked-eye evidence of disease have occasionally shown the presence of tubercle bacilli. Baumgarten considers long dormancy of tubercle bacilli in lymphatic glands, the medulla of bone, etc., as common, the young tissues of growing animals having special resisting power against the bacilli. His view involves the unlikely supposition that a very large part of the human race carry within them tubercle bacilli at birth. At the same time the analogous case of congenital syphilis, with long latency of an infection acquired before birth, indicates that congenital tuberculosis is within the range of possibility. It is possible, as J. K. Fowler has suggested, that evidence will accumulate in favour of the view that sometimes tuberculosis of the glands, joints, and bones in children may have been transmitted from the parent and remained dormant for several years. To prove such cases it would be necessary to show that the mother was tuberculous, and that there had been no exposure to infection after birth. In the absence of evidence on the latter point, either the ordinary view of infection after birth, or the view that infection was acquired before birth, would be tenable.

The fact that visible tuberculosis is more commonly found

TABLE XXXVIII

	Still Births and 1 Day Old.	1 Day to 4 Weeks.	1 to 2 Months.	2 to 3 Months.	3 to 6 Months.	6 to 9 Months.	9 to 12 Months.	1 to 2 Years.	2 to 3 Years.	3 to 4 Years.	4 to 5 Years.	Total.
Number of autopsies .	184	250	52	33	76	88	65	311	189	160	134	1542
Number with tuberculous changes .	...	...	...	2	8	15	18	83	56	51	30	263
Per cent. of total .	...	...	...	6·1	10·5	17·0	27·7	26·7	29·6	31·9	22·5	17·0

with each additional month after birth, may be explained either
on the supposition that early-life tuberculosis is in the main
acquired after birth ; or by assuming that ante-natal tuberculosis remains long latent so far as symptoms are concerned.
The following illustrations on this point will suffice. Cornet
(1904, p. 307) gives the figures on the preceding page relating to
a number of autopsies made on children under 5 years old dying
in children's hospitals in Berlin.

These figures clearly show that whether infection is received
before or after birth, visible changes are not usually shown in
the body until some months later. (The figures in the above
table must not be regarded as giving any indication of the true
frequency of fatal tuberculosis in children. To do this it would
be necessary to compare the deaths from this disease with the
number of children living at the same ages. The figures do,
however, show its rarity in the first few months of life.)

Veterinary results are to a like effect. Thus Cornet (1904,
p. 308) gives the distribution of tuberculosis among cattle in
Saxony, where the inspection of meat is compulsory, as follows :—

Of 120,490 calves up to 6 weeks of age	.	.	3, or	0·002	per cent.
,, 665 cattle from 6 weeks to 1 year	.	.	1, ,,	0·15	,,
,, 6,328 ,, ,, 1 to 3 years old	.	.	440, ,,	6·9	,,
,, 13,307 ,, ,, 3 to 6 ,, ,,	.	.	1,285, ,,	9·7	,,
,, 11,101 ,, over 6 years old	.	.	1,881, ,,	16·9	,,

The most probable interpretation of the preceding facts is
that post-natal infection is the usual source of tuberculosis,
though ante-natal infection occasionally occurs, and it may be
somewhat more frequent than is generally recognised.

HEREDITARY PREDISPOSITION.—Phthisis is usually regarded
as a typically hereditary disease, in the causation of which
family predisposition plays a large part. The extent to which
heredity is held to operate has diminished as our knowledge of
the causation of tuberculosis has become more exact. The most
prevalent view is contained in the following statement by Drs.
C. J. B. and C. Theodore Williams (1887, p. 58) :—

Family predisposition has by general consent held a very prominent
place, but the value of its influence in the causation of phthisis has been
modified of late years by the fuller recognition of other causes which had
been to some extent overlooked—such as damp, inflammatory attacks,
etc. These and other direct sources of phthisis must exercise in our calculations a depreciatory influence on the amount we assign to hereditary

transmission, and numerous cases of this disease which have hitherto been held to originate in a consumptive ancestry, will now be traced to a nearer and more direct cause. Nevertheless, no small number of cases owe their origin to hereditary predisposition, though it is not always easy to demonstrate their hereditary character. Its exact value as a predisposing agent, its mode of transmission, the varieties of the disease in which its influence is most apparent,—all these and other points of interest are by no means settled questions, but still open to further inquiry.

Similarly Dr. S. West (1902, vol. ii. p. 449) states that " recent additions to our knowledge of tuberculosis have greatly modified the views held as to the influence of inheritance in phthisis "; but after giving statistics he concludes that " family predisposition is an essential factor in phthisis, though probably not exerting so important an influence as has been hitherto believed."

The evidence on the strength of which it is considered that hereditary predisposition forms an important factor in the causation of phthisis consists usually in showing that a large percentage of the parents and other relatives of the total consumptives had also suffered from the same disease. West (p. 449) says that about 28 per cent. of the total cases taken at random yield, on an average of a large number of cases, a history of phthisis in the parents, and about 25 per cent. more in collateral relatives. Walshe (1871, p. 461) in a careful investigation of 162 cases found that 26 per cent. of them had one or both parents similarly diseased. J. E. Squire (quoted by Fowler, p. 312) gives 12,509 cases of phthisis, showing in 24·8 per cent. of these cases that one or both parents had been consumptive. When grandparents and collaterals were included, the percentage of heredity became 62·3. Williams (1887, p. 63) thinks that " an average of 12 per cent. for direct hereditary transmission, and of 48 per cent. for family predisposition, are not unfair estimates for the upper classes." Wilson Fox found a history of direct inheritance in 33 per cent. of hospital cases.

Facts like the above, although they are commonly regarded as good evidence of hereditary influence, are almost valueless unless further tested. This was realised long ago by Walshe (p. 461), who observed about his own results :—

Does this result, that about 26 per cent. of my tuberculous patients came of a father or mother, or of both parents, similarly diseased, prove, even in this limited proportion, the reality of *hereditary influence* in the production of the disease? I think not. It shows that of a given generation (*b*) about 26 per 100 came under ascertainable conditions of a tuberculous parent (generation *a*). But this ratio of 26 per 100 might be, and probably is, no higher than that of the tuberculised portion of the population generally.

In another paragraph (p. 54) he says :—

If it be true, as always taught, that one in every three persons dying from all diseases indiscriminately in the Paris hospitals has tubercle in the lungs, the existence of an almost universal family taint becomes an unavoidable inference.

Phthisis, like scarlet fever, is a common and an infectious disease, and the futility of depending on statistics like those already quoted, as evidence of hereditary predisposition, may be illustrated from the latter disease. For some years past I have ascertained in the course of my official experience the family experience of households invaded by notifiable infectious diseases ; and I recently abstracted 100 family histories of scarlet fever in which the records were sufficiently complete to be trustworthy. Out of every 100 patients belonging to different families, both parents of seven patients had suffered from scarlet fever previously, the fathers only of sixteen patients and the mothers only of nine patients had suffered from scarlet fever, while in 68 per cent. neither parent had suffered from this disease. The resemblance to the percentages for tuberculous families is. striking, and both sets of figures alike fail to prove any true hereditary predisposition.

HEREDITARY PREDISPOSITION OR INFECTION.—It is easy to prove heredity in the case of a disease like hæmophilia, where (*a*) the disease is rare and presumably not infectious, and (*b*) either all or almost all the cases occur among those whose ancestors had the same disease. But in phthisis we have to deal with a disease which in the first place is infectious, and would therefore give no such clear evidence of heredity, even if heredity were potent ; and which, in the second place, is very common, causing in the general community about one out of every twelve male and one out of every seventeen female deaths from all causes. Since it is infectious, one cannot expect all the cases to be limited to families with hereditary taint, however strong this influence may be, and in actual fact it is not so limited.   Finally, even if it be shown that the number of adult deaths from phthisis amongst those with a tuberculous family history is in that class much greater than the number among a corresponding number of the general population similarly situated as to age and sex, it does not necessarily follow that this is due to hereditary predisposition. It may result from greater exposure to infection.   There cannot be said to exist satisfactory data enabling this doubt to be cleared up.   The nearest approach to such data is embodied in a " first study " of the statistics of phthisis by Professor Pearson, in which the family history of a hypothetical random sample of the general community is compared with that of consumptives.   Even these, however, fail to distinguish between family infection and the inheritance of family predisposition. An examination of the mathematical method used by Professor Pearson would be outside the scope of the present discussion ; but it is important to note as a matter involving no criticism of method, that his results depend in part upon hypotheses which may not be accepted generally as justified, and upon ascertained data which may be regarded as too few to warrant conclusive inferences.   Indeed he himself states : " This investigation does not profess to be more than preliminary, and its results need confirmation when much more numerous data are available."   He proceeds, however, to state that : " I feel fairly confident that for the artisan class the inheritance factor is far more important than the infection factor."   This statement goes beyond Professor Pearson's data, and his assumption that in towns the artisan classes can scarcely escape infection, except by the absence of the tuberculous diathesis is unproven. By infection he doubtless means efficient infection, and no point is clearer in the pathology of tuberculosis than that efficient infection depends largely on the dosage of infective material. The considerations in Chapter XIII. indicate that infection is much more limited and localised than is usually supposed. It is to be hoped that Professor Pearson's most interesting researches may be continued, and that he may receive in the future more ample and more complete data from physicians than he has hitherto had placed at his disposal.   It would be a great advantage if, in such a research on a larger scale, consumptive families could be classified into groups according to the length of interval between the termination of one case and the earlier symptoms of successive cases in the same family.

The question asked by Burton-Fanning (1904, p. 22) cannot be regarded as a serious contribution towards the solution of the problem, without further detailed evidence than is given. He asks :—

> If it is entirely a matter of infection and not of heredity, why are the members of the family picked out, and other occupants of the house, such as the servants, avoided ?

In the context this writer gives no evidence to show that the servants actually escape. Instances are on record in which they are known to have fallen victims after prolonged un-skilled attendance on consumptives, though the frequent migrations of servants render it difficult to obtain such evidence. Before importance can be attached to this question, there must be evidence on a considerable scale that with fairly equal degrees of exposure to infection (both as to duration and intimacy) servants escape when relatives suffer. The remarks in Chapter X. on long latency have also to be borne in mind in interpreting results.

On the whole, we shall probably not err greatly if we agree with Koch's statement (1901, p. 26) that

> great importance used to be attached to the hereditary transmission of tuberculosis. Now, however, it has been demonstrated by thorough investigation that, though hereditary tuberculosis is not absolutely non-existent, it is nevertheless extremely rare, and we are at liberty, in considering our practical measures, to leave this form of origination entirely out of account.

THE PRACTICAL ASPECTS OF HEREDITY IN TUBERCULOSIS. —The statement last quoted from Koch must command par-ticular approval, when considered in relation to administrative measures. From the standpoint of practical public health administration, if it were ultimately to be established that heredity exercises a greater effect on the transmission of tuber-culosis than has hitherto been attributed to it, the measures of precaution indicated by this result might be increased in number, but none of those of which the adoption is recommended on other grounds would become more safely negligible than they are now considered to be. The inheritance of a disposition to tuberculosis if demonstrated as a general phenomenon would show the presence in the community of a larger number of susceptible persons than could be inferred from other considerations. The existence of this larger number of susceptible people would call not for the neglect but for the more careful enforcement of the precautions by means of which susceptibility is prevented from developing into actual infection. The logical alternative is to kill off the susceptible stock or, as has been suggested, to allow them to infect their susceptible brethren and together with them perish of their disease. Such proposals have only to be stated in their crude terms in order to be apprehended and reprehended as an unsocial negation of civilisation.

MARRIAGE OF AND BETWEEN CONSUMPTIVES.—As the matter is not separately dealt with in Part III. of this book, it is convenient to add here a note as to the practical bearing of the preceding facts and considerations on the marriage of, and particularly on the marriage between, consumptives. Assuming that advice based on physiological and medical considerations will be allowed to carry weight in a matter in which the affections alone as a rule are allowed control, it is evident that in many instances the marriage of those of consumptive stock is to be deprecated, especially when both parties come of such stock. On the other hand, when it is remembered that in at least 30 per cent. of the adult population there is a history of consumption in the antecedents, a sweeping condemnation of such marriages can be justified only if it is shown that this percentage is made up by a much higher percentage in a relatively small portion of the total population. The measure of the actual danger in any given instance would be made on the strength of a number of facts :—

(1) At what age did phthisis show itself in the preceding generation ? Has the man or woman now concerned passed that age ?

(2) What is the interval since the man or woman now concerned was last exposed to infection from the consumptive

relative ; and prior to that what was the duration and extent of exposure ?

(3) Are the circumstances of the person now being advised such as are likely to call into activity any latent infection ?

CHAPTER XXVI

CONDITIONS OF ENVIRONMENT LOWERING RESISTANCE TO INFECTION; SOCIAL MISERY; AND INSANITARY CIRCUMSTANCES

TUBERCULOSIS is most prevalent and most fatal under conditions of social misery, and when the surroundings of the patient are insanitary. It is not surprising, therefore, that it is frequently regarded as due to social misery, and that for its prevention many reformers are satisfied with an appeal for general social reform, without attempting to analyse the constituents of social misery which in particular favour tuberculosis. Without attempting any complete analysis of social misery and of the insanitary circumstances so closely associated with it, it may be said that in it are united in a vicious circle, ignorance, privation, and suffering, and that efforts against any of these will undoubtedly help to reduce the amount of tuberculosis. These factors are in themselves complex. Thus privation involves the operation of several influences, to each of which it is difficult to apportion its true weight. Underfeeding and defective nutrition (pp. 179 and 230) undoubtedly play a part in producing the excess of tuberculosis found in the poor, though only a relatively small part. Neglect of the ordinary rules and precautions of a hygienic life, as to cleanliness, wearing of suitable apparel, precautions after exposure to rain and weather, and so on, doubtless also favour tuberculosis, though no preponderant weight in the balance can be ascribed to them. Unfavourable sanitary circumstances of the poor, especially housing, play their part ; this is gauged in relation to other factors—so far as the data permit—on pp. 224 to 229. Domestic overcrowding has already been fully considered on pp. 146 to 149. It undoubtedly plays a very large share in the production of tuberculosis ; and to this factor more than to any other attention is required, if the decline in the death-rate from tuberculosis is to be made more rapid than at present.

As no special chapter in Part III. is devoted to ordinary sanitary measures in relation to the prevention of tuberculosis, it is convenient to consider here the measures practicable against it. There are two ways in which overcrowding can be abated : one is the slow measure of official inspections, followed by official notices in the instances in which overcrowding is detected. Those who have official experience know the limitations of this method, valuable though it is. Before the limit of legal over-crowding (about 350 cubic feet for each person) is reached, there may be social overcrowding of a most objectionable character, over which official inspection can exercise no control. Even when there is suspicion of legal overcrowding, it is very difficult to obtain conclusive evidence of its existence, except in lodging-houses in which night inspections are possible. Under these circumstances official remedies against overcrowding are bound to operate slowly, although much improvement has already been accomplished.

The alternative remedy is the removal from the congested dwelling of those liable to convey infection. This has been done for typhoid and typhus fevers and for small-pox, and has led to an immense reduction in their prevalence. In scarlet fever and diphtheria similar measures have not been successful to an equal extent, because of the failure to track slight cases of these diseases, which remain at home or in school spreading infection. In phthisis, as shown in Part II., the evidence indicates that similar removal of advanced cases from the poorest homes has been a predominant cause of the great decline in the death-rate from that disease already secured.

Overcrowding is nearly always associated with other evil house conditions—such as defective light and air and absence of thorough ventilation—which undoubtedly protract the extra-corporeal life and retard the destruction of the tubercle bacilli. Do they do more than this ? Some experimental results appear to indicate that they may. Thus Trudeau inoculated a number of rabbits with equal doses of tubercle bacilli ; half of these were allowed to run free in the open air, and the remainder were placed in a damp hole to which sunlight had no access. Both sets of rabbits were killed at the same time, and it was found that the first had recovered or only had slight lesions, while the second had extensive tuberculosis.

Ransome's experiments (1895, p. 15) point in the same direction. In 1889–90, experimenting with Dreschfield, he showed that

the air of a poor cottage in Ancoats, with poor ventilation and undrained basement, in which several cases of phthisis had occurred, was able to preserve unchanged the virulence of tuberculous sputum for two or three months at least, but that the same sputum exposed freely to air and light in a hospital for phthisical patients and also in a well-lighted, well-drained, and well-ventilated house entirely lost the power of communicating the disease to guinea-pigs by inoculation. A further research carried on in 1894 in conjunction with Professor Delépine proved that less than two days' exposure to air and light with only one hour of sunshine was sufficient to destroy the virulent power of tuberculous sputum when it was exposed in a clean, well-drained, well-lighted house. Evidently in the air of the Ancoats cottage there must have been some form of organic impurity favourable to the life of the bacillus.

Whatever be the interpretation put upon these experiments, there can be no difference of opinion as to the ill-effects of overcrowding, defective light and air, absence of thorough ventilation, and still more of domestic uncleanliness in favouring the occurrence and spread of tuberculosis. Probably these factors operate chiefly by facilitating the spread of infection ; but it is possible that they also tend to devitalise the occupants of such houses and render them more ready victims of infection. Whatever opinion be held on this point, the indication clearly is to adopt the most strenuous efforts to remove these evil conditions, wherever found.

CHAPTER XXVII

CLIMATE AND SOIL

CLIMATE.—The anxious inquirer after indications as to the climate associated with the lowest death-rates from tuberculosis would not obtain any satisfactory hints from the statistics scattered throughout this book, or found elsewhere. It may be said in brief that there is scarcely a climate which has not been looked upon at one time as predisposing to this disease, and at another as curing it. There is no certain evidence that it is less prevalent at high than at low altitudes, except in so far as the former are usually more isolated and less densely populated than the latter. Hirsch (vol. iii. pp. 197–8) has said :—

> The disease occurs *cæteris paribus* in all geographical zones with uniform frequency; equatorial and subtropical regions are visited with consumption not less than countries with a temperate or an arctic climate. . . .

The only statements that can be made in this connection with absolute certainty are that

1. Anything favouring an open-air life diminishes tuberculosis.

2. Tuberculosis is less prevalent in the less densely populated and more isolated communities.

SOIL.[1]—In regard to soil, there is almost equal uncertainty. Thorne is quoted by Roberts (1902) as saying that in the prevention of pulmonary tuberculosis " nothing would do good unless people refused to live on a damp subsoil." A damp subsoil is stated in all text-books of hygiene to be a most important cause of phthisis.

The proved infectivity of the disease makes it somewhat difficult to adjudge what importance should still be attached to soil in relation to its causation. It is therefore desirable to

---

[1] The greater part of the rest of this chapter appeared as an article on " The Influence of Soil on the Prevalence of Pulmonary Phthisis "(*Practitioner*, February 1901).

summarise the evidence and to discuss it in the light of modern pathology.

In order of time, the first observations on the subject were made by Dr. H. I. Bowditch (1862). He laid down the " Law of Soil Moisture " in the following two propositions :—

(1) A residence on or near a damp soil, whether that dampness be inherent in the soil itself, or caused by percolation from adjacent ponds, rivers, meadows, marshes, or springy soils, is one of the primal causes of consumption in Massachusetts—probably in New England, and possibly in other portions of the globe.

(2) Consumption can be checked in its career, and possibly—nay, probably—prevented in some instances by attention to this law.

Dr. Gavin Milroy in the Seventh Annual Report of the Registrar-General for Scotland (pp. xlvii–xlviii) quoted Dr. Bowditch's conclusions drawn " from a very thorough inquiry into one of the causes of consumption in Massachusetts." He then proceeded to investigate the law. Such an explanation he found would agree with the very different proportion of deaths from consumption occurring in the eight principal towns of Scotland. Taking a five-yearly average (1857–61) the death-rate from consumption per 100,000 of population was found to be 206 in Leith, 298 in Edinburgh, 310 in Perth, 332 in Aberdeen, 340 in Dundee, 383 in Paisley, 399 in Glasgow, and 400 in Greenock. Attention was then drawn to the fact that if each town had been arranged in the order of comparative dryness of its site,

they would almost have arranged themselves in the above position—Leith and Edinburgh the most free from consumption, and also having the driest sites ; Glasgow and Greenock the most ravaged by that disease, and beyond all comparison situated on the dampest sites.

Dr. G. Buchanan's investigation of the same subject was embodied in two reports, which were written before he had seen the remarks summarised above from the Seventh Report of the Registrar-General for Scotland, or Dr. Bowditch's essay on the subject. He adds :—

I should not insist on this point, except for the purpose of giving to the conclusions which Dr. Bowditch and myself have obtained, the additional weight that they deserve from having been arrived at by a second inquirer, wholly ignorant of and therefore unbiassed by the work of the first.

Dr. Buchanan's first report is contained in the Ninth Report of the Medical Officer of the Privy Council (1866). This report summarises the improvements carried out in 25 towns visited in the course of 1865–66, in which the authorities had carried out works designed for the improvement of the public health. The towns were selected as being places where structural sanitary works had been most thoroughly done, and were not chosen for any previously ascertained improvement in their health. The general result of the inquiry, so far as phthisis is concerned, was that when the sanitary improvements carried out had been associated with drying of the subsoil, the phthisis mortality had declined, sometimes to one-third or even one-half of its previous amount. Great difficulty was experienced in ascertaining the degree of drying of the soil, as sewerage works were not executed with this direct object in view. It became necessary therefore to indicate the degree of drying " in as accurate general terms as may be." In the table on the following page I have set forth the main results of Dr. Buchanan's research, arranging the towns according to the stated influence of sewerage works on the subsoil.

Thus in the 6 towns in which " much drying " of the subsoil followed the carrying out of works of sewerage, the mortality from phthisis declined to degrees varying from 49 to 17 per cent. ; in 4 of the 5 towns in which " some drying " occurred a decline of from 43 to 19 per cent. occurred, but at Ashby-de-la-Zouch an increase of 19 per cent. occurred ; in 5 of the 7 towns in which " minor degrees of drying " occurred, the reduction was from 1 to 32 per cent., in Chelmsford the death-rate from phthisis remained stationary, and in Carlisle it increased by 10 per cent. ; while in 3 of the 5 towns in which " no change in the subsoil " occurred, it was reduced from 5 to 8 per cent., and increased at Brynmawr to the extent of 6 per cent., and at Alnwick to the extent of 20 per cent. Dr. Buchanan notes in his report that at Leicester a greater reduction of mortality from phthisis occurred during the carrying out of the sewerage works than was subsequently maintained ; and that at Stratford " a large reduction of phthisis was for the time observable," although the subsequent decline was only 1 per cent. It is noted also that towns which like Salisbury made special arrangements for drying their subsoil improved conspicuously, as did also those towns with large sewers and those with deep storm culverts. Failure to reduce phthisis is also stated to be most observable where, as at Penzance and Brynmawr, the soil already contained little water, or where the storm water was not properly treated, or where the deep drainage consisted of impervious pipes laid down in compact channels, as at Penrith and Alnwick.

Four exceptional cases are pointed out by Dr. Buchanan: Chelmsford and Carlisle, which had more lowering of subsoil

TABLE XXXIX

	Much Drying of Subsoil.			Some Drying of Subsoil.	
	Previous Phthisis Death-rate (all Ages) per 10,000 Living.	Degree of Change in Phthisis Death-rate.		Previous Phthisis Death-rate (all Ages) per 10,000 Living.	Degree of Change in Phthisis. Death-rate.
Salisbury	44⅓	− 49 per cent.	Rugby	28½	− 43 per cent.
Ely	32	− 47 ,,	Worthing	30½	− 36 ,,
Banbury	26⅔	− 41 ,,	Cheltenham	28¾	− 26 ,,
Macclesfield	51½	− 31 ,,	Bristol	33½	− 22 ,,
Croydon	(59½)¹	(− 17)¹ ,,	Warwick	40	− 19 ,,
Cardiff	34¾	− 17 ,,	Ashby	25½	+ 19 ,,

	Various Minor Degrees of Drying of Subsoil.			No Change in Subsoil.	
	Previous Phthisis Death-rate (all Ages) per 10,000 Living.	Degree of Change in Phthisis Death-rate.		Previous Phthisis Death-rate (all Ages) per 10,000 Living.	Degree of Change in Phthisis Death-rate.
Leicester	43⅓	− 32 p.c.	Doubtful amount of drying.	Penzance	30¾	− 5 p.c.
				Brynmawr	28⅓	+ 6 ,,
Newport	37	− 32 ,,	Local drying.	Morpeth	30½	− 8 ,,
Dover	26⅔	− 20 ,,	Do.	Penrith	39½	− 5 ,,
Merthyr	38¼	− 11 ,,	Some recent drying.	Alnwick	28⅓	+ 20 ,,
Stratford	26⅔	− 1 ,,	Some local drying.			
Chelmsford	32½	nil	Slight drying.			
Carlisle	32	+ 10 ,,	Drying with local defects.			

¹ Phthisis and lung diseases together.

water than some towns which stood well as regards reduction of phthisis; and Worthing and Rugby, which, on the other hand, experienced a greater reduction of phthisis than other towns in which there occurred a more complete drying of the subsoil. The following remark by Dr. Buchanan on this point deserves quotation :—

Perhaps it had better be confessed that there are exceptions to the rule of subsidence of phthisis after drying of subsoil ; or the suggestion may be allowed that the nature of the change in climatic conditions, produced by drying the subsoil of a locality, is not everywhere the same (the environs of Chelmsford, for example, still get flooded through the action of a mill-dam), and that different degrees of effect may hence be produced on consumption.

Before discussing the facts above summarised, it is desirable to summarise Dr. Buchanan's second report made in the following year, in which he proceeded to examine the apparent relation between wetness of soil and prevalence of consumption, " with direct reference to geological considerations." The necessity of taking into account surface peculiarities quite as much as the great divisions of the geologist is pointed out. The statistics of 58 registration districts in the counties of Surrey, Sussex, and Kent, embracing a population of 1,118,372, living on 3812 square miles, were taken, the registered phthisis mortality at ages 15–55 being calculated for each district. On tabulating these it soon appeared that " the districts arranged in the order of the prevalence of consumption in them are also to a very large extent arranged in the order of the dryness or wetness of their soils." Although this was so, the difficulties in classifying districts properly were very great, owing to the fact that one section of the population of a district might be living on pervious and

TABLE XL

Groups of Districts.	Percentage Proportion of Population.	
	On Pervious Soils.	On Retentive Soils.
A. With least phthisis	90·9	9·1
B. With next least phthisis	87·7	12·3
C. Middle as to phthisis	79·5	20·5
D. With still more phthisis	79·2	20·8
E. With most phthisis	64·2	35·8

another on impervious strata. In such a district the number living on each kind of soil was estimated, and from the results thus obtained and the mortality statistics the groups on the previous page were derived.

The preceding classification is, as explained by Dr. Buchanan, open to objection, because, for instance, in group D. low plains of gravel - covered chalk are reckoned under pervious soils, " which might, so far as their water-holding faculty goes, as fitly find a place among the retentive formations."

The alternative plan of classifying districts according to their geological conditions brought out more certain conclusions : (a) On examining the prevalence of phthisis upon pervious soils from which water can drain away, as compared with its prevalence upon retentive soils, it was found that " the descending series of the percentage numbers on sands and the ascending series of those on clays was wonderfully nearly regular for the districts arranged in the order of their consumption ; so much is this the case, indeed, that they could not be expected to be more regular unless one should go the length of contending that phthisis was a disease influenced by no other circumstance than the one condition of soil."

(b) Within the limits of " pervious soils " may be included great ranges of wet and dry soils, according to the elevation of the ground and the dip of subjacent impervious beds. Thus, Chichester, situated on low-lying gravel over London clay, had a very unfavourable position for pulmonary tuberculosis, while districts on the same gravel, with a sloping clay under it, as at Croydon, Epsom, Richmond, occupied a more favourable position. In chalk areas again, for similar reasons, there was least phthisis on the more elevated portions. On the other hand, low-lying districts on gravel and chalk near the sea, e.g. Dover, had a favourable phthisis mortality.

(c) When comparing impervious districts differences were seen. London clay had commonly a much less degree of wetness than the Weald clay, and there appeared to be a corresponding difference in the phthisis mortality. The general results from this inquiry are so important that they deserve complete reproduction:—

(1) Within the counties of Surrey, Kent, and Sussex, there is, broadly speaking, less phthisis among populations living on pervious than among populations living on impervious soils.

(2) Within the same counties, there is less phthisis among populations living on high-lying pervious soils than among populations living on low-lying pervious soils.

(3) Within the same counties, there is less phthisis among populations living on sloping impervious soils than among populations living on flat impervious soils.

(4) The connection between soil and phthisis has been established in this inquiry—

(a) by the existence of general agreement in phthisis mortality between districts that have common geological and topographical features, of a nature to affect the water-holding quality of the soil ;

(b) by the existence of general disagreement between districts that are differently circumstanced in regard of such features; and

(c) by the discovery of pretty general concomitancy in the fluctuation of the two conditions, from much phthisis with much wetness of soil to little phthisis with little wetness of soil.

But the connection between wet soil and phthisis came out last year in another way, which must here be recalled,

(d) by the observation that phthisis had been greatly reduced in towns where the water of the soil had been artificially removed, and that it had not been reduced in other towns where the soil had not been dried.

(5) The whole of the foregoing conclusions combine into one—which may now be affirmed generally, and not only of particular districts—that WETNESS OF SOIL IS A CAUSE OF PHTHISIS TO THE POPULATION LIVING UPON IT.

(6) No other circumstance can be detected, after careful consideration of the materials accumulated during this year, that coincides on any large scale with the greater or less prevalence of phthisis, except the one condition of soil.

(7) In this year's inquiry, and in last year's too, single apparent exceptions to the general law have been detected. They are probably not altogether errors of fact or observation, but are indications of some other law in the background that we are not yet able to announce.

The independent generalisations of Bowditch and Buchanan have been generally accepted, and have formed the basis of advice which has determined changes of residence for thousands of phthisical patients. There have been, however, attempts made to minimise or rebut their conclusions. Thus it was pointed out by Pearse that in several rainy districts of Devonshire phthisis was but seldom a cause of death ; and that the mortality from phthisis was less at Wisbeach, in the fen district, than at Axminster on the red sandstone (*Lancet*, 1876, December, p. 833). In Holland, again, there is less phthisis than in France, and " the more elevated provinces with diluvial soil suffer more than the deep depressions with an alluvial soil,

such as Zeeland, which has the smallest phthisical death-rate "
(Hirsch, p. 203).

In this country, the late Dr. C. Kelly, Medical Officer of
Health of the combined district of West Sussex, a portion of the
special area investigated by Buchanan, published statistics
which are not confirmatory of Buchanan's results. In his report
for 1879 he showed that the phthisis death-rate had been distinctly lowered in that district in recent years, " while very little,
if any, change has taken place during the same period in the
drainage of the soil." Sir R. T. Thorne (1888, p. 51) commenting
on this statement, said that the large amount of agricultural
drainage which had then already been effected throughout
the kingdom would be expected to have produced a result in rural
districts very similar to that brought about by sanitary drainage in towns. On this point further evidence appears desirable.
Dr. Kelly gave the following statistics for West Sussex. This
is a district which covers an area of 335,492 square acres, or
about 524 square miles, with a population in 1887 of 105,520.
The different soils found in this district are (1) pervious soils,
which include the upper and lower greensands, the chalk and
the lower Tunbridge Wells sands; (2) the retentive soils, which
include the Weald clay, the clayey beds of the lower greensand
and the gault; and (3) moderately pervious soils, sloping from
the sea to the South Downs, where the chalk is covered for a
depth of 15 to 50 feet with loam and brick-earth.

TABLE XLI

Nature of Soil.	Population.	Death-rate per 1,000,000 Living at all Ages from		
		Phthisis.	Lung Diseases.	All Causes.
Pervious	33,820	1514	2131	14,852
Moderately pervious . .	29,640	1467	1892	14,463
Retentive	23,530	1542	2583	14,942

It will be observed that the amount of phthisis is not appreciably greater among populations living on a retentive than
among populations living on pervious soils, although other
respiratory diseases are in excess on the former soil.

In view of the discrepant results indicated in the preceding statistics we may ask whether there is an essential relationship between wetness of soil and phthisis mortality among the population living on such a soil, or whether the commonly experienced excess of phthisis on wet soils is not due rather to the fact that those who are found dwelling on a wet soil are likely to be of a lower class of the community, worse housed, and more exposed to the infection of phthisis. Buchanan himself agrees that there are exceptions to the law, and suggests that " they indicate the presence of other influences in the subsoil, which have hitherto escaped detection." Hirsch suggests, as a more probable explanation, that other etiological factors besides the influence of soil come into force under the given circumstances, and serve to neutralise the benefits even of the most favourable conditions of soil ; and with this suggestion I agree. It appears probable that much of the benefit ascribed to drying the soil has been due really to other factors of improvement which commenced to operate about the same time as the former.

It is difficult to fit in our present knowledge, that the essential cause of tuberculosis is the tubercle bacillus, with the wet soil theory. It cannot be maintained that such a soil favours the growth of the tubercle bacillus, an organism the extra-corporeal cultivation of which is beset with difficulties. We can only conclude that the wet soil operates merely as a predisposing cause. It implies greater loss of heat by evaporation, more easy provocation of catarrhs, especially when, as would commonly happen, it is associated with cold and wet houses. Against these factors a house even on a wet soil can in a large measure be protected.

The wet soil must be placed, like overcrowding and insufficient nutrition, among predisposing causes, infection being the chief and essential cause. It must be placed furthermore in a lower place than either overcrowding or underfeeding.

Consumption is essentially a disease of crowded populations, of indoor occupations, transmitted by infection, favoured by the rebreathing of respired air, and by organic filth of all kinds. Crowding, especially crowding of the sick, has greatly declined, and was already in the process of declining, while the sewerage works referred to in Table XXXIX. were being effected.

PART II

THE INCIDENCE OF TUBERCULOSIS UPON COMMUNITIES

CHAPTER XXVIII

INTRODUCTORY

ACTUAL experience on a large scale is the final test of hypothesis and the surest basis for action. This maxim is particularly applicable to public health administration. The study of communal experience is therefore of the utmost help to the public health service ; but for trustworthy results this study must be conducted with a clear recognition of the complexity of the material to be examined. With no statistics of disease is this caution more necessary than with those relating to tuberculosis.

In the foregoing chapters tuberculosis has been seen to be an infectious disease having a variable period of incubation, and a course which may extend intermittently or continuously over many years. Its prevalence and the death-rate due to it may be favoured or hindered by a great variety of personal, economic, and sanitary conditions affecting the populations at risk. Many of these conditions are themselves composite and of great complexity ; and during a considerable part of their infective sickness most patients are able wholly or partially to keep at work and to migrate from one district to another. Without detailing the difficulties which these characters of tuberculosis introduce into· statistics measuring the prevalence of the disease in different communities, or the errors which may arise from applying to such statistics the methods appropriate to acute disabling infectious diseases, it suffices for the present purpose to recognise that the causation of tuberculosis in communities has all the complexity of its causation in the individual, with the added complexity due to variations in economic and sanitary environment and to the migration of infected persons.

To obtain the best practical results we must simplify this complexity. As already seen, a considerable number of influences either promote or hinder the spread of tuberculosis ; but the preceding chapters could afford little information as to their relative importance. Were it possible to adopt all known measures of precaution and all the methods of treatment, this absence of quantitative information would have merely academic interest. Practical administration, however, can afford no such wholesale reproduction of laboratory conditions. The amount of money and energy available for the public health service, though it may fluctuate from generation to generation, is always limited ; and of the measures that would aid in the prevention or cure of disease only a portion can be put into simultaneous operation. Thus any such measure yielding less than the utmost value for the resources expended represents an amount of avoidable and permitted disease proportionate to the relative inefficiency of the measure. It will be seen, therefore, that the rational as opposed to the capricious or random selection of measures is supremely important to the public health service ; and where it can be had, actual experience is the safest and final guide. The chief purpose for which the incidence of tuberculosis upon communities must now be studied is to learn, if possible, from actual experience the relative extent to which any or all of the elements of economic and sanitary environment have promoted or hindered the spread of the disease.

Such study is of course beset with the ordinary dangers of statistical reasoning, which are much the same as those of any edged tools in unskilled hands. In order to learn the causes of variations in the incidence of a disease upon communities, any sets of figures intended to measure this incidence must in particular be free from the fallacies due to migration of patients, whereby an infection may be acquired in one district and be chronicled as disease or death in the statistics of another. For this reason among others local statistics have to be handled with caution even when they concern acute infectious diseases of only a few weeks' duration. Tuberculosis is not only an infectious but also a chronic disease, which on the average probably extends over years and often escapes recognition during a large part of the time. Fallacy is almost inevitable in such a case if inferences as to causation are sought from individual groups of local statistics.

If, for example, sanatoria for consumption were established

in certain towns or counties of a country otherwise poorly provided with them, merely elementary statistical reasoning would prevent a comparison between the death-rates of such towns or counties, which would attract consumptives beyond from outside their bounds, and those of towns or counties without sanatoria, with any idea that the comparison could give information as to the effect of sanatorium provision upon the general prevalence of phthisis. Similarly the figures of a small rural county with a population less than that of many single towns, could only be used for inference as to the causes of variations in its tuberculosis death-rates if correction were made for the migration of healthy persons to towns and of sick persons to their country homes, where they can live at a smaller cost and nearer their own people.[1]

Nor is it merely its long activity nor its still longer latency which demands a wide basis of observation before conclusions can be drawn as to the causation of tuberculosis. Its endemic prevalence is affected, as we have seen, by factors of sanitary,

---

[1] The difficulty of forming non-fallacious conclusions from " parochial " statistics concerning an infective disease of protracted latency and protracted duration may be further illustrated by the phthisis death-rates in tenement houses and in the different districts of a large town. It is well known that the phthisis death-rate is higher in populations inhabiting one room than in those inhabiting dwellings with two or more rooms ; and is greatest in overcrowded dwellings of any given size. The association between the phthisis death-rate and size of dwelling and overcrowding is complex, and before drawing inferences as to the effect on phthisis of the increased infection and lowered resistance accompanying overcrowding, we should ascertain among other things to what extent the inhabitants of these overcrowded tenements drifted into them after and perhaps because they had become consumptive. Similarly, in comparing different districts of a large town or even small towns with each other, allowance has to be made for the influx of consumptives into poorer districts as they go down in the social scale. If this can be done,—and it implies a complete knowledge of each patient's history and of the duration of the latent period of his disease,— it has further to be noted that inasmuch as the opportunities for infection by phthisis vary enormously in different districts, the effect of measures against infection must correspondingly vary. We must therefore either compare the influence of such measures on large masses of population in whom this source of error is likely to be equalised, or on small aggregations having a like composition. It is evident, for instance, that efforts against infection may have had a greater effect on the death-rate from phthisis in a district whose death-rate from this disease is still 2 per 1000 than similar efforts in another district of a different social stratum whose death-rate from phthisis is only 1 per 1000. For the above and other reasons, local statistics of phthisis cannot be used without fallacy, unless corrections are made which only the most intimate investigation will render practicable.

including social and economic, environment, which themselves
are of high complexity and largely interdependent. Such
phenomena may be unrecognisable in experience on a small
scale.

To eliminate or minimise the effects of migration and complexity we must study communities in which the balance between
immigrant and emigrant cases is small relatively to the total
volume of disease, and which are so large as to allow the operation
of complex phenomena to become evident. The use of figures
relating to large communities is further commended for the
study of tuberculosis because their size reduces the chance
of the results being determined by some local or accidental
feature among the complex relevant conditions of environment.
The experience of smaller communities can only be taken either
as hints which may possibly be confirmed by other information,
or as illustrations of the manner of action of influences of which
the existence has been demonstrated independently.

In the investigation which is summarised in the following
pages it has been found possible to obtain significant results
as to the causes of the variation in death-rates from tuberculosis by grouping these rates for given communities and
periods with the figures which represent for the same communities and periods the variations of sanitary and economic
environment, thus disclosing what the figures can tell of the
relationship between the two sets of phenomena. The following
chapters include the results of the comparison of such of these
data as are available. It will be found that improvement
in general communal health and in the individual factors
affecting it has not always corresponded with the reduction of
tuberculosis, although the statistical evidence shows a probable
connection between most of these factors and the disease. If
no constant correspondence had appeared between the course of
tuberculosis and any element of environment, no conclusion
could have been obtained from the statistical study of communal
experience, and we should have been left to draw the most
probable inferences we could from the facts stated in Part I.
Such a result would not have been surprising. Communal
experience has to be studied not in the orderly sequence of
individual influences provided in laboratory experiment, but in
the simultaneous and highly complex combinations of influences

found in communal life. In these combinations nothing is more common than to find that the number of unknown quantities is too great and the facts too few to permit of an approximate estimate of the respective values of the unknowns. It will be found, however, that the course of tuberculosis has followed that of one element of sanitary environment, namely, the institutional segregation of tuberculous patients. From an administrative standpoint, this result has considerable consequences. It is desirable therefore to examine in detail the evidence as to each of the elements of sanitary environment concerned.

In most cases the figures relating to phthisis have been taken as representing tuberculosis, as they are recorded more fully, and are based on diagnosis which is more accurate than that of total tuberculosis. In almost all cases the incidence of the disease has had to be measured by its death-rate.

CHAPTER XXIX

TUBERCULOSIS AND GENERAL HEALTH IN VARIOUS
COMMUNITIES: VIRULENCE, NATURAL SELECTION,
AND DECADENCE

THE first teaching of communal experience on this subject,
the evidence for which will be outlined in the present
chapter, is that the control of tuberculosis is not merely a
question of the improvement of general health and of sanitary conditions. No result could be more important or more encouraging
for practical purposes. Those concerned in the service of public
health know how much remains to be done before it can be said
to have done its best. If general sanitary conditions are understood—as they are in this connection—to include all those conditions which affect general health, the task that remains to be
done is indefinitely great. The improvement of conditions of
housing, abolition of overcrowding, the enforcement of a higher
standard of specific and general cleanliness, the removal of
injurious conditions of work, whether in mine, factory,
workshop, shop, office or home, the promotion of reasonable recreation in our towns, the removal of hindrances to
temperance and thrift, all of which come within the range of
the task, illustrate the vastness of the physical, economical,
and even moral problems involved, and of their importance
to national life, happiness, and efficiency. The cultivation of a
popular sanitary conscience is therefore an object of supreme
importance to the well-being of any community, and the connection between tuberculosis and bad general sanitary conditions
can be utilised to the full extent in stimulating this conscience.

But though this connection is far-reaching and intimate, it
must not be allowed to obscure other influences which have
had more direct effect on tuberculosis. There are few sanitary
improvements that do not in some measure tend to hinder the
spread of tuberculosis. This fact is evidenced so strongly and

in so many ways, that the doctrine that the control of tuberculosis must be sought not by measures specially directed against the disease, but by improvement in general sanitary environment, has been adopted by many as the final formula on which the control of tuberculosis must be based.   The correctness of such a doctrine does not follow necessarily from the many facts illustrating the connection between tuberculosis and sanitary environment ; and an examination of the actual experience of large communities shows that it is contradicted by the facts.   To those who hope for the extirpation of the disease, this result is a matter of congratulation.   The demonstration of the formula which says that tuberculosis is to be conquered mainly through improvement in general sanitary conditions, and not through special measures acting in conjunction with them, would have been full of profound discouragement and the sickness of hope deferred.   If the control of tuberculosis must await the general perfection of sanitary conditions, including the economic and moral circumstances which form an essential part of them, no reasonable limit could be put to the time which must elapse before tuberculosis disappears.

The belief that no practicable special measures exist by which the disease can be controlled more rapidly and directly than by measures of general sanitary reform, is not supported by past experience in regard to other infectious diseases which have been extirpated wholly or in part.   Cholera, typhus and enteric fever in England, and small-pox in Germany have been stamped out or greatly diminished by adding to the necessarily partial measures of general sanitary reform a complete application of such special measures as actual experience has shown to be efficient. Tuberculosis can be extirpated similarly, if similarly the slow effect of only gradually improving sanitary circumstances be supplemented by special measures having a more rapid and specific effect on the disease.   If such measures are contained in the general body of sanitary improvement, they require to be dissected out and identified before they can be applied with rapidity and completeness.

There has been no constant relation between improved general sanitary circumstances and reduction in tuberculosis. The most definite expression of the course of general sanitary (including social) improvement in the gross and of tuberculosis is to be found in the course of the death-rate from all causes other than tuberculosis and the death-rate from tuberculosis. For the reasons explained previously, the death-rate from tuberculosis will be taken to be measured by that of phthisis.

In Table XLII. the death-rates from pulmonary tuberculosis and from all other causes in various countries and capital cities are given for 1881–85 and for 1901–03 or 1901–02. These relatively recent periods are taken for comparison, because in some instances earlier figures are unobtainable.

TABLE XLII

	A.		B.			
	Death-rate from all Causes except Phthisis.		Death-rate from Phthisis.		Percentage Change in	
	1881–85.	1901–03.	1881–85.	1901–03.	A.	B.
England and Wales .	17·97	14·94	1·83	1·23	− 17·0	− 32·7
Scotland. . .	17·45	15·76	2·11	1·47	− 9·9	− 30·3
Ireland . .	15·90	15·45	2·08	2·15	− 2·8	+ 3·4
Norway . . .	15·75	12·58	1·39	1·92	− 20·4	+ 38·1
Prussia . .	22·29	17·90	3·11 [1]	1·93 [1]	− 19·7	− 37·9
Massachusetts .	16·68	14·77	3·14	1·67	− 11·5	− 46·8
Paris . .	19·99	14·15	4·41	3·65	− 29·3	− 17·2(?)
Berlin . .	21·38	13·76	3·32	2·04	− 33·7	− 38·5
Copenhagen .	19·38	14·81	2·89 [2]	1·38	− 23·7	− 52·2
London . .	18·78	15·38	2·20	1·65	− 19·2	− 25·0
Manchester .	18·76	16·34	2·42	2·01	− 13·1	− 16·9
Edinburgh .	16·34	14·74	1·89	1·51	− 9·5	− 20·1
Glasgow . .	22·34	17·83 [3]	3·14	1·68 [3]	− 20·0	− 46·5
Dublin . .	24·25	23·02	3·55	3·28	− 5·2	− 7·6
Belfast . .	20·32	18·32	3·78	3·08	− 10·2	− 18·5

[1] Tuberculosis.   [2] 1880–84.   [3] 1901–04.

It will be noted that in all cases the general death-rate apart from phthisis has declined ; as has also the phthisis death-rate in all except Ireland and Norway.

The increase in Ireland is really greater than it seems. Emigration, as will be seen later (p. 217), has altered the age and sex distribution of the population by removing a large part of the young and middle-aged, among whom most deaths from phthisis occur ; and when the figures are corrected for age and sex distribution, the true increase of phthisis on the assumption of constant age and sex distribution is seen to be really larger than the figures show. Thus when the crude phthisis death-rate in Ireland for 1891, which was 19·3, is corrected for age distribution of population so as to make it comparable with that for 1901 (21·5), it becomes 17·7 per 10,000 ; and the crude increase of 12 per cent. becomes a corrected increase of about 22 per cent.

A very high decrease of general death-rate apart from phthisis is shown by Norway, which shows increase of its phthisis rate.[1] It will be noted also that in every country and city in which a decrease of phthisis has been shown this decrease is greater than that of the death-rate from all other causes. This disparity is of very variable extent, but except in Dublin and Manchester the disparity between the two diseases is always great. Table XLIII., calculated from Dr. Tatham's data for England and Wales, makes a similar comparison analysed in detail into sexes and ages.

TABLE XLIII.—ENGLAND AND WALES

Percentage Decline or Increase of Death-rate when the experience of 1861–70 is compared with that of 1896–1900

At Ages	Males.		Females.	
	General Death-rate *minus* Phthisis.	Phthisis.	General Death-rate *minus* Phthisis.	Phthisis.
0–	– 14	– 60	– 16	– 65
5–	– 49	– 67	– 45	– 58
10–	– 46	– 68	– 42	– 61
15–	– 32	– 59	– 40	– 63
20–	– 34	– 52	– 36	– 62
25–	– 28	– 43	– 29	– 58
35–	– 15	– 25	– 14	– 46
45–	– 1	– 17	0	– 44
55–	+ 6	– 19	+ 2	– 40
65–75	+ 3	– 24	0	– 36
All Ages	– 13	– 38	– 14	– 54

[1] The official figures relating to Norway, by reason of the increased completeness of certification, show a higher increase than is likely to have occurred in fact; but no reasonable correction in this respect would show decline of phthisis during the period in question; and the argument developed in the text—which would remain the same if even a stationary death-rate from phthisis were substituted for the increase shown by the official figures—is unaffected. So far as England and Ireland are concerned the figures may be accepted within narrow limits of error.

It is clear from this table that in England, as in the instances in Table XLII. to which reference has been made, the reduction of the phthisis death-rate is enormously greater than that of the general death-rate from all other causes ; and the discrepancy is especially great at the working years of life in which phthisis causes its heaviest death-rate. If phthisis had shared only to an equal extent in the general reduction of mortality, a presumption would have arisen that the improvements in general sanitary conditions which have been operating to reduce the general death-rate, such as higher wages, cheaper food and clothing, improved sanitation, and other allied influences, are in themselves a sufficient explanation of the reduction of phthisis. The above figures show that, however much these influences have contributed to the reduction, they do not explain it sufficiently, unless it be assumed that phthisis is far more susceptible to the operation of these influences than other diseases. For this view there is no evidence, and I am not aware that it has been put forward. On the English figures, therefore, the variation in the phthisis rate must accordingly be taken to have involved co-variations in some phenomenon or group of phenomena which have had no material effect on the general death-rate.

The same conclusion results from the figures of other countries. Where phthisis has been reduced, the reduction has been not at the rate of the reduction of the general mortality but at a much faster rate. The extra rapidity of the decline of phthisis is not a fixed part of the reduction of the general mortality, but a part which varies widely from country to country ; in two countries an improvement in general mortality has been accompanied by an actual increase in mortality from phthisis, and in one of them both the improvement in general sanitary conditions and the increase in the death-rate from phthisis have been exceptionally large. Thus in the experience of a considerable number of countries, the conditions improving general health have not had any constant effect on the prevalence of tuberculosis, and in Norway, in which an exceptional improvement in general health has occurred, it has been accompanied by increase in mortality from tuberculosis. It follows therefore that, whatever may have been diminishing tuberculosis, improvement in general sanitary and social circumstances has not been the principal cause, and that an influence or influences of more powerful and rapid operation must have been at work in the communities examined.

So far as this comparison carries us, variations in the death-rate from tuberculosis might be wholly independent of any sanitary conditions. From what has been seen in Part I., this alternative is clearly incorrect, seeing that many conditions affecting general health are known independently to have a powerful and direct effect on tuberculosis. Simultaneously, however, with the operation of general sanitary improvement other influences may have been at work independent of sanitary conditions or not dependent on them directly ; these influences may have done more to modify the prevalence of tuberculosis than any influences of sanitary environment, and it is conceivable that the control of tuberculosis is not to be expected primarily through measures of further sanitary reform, whether general or special.

The three influences not necessarily associated with general sanitary environment which have been suggested as having possibly operated in different communities to produce the recorded variations in the death-rate from tuberculosis are : an attenuation of the virulence of the infecting organism ; a process of weeding-out of the more susceptible population ; and an exactly contrary process of survival of the unfit and consequent decadence of the average population.

Variations of virulence in the specific micro-organisms are known to have occurred with some infectious diseases. They have been demonstrated by variations in the type as well as the severity of the clinical symptoms, and hitherto only when such variations have been demonstrable has a variation in the virulence of the disease been suggested. There is no evidence that such a variation has occurred in the case of tuberculosis ; and the suggestion is made in the teeth of a considerable volume of evidence to a contrary effect. The clinical types of the disease, as recorded in the contemporary descriptions of Graves, Watson, Walshe, Flint, and others at the beginning of the period, show the same varieties of type and duration as are now seen. No well-marked distinction has been established between the types of tuberculosis in different countries. Though consumptives probably live longer now than they did formerly, it must be remembered that the rational treatment of the disease has only become general in recent years. The assumed attenuation of virulence which is held to be displayed in one country because its tuberculosis bill has decreased, can scarcely be assumed to have existed simultaneously in neighbouring and inter-communicating countries in which the disease has increased, notwithstanding the fact that the clinical types of the disease, so far as can be ascertained, have remained unchanged in both countries during the whole period under examination. All the evidence available tends therefore to show that outside bacteriological laboratories no change of virulence has occurred in the bacillus of tuberculosis, and the only evidence from which it has been sought to infer such a change is the decrease of the prevalence of tuberculosis in certain countries, the actual phenomenon to explain which this otherwise unsupported assumption has been made.

The hypothesis that the reduction of the disease may be due to elimination of susceptible strains of human beings depends similarly on the mere fact that it is consistent with the decrease which has occurred. The evidence of the transmission of sus-ceptibility has not been sufficient to show that this transmission occurs so frequently as to be a predominant factor in the transmission of the disease. On the other hand, there is abundant evidence to show the existence of susceptibility, not inherited and permanent, but temporary and acquired through circumstances of environment. It is equally clear that the liability to infection is affected by extent of dose, and that a considerable proportion of the population in contact with tuberculous patients is exposed to extreme and prolonged infection. Persons placed in these circumstances would acquire infection with greater certainty than others, and when they were children of tuberculous parents this occurrence would be practically indistinguishable from inherited susceptibility, and has doubtless often been regarded as such. Even if the inheritance of susceptibility had been demonstrated as a common occurrence, it could only explain the decreases that have occurred in most countries on the assumption that the susceptible victims had a special infertility. The mere death of susceptible patients at the end of a chronic infectious disease of long duration and extending most often into middle life can have had little or no effect on the susceptibility of the children of these patients, unless these children are on the average much less numerous than the children of entirely healthy stocks. Although there appears to be a difference between the two stocks in this respect, it does not suffice to explain results already obtained.

In considering the suggestion that decadence has been responsible for the increase of phthisis, where this has occurred, we may turn again from the discussion of interesting but quite unverified hypotheses to the more sober study of actual experience. The country in regard to which this has been oftenest urged is Ireland. The undoubted general poverty of the country makes the suggestion *primâ facie* plausible ; and unhappily plausible hypotheses whose face is their fortune are often accepted because no one is concerned to ask for more solid credentials. If the instructive experience of Ireland in regard to phthisis is to be explained by an ill-defined influence of which the control is hard and uncertain, the prospect of mastering the endemic prevalence of phthisis in Ireland would be postponed to an extent that would discourage administrative reform directed against more definite causes. In itself, therefore, the alleged decadence of the Irish people in Ireland deserves careful consideration ; and the study is not the less desirable because, as we shall find, the existence of a general average decadence of population in Ireland is, so far as phthisis is concerned, a wanton speculation contradicted directly by the facts.

The suggestion is that the long stream of emigration from Ireland has left behind it a physically inferior population of excessive susceptibility to phthisis. This emigration reached its height in 1851, when over 34 per 1000 of the entire population left their country ; but it has continued up to the present time, still averaging 9 per thousand per annum during the present century. That the effect of this emigration has been to leave a decadent residual population is merely an assumption, which at the outset is discredited to some extent by the fact that the birth-rate in Ireland (corrected for the number of women at child-bearing ages and for the number of married women) has increased from 35·2 in 1881 to 36·1 per thousand in 1901, against a decrease in England from 34·7 to 28·4. It is discredited further by the fact that the majority of those driven from Ireland were among the poorest, and these through their poverty must have been the least fit. The cottiers and farm labourers on the smallest holdings emigrated in the largest numbers ; those who remain are children of the families who could resist the stress of famine and evictions, and who in recent years have been living in progressively better conditions than their predecessors. Even a comparative examination of the present population does not show an appreciable difference in the communal susceptibility to phthisis between rich and poor towns. Belfast is the part of Ireland which probably has suffered least from emigration, and is commercially the most prosperous. Yet its death-rate from phthisis was 307 per 100,000 in the five years 1901–06, as compared with 315 in the much poorer and more crowded city of Dublin.

These considerations, though much more weighty than the general speculation by which decadence in the Irish population is alleged, are still to some extent inferential. Fortunately it is possible to settle the question definitely by actually following the emigrated population and comparing their susceptibility with that of the residual Irish.

The chief emigration from Ireland has been to the United States. If the cause of the increased death-rate from phthisis in Ireland is the physical inferiority of its residual population, the death-rate from phthisis of the Irish population in the United States ought to be lower than that in Ireland. It is practically certain that no disturbing influence in such a comparison is exercised by greater well-being or better sanitation or housing in Ireland than in the United States. The American Census Report for 1900 gives the death-rates from phthisis in the registration area and its subdivisions among whites in the census year, classified according to the birthplaces of the mothers of the deceased. For all inhabitants of these States the phthisis death-rate in 1900 was 113, for English (defined as above) 135, for Scotch 173, for Germans 167, for Irish 340. The difference is seen both in cities and in rural districts, the phthisis death-rate of the Irish in rural districts being 239, as compared with a general rate of 108. In Ireland in the same year the phthisis death-rate was 226 and in Dublin 346. These are death-rates uncorrected for age distribution. For such correction we turn to the vital statistics for the city of Providence, Rhode Island, which are well known to be among the most trustworthy in the United States. Dr. Chapin, the city registrar and medical officer of health, has published statistics corrected for age distribution which enable a corrected comparison to be made. He applied the death-rate from phthisis in Ireland in 1901 for sex and age periods to the population of Providence in 1900 born of Irish mothers. "It was found that the theoretical mortality from phthisis of this element of the population (of Providence) according to these (the Irish) data was 258 per 100,000 living. The actual rate for the period 1896–1905 was, however, 339. The mortality from phthisis of the Irish in Providence is therefore 81 per 100,000, or 31·4 per cent. more than the mortality of the Irish in Ireland."

It is clear therefore that, so far from emigration having increased the communal susceptibility of the residual Irish population to tuberculosis, the Irish in Ireland have a substantially less susceptibility than their emigrated brethren, and that this difference is not due to any inferiority in the environment of the emigrated population. The inability of extreme poverty to produce a high death-rate from phthisis in a rural population is strikingly shown in the County of Mayo (p. 180).

CHAPTER XXX

TUBERCULOSIS IN URBAN AND IN RURAL COMMUNITIES

IN the present and the succeeding chapters we have to consider the experiences of large communities over long periods of time, and to compare the variations in the figures measuring the incidence of tuberculosis and those, where they can be obtained, which measure the variations in the element of experience under consideration.

To avoid misapprehension, a preliminary remark is necessary as to the years which should be compared. The effect of alteration in environment does not begin to appear till after a certain interval. If the element in question operates solely by diminishing infection, the interval must be that which represents the minimum period of incubation and latency. This interval cannot be stated with any exactness, and it is still less possible to state the interval which would have to elapse before an alteration which modified resistance of the community to infection would produce an evident effect. Strictly speaking, the figures which represent alteration in environment should be compared with those which represent incidence of tuberculosis at a period later by this interval. It is fortunate that the run of these figures in the present inquiry, as might be expected with a disease of long incubation and latency such as tuberculosis, is such that changes from one quinquennium to another are not abrupt; and in a sufficiently long series of pairs the results of identical quinquennia can therefore be grouped with substantially the same result as if the element of environment were represented by the figures of the next quinquennium or the next but one.

Communities may be grouped most broadly according as they are urban or rural, and the experience now to be examined shows the remarkable result that while urban conditions have promoted the prevalence of tuberculosis, they have rarely sufficed to prevent extraordinary decreases in the disease, nor in all cases have rural conditions sufficed to prevent increases. Town life on the whole is less healthy than rural life. Some evidence of the unquestionable correctness of this belief may be gathered from an inspection of Table XLII., p. 212 ; and this difference to the disadvantage of the towns is seen in tuberculosis as well as in other diseases. This result may be checked with the help of two valuable tables by Dr. Tatham, published in the Registrar-General's Report for 1904, from which the following table is extracted and calculated. This table deals with an estimated urban population of 18,262,173, including the chief industrial centres, and a rural population of 4,327,835, including only a few unimportant towns and villages. The death-rates have been corrected for variations in the age and sex distribution of the respective populations.

TABLE XLIV.—ENGLAND AND WALES

Selected Urban and Rural Counties of the Registrar-General, 1898–1903

	Corrected Death-rates per 1000 of Population.			
	Males.		Females.	
	All Causes except Phthisis.	Phthisis.	All Causes except Phthisis.	Phthisis.
Urban Counties .	18·4	1·66	17·5	1·11
Rural ,, .	13·5	1·27	13·2	1·07
	Proportional Figures (Rural rates = 100)			
Urban Counties .	137	131	133	104
Rural ,, .	100	100	100	100

These collective results show no less strongly than those of individual countries and towns that town life is unhealthy as a whole, and is favourable to the prevalence of phthisis. If they could be corrected for the fact that the towns attract the robust and strong, while the weakly tend to remain in and return to rural districts, the extent of this mischief would be exhibited more strikingly and even more accurately. In the absence of powerful countervailing influences, those countries would therefore be expected to have suffered most from phthisis and to have shown most marked increase in the disease in which the excess of urban over rural population has been the largest and the most progressive.

An examination of the facts shows, however, that the exact contrary has occurred.

Table XLV. exhibits for certain countries the distribution of the population between town and country at or near the beginning and end of the period under review. The definition of " urban " varies somewhat in different countries, but in each country remains the same throughout the period under examination, so that the results are comparable. The corresponding phthisis rates are included in the table, and the changes in the death-rates are expressed as percentages of the earlier figures.

TABLE XLV

	Percentage of Total Population who were Urban in		Phthisis Death-rate.		Percentage Increase in Urbanisation.	Relative Amount of Urban Population in most Recent Period, that of England being taken as 100.	Percentage Reduction or Increase of Phthisis.	Phthisis Death-rate, 1901–03, that of England = 100.
	1861.	1901.	1866–1870.	1901–1903.				
England and Wales .	63	77	2·45	1·23	22	100	− 50	100
Scotland . . .	52	70	2·59	1·48	35	91	− 45	120
Ireland . .	20	31	1·82	2·15	55	40	+ 18	175
	1864.	1895.						
Prussia . .	30	41	3·20[1]	1·94[1]	37	53	− 39[1]	?
	1865.	1891.						
France . . .	29	38	4·57[2]	3·65[2]	31	48	? none	297
	1840.	1890.	Mass.					
United States . .	8	29	3·65	1·67	262	38	− 50	136
	1865.	1891.						
Norway . . .	16	21	1·32[3]	1·92	31	27	+ 46	156

[1] Between 1877–80 and 1901–03.   [2] Paris.   [3] In 1876–80.

More recent data as to urbanisation are contained in Table XLVI. from Dr. Shadwell's work (1905, vol. ii.).

TABLE XLVI

*Percentage of the Population of Great Towns having over 100,000
Inhabitants to the Entire Population of each Country*

England.		Germany.		United States.	
1881.	1901.	1880.	1900.	1880.	1900.
31·6	35·0	7·2	16·2	14·6	18·8

In context with these results reference may be made again to
Table XLIV. It will be noticed that the excess of the general
death-rate in urban counties over that in rural counties is
approximately equal for males and females (37 and 33 per cent.),
while the excess of phthisis in urban counties is 37 per cent.
among males and only 4 per cent. among females. In Birmingham
and Sheffield the female death-rate from phthisis, as shown in
Fig. 13, p. 166, is actually lower at most ages than that in England
and Wales as a whole. When it is remembered that women
spend much more time at home than men, and that their experience must reflect more than that of men the influence of home
environment, it becomes clear that the influence of urban life
on phthisis is specifically different from its effect on other causes
of mortality in the aggregate.

The experience summarised thus shows that enormous changes
have occurred both in the extent of urbanisation and in the prevalence of phthisis in each of the countries examined, and that
in every country town life has been associated with a greater
prevalence of tuberculosis than has country life. There has
been everywhere a heavy increase of urbanisation, which in
spite of the larger amount of phthisis in towns has been accompanied in most countries by a large reduction in the prevalence
of phthisis both in town and in country; indeed, the countries
with the most town life have suffered actually the least from
phthisis. It follows therefore that, powerful as has been the
influence of town life in assisting the prevalence of tuberculosis,
some other more powerful influences have been in operation in
most countries to restrain the disease.

CHAPTER XXXI

TUBERCULOSIS IN OVERCROWDED COMMUNITIES

THE next fact to be extracted from communal experience is that even overcrowding has been unable to exert a predominating influence on the course of tuberculosis. Overcrowding is the most mischievous factor of town life. Its operation even in country districts must be detrimental; and in towns the privation of light and air which it usually entails must add greatly to its depressing effect. So much is certain from general considerations, and it is equally certain that tuberculosis as well as other diseases must be susceptible to the influence of overcrowding. In the last chapter we found as a fact in international experience that town life, though tending powerfully to increase the prevalence of tuberculosis, has not sufficed to cause an increase in the face of other countervailing circumstances to be considered subsequently. It is unnecessary or impracticable to examine separately certain of the factors of town life. We have seen in Part I. that subsoil drainage is not likely to have been a factor of primary importance for this purpose. The substitution in town life of industrial for agricultural conditions is so essential a part of urbanisation that a separate investigation of its changes could give no different results from those obtained in the last chapter. The amelioration of industrial conditions in regard to dust, ventilation, etc., is not expressed directly in any recorded figures; to some extent an indirect expression may be found in the evidence which will be considered as to sanitary education. Neither can a direct expression be obtained for the changes in provision of light and air; but indirectly they are covered by the changes in overcrowding, which fortunately are recorded sufficiently for the present purpose. It is in overcrowding that the most vicious results of town life must be sought: and they deserve very careful consideration.

The difference in total housing accommodation between urban and rural communities in England and Wales may be seen broadly in Table XLVII.

TABLE XLVII

1901.—*Of the Total Population in Urban and Rural Districts respectively, the Percentage living in each Class of House was as follows :—*

	Tenements containing					
	One Room.	Two Rooms.	Three Rooms.	Four Rooms.	Five or more Rooms.	Total.
Urban Districts .	2·0	7·4	10·3	21·2	59·1	100·0
Rural ,, .	0·2	3·9	8·1	24·0	63·8	100·0

Thus, compared with rural districts, ten times as large a proportion of the total population lived in one-roomed tenements in urban districts, and nearly twice as large a proportion lived in two-roomed tenements.

The difference in overcrowding between urban and rural communities in England and Wales is shown in Table XLVIII. A tenement is reckoned as overcrowded in which on an average each room, whether bedroom or living room, is occupied by more than two persons.

TABLE XLVIII

1901.—*Of the Total Population in Urban and Rural Districts respectively, the Percentage Overcrowded in Tenements of four Rooms and under was as follows :—*

	Tenements containing			
	One Room.	Two Rooms.	Three Rooms.	Four Rooms.
Urban Districts	0·95	3·07	2·63	2·25
Rural ,, ...	0·09	1·54	1·98	2·23

This table shows that ten times as many one-roomed

tenements, and twice as many two-roomed tenements were overcrowded in urban as in rural districts.

Nothing could be more conclusive than these results as to the difference both in housing and in overcrowding between urban and rural districts. Compared with rural districts, towns in 1901 had ten times as large a proportion of the total population housed in one-roomed tenements ; and of the population so housed in one-roomed tenements, ten times as many were overcrowded in towns as in country. Nearly double the proportion of town population inhabited two-roomed tenements as of country population, and of these twice as many were overcrowded in town as were in the country. Compared with 1891 marked improvement had occurred in overcrowding in towns, but very much more in the country districts. By the side of these improvements have gone, as we have seen, marked decreases in the prevalence of phthisis, and by the side of the disparity in housing between town and country there is the disparity already shown in the urban and rural phthisis death-rate for males. The female death-rate, which would be most strongly affected by home conditions, is substantially the same for towns as for country, in spite of the enormous difference in housing and overcrowding.

In the case of Ireland, the relations between overcrowding and tuberculosis are masked completely.

It has already been seen (Fig. 31 and Table XLII.) that the death-rate from phthisis in Ireland has increased. This higher death-rate has been associated with a progressive improvement in conditions of housing. The facts on which this statement is

TABLE XLIX

Percentage of Different Classes of Houses in Ireland

	1841.	1861.	1881.	1891.	1901.
1st class . . .	3·0	8·3	9·7	10·5	11·2
2nd ,, . . .	19·9	37·6	46·9	53·6	59·3
3rd ,, . . .	40·1	45·7	39·2	33·8	28·4
4th ,, . . .	37·0	8·4	4·2	2·1	1·1
	100·0	100·0	100·0	100·0	100·0

based (Table XLIX.) are taken from a paper by Dr. (now Sir T.) Matheson, Registrar-General for Ireland (1903).

The fourth class of houses comprises chiefly houses of mud or other perishable materials, having only one room and window ; the third class, a rather better class of house, having two to four rooms and as many windows ; the second class is equivalent to what would be considered a good farmhouse having five to nine rooms and windows ; and the first class comprises all better houses. The changes in the proportion of these different classes of houses are set forth more clearly in Fig. 19.

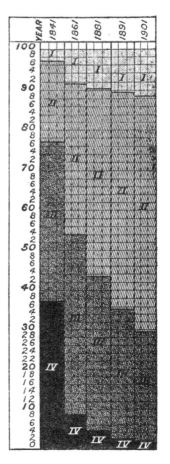

Sir T. Matheson's conclusion is that "the material improvement in the housing of the people of Ireland since 1841 is very satisfactory, but that there is still much to be accomplished."

Comparing Ireland with England and Scotland, Sir T. Matheson finds that in 1901 in England 3·6 per cent., in Ireland 8·7 per cent., and in Scotland 17·5 per cent., of the total dwellings consisted of only one room ; further, that the percentage of the total population living in these one-roomed tenements and having five or more persons in each tenement was 0·15 in England, 1·78 in Ireland, and 3·27 in Scotland. Thus Scotland has more than double the proportion of one-roomed tene-

FIG. 19. — Showing steady improvement in Housing Conditions in Ireland.

ments that Ireland has, and in nearly twice as many of these the number of occupants exceeds five.

Contrasting these facts with the corresponding phthisis death-rates, we see that some counterbalancing influence or influences have prevented Ireland from obtaining any lowering of its phthisis death-rate along with its improvement of housing, and have enabled Scotland with a larger proportion of single-roomed tenements and more overcrowding than Ireland to secure a lower death-rate than the latter country.

In Paris the conditions of housing are extremely bad, and the phthisis death-rate is high and probably almost stationary. Over one-fourth of the total families were housed in single rooms, and nearly one-third in tenements of two rooms, and more than three-fourths in three rooms or less.

Official figures are available for Berlin for every five years from 1861 to 1895. From these we learn that the number of one-roomed tenements out of every 100 tenements of all sizes has been about 50 throughout these forty-five years, while the number of two-roomed tenements in the same interval has only varied from 24 to 27 per cent., of three-roomed tenements from 10 to 12 per cent., and of larger tenements from 11 to 12 per cent. of the total number. A very large proportion of the population of Berlin live in block-dwellings, and the average size of these block-dwellings has increased. Doubtless the standard of these dwellings as to cleanliness, as elsewhere, has improved; but it is a remarkable fact that although half the families in Berlin live in single rooms, the death-rate from phthisis in that city has declined 45 per cent. between 1876–80 and 1901–03.

In Norway the census returns for the towns show that in 1891 the proportion of dwellings comprising one room was 42·4, and comprising two rooms was 27·6 per cent. of the total dwellings, while in 1900, the proportion of one-roomed dwellings had decreased to 28·1 per cent., and of two-roomed dwellings had increased to 34·5 per cent. of the total dwellings.

In New York a similar story has to be told. Dr. Hermann Biggs (1903–04, p. 191) says :—

There has been a more rapid fall in the tuberculosis death-rate in New York City than in any great city in the world, and this notwithstanding the fact that the conditions in many respects are much more unfavourable, because of the very dense population in the great tenement-house districts of the city, and the large element of foreign born population. It should be remembered that in no city of the world is there such a density of population as exists in many of the wards of the borough of Manhattan.

As illustrating Dr. Biggs' observation it may be stated that the phthisis death-rate was 4·27 in 1881 and 2·40 in 1903, a fall of 44 per cent. ; the corresponding rates in London being 2·18 and 1·60 and its fall 26 per cent.

Further figures comparing the conditions of housing in different countries are summarised by Dr. Shadwell (1905, vol. ii. p. 198) in the following sentence : " In England the industrial classes live in separate houses or cottages, in Germany they live in barracks, and in America in larger houses which are shared by more than one family." He adds : " We have nothing. to compare in England to the house famine which prevails in Germany."

The outcome of the available figures is to show improvement of housing associated with

(*a*) decrease of phthisis (England, Scotland),

(*b*) stationary or increasing phthisis (Ireland and Norway);

and heavily and increasingly congested housing associated with

(*a*) high and almost stationary phthisis death-rate (Paris),

(*b*) great decrease of phthisis death-rate, which is still high (Germany, Berlin, New York).

It is highly probable that neither the association between improved housing and reduced phthisis in Great Britain, nor that between very congested housing and high phthisis rates in the foreign countries quoted is accidental. In view of the known pathology of the disease, no circumstance could be more calculated to exercise a uniformly adverse influence on this disease than overcrowding. Clearly, however, abnormally high congestion of housing has been unable in most of the above countries to prevent immense decrease in the phthisis rate ; and marked improvement in housing in Ireland, which has brought it well above the level of Scotland as to average number of rooms per dwelling for the very poor, has not sufficed to prevent the rise of the phthisis rate. Overcrowding must therefore be classed with urbanisation as a factor which, though of proved effect on the phthisis rate, has usually been unable to overcome counteracting influences by which the phthisis rate has been diminished.

CHAPTER XXXII

TUBERCULOSIS IN COMMUNITIES OF VARYING WELL-BEING

THE influence of well-being on the phthisis death-rate has never been questioned, and in the judgment of many authorities it is the most important factor. Thus Sir Hugh Beevor (1901, p. 158) says :—

> As the wages rise, phthisis rate falls; this fall affects especially the young ; it is due to food supply.

In another place (1899) he says :—

> The British public eat more and more. Agricultural returns declare that in the last twenty years, the yearly ration per head of the public had increased 10 per cent. in both bread and meat. . . . Nowadays, patients at Nordrach rightly hold that their extra feeding is a great means of cure ; nutrition is equally a means of prevention.

Sir Douglas Powell (1904) gives expression to the same view in the following statement :—

> The prevention of consumption involves a much wider issue than the circumvention of the bacillus. . . . The abolition of the Corn Duties and other Free Trade legislation, and improved rates of wages, have done more than any notification law against the disease would have been likely to have effected.

It may be assumed that, in the above extract, the action which in a well-regulated district would follow on notification is indicated.

Well-being is, of course, a very complex condition, which cannot be measured completely by any single element. No factor, however, more deserves careful attention, and in the following pages its course is measured independently by the price of wheat, the cost of total food, the total cost of living, wages, the amounts of food consumed, and the amount of pauperism.   In considering those elements which relate to food it must be remembered that we are dealing not with the therapeutic effect of these elements on tuberculous patients on whom they are applied under exceptional conditions and in some excess, but with their prophylactic influence taken in normal quantities and in the circumstances of ordinary life.   Much clinical experience appears to indicate that high feeding, especially with proteids, has a marked beneficial effect in the treatment of tuberculosis ; and although, so far as I know, there is no record of its value apart from open-air treatment, and the latter may therefore possibly be partially responsible for the beneficial results ascribed to the former, it is likely that the high diet has been at least an important factor in the therapeutical effect.   It is, of course, quite possible that food in no more than ordinary amounts, and especially proteid food, may exert in health a prophylactic influence against tuberculosis similar to the therapeutic effect on the consumptive exerted by abnormally high amounts under open-air conditions.   On existing evidence, however, it is equally possible that a certain minimum excess is necessary for producing the predominant therapeutic effect which has been remarked ; and a similar excess may conceivably be necessary to the production of the fullest prophylaxis that can be obtained by diet.   There is, so far as I know, no evidence to enable one to decide between these possibilities.

In using the figures which express the extent to which the countries under comparison have enjoyed the several elements of well-being, no correction is made for the varying benefit which different persons and possibly different nations will have derived from equal amounts of commodities.   The absence of such correction in the present inquiry is without serious importance. The nation in whom thrift or superior efficiency in utilising their means might have been supposed to have produced the decrease in phthisis is Germany ; and if it were in fact shown that Germans had such superiority over the other nations in question, then the bare comparison of their means with those of less thrifty nations would be inconclusive.   In the present discussion, however, the inclusion of France and Norway, whose figures for phthisis are very different from those of Germany and whose reputation for thrift is equally high, avoids the difficulty.

PRICE OF WHEAT

In Table L. the proportional prices of wheat and the death-rates from phthisis in several countries are given relatively to the corresponding prices or rates in 1901–02, which are stated as 100.

TABLE L

Relative Figures for Wheat and Phthisis

	Wheat.				Phthisis.						Tuberculosis in Prussia.	
	United Kingdom.	France.	Germany.	United States.	England and Wales.	London.	Scotland.	Ireland.	Paris.	Massachusetts.		
1841–50 .	197	125	116	143	...	...	...	...	...	...	...	
1851–60 .	201	140	147	186	229 / 209	206 / 169	162	...	...	246 / 233	...	{ 1851–55 / 1856–60
1861–70 .	188	137	132	228	208 / 200	170 / 173	172 / 176	83 / 85	124 / 168	219 / 201	...	{ 1861–65 / 1866–70
1871–75 .	201	151	145	206	181	152	169	89	110	207	...	
1876–80 .	175	139	130	164	166	146	157	93	111	186	165	
1881–85 .	148	120	113	140	149	128	144	97	121	189	163	
1886–90 .	116	114	107	112	134	114	128	99	121	164	145	
1891–95 .	103	108	103	91	119	113	120	99	112	140	121	
1896–1900 .	105	104	100	105	108	109	114	99	104	119	104	
1901–02 .	100	100	100	100	100	100	100	100	100	100	100	
	326	440	426	328	123	165	147	215	365	167	193	

Absolute price in pence per imperial gallon in the years taken as standard.   Death-rates per 100,000 from Phthisis or Tuberculosis in 1901–02 or 1901–03.

In Figs. 20 to 23 the facts of Table L. are shown diagrammatically. By the use of proportional figures the curves of prices and phthisis rates are reduced to the same scale, and can be exactly compared.

Fig. 20 shows the phthisis and wheat curves for the United Kingdom. As previously shown by Sir Hugh Beevor, there is a fairly close relationship in Great Britain between the phthisis and wheat curves. There is one important exception to this statement.   Prior to 1875 a great reduction of phthisis had occurred, without cheapening of wheat.

In Ireland, which has shared the benefits of cheaper bread, there is obviously no relation between the price of wheat and

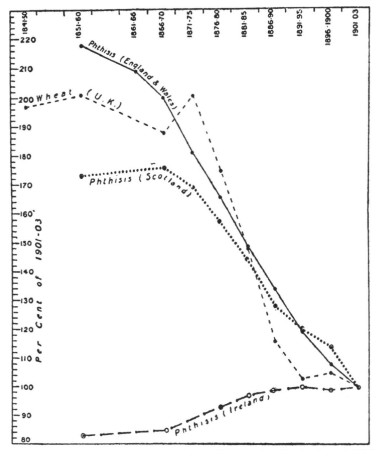

FIG. 20.—Proportional Death-rates from Phthisis in England and Wales, Scotland, and Ireland, and Price of Wheat in the United Kingdom, 1841–50 to 1901–03

Note.—The curves in Figs. 20 to 26 do not show actual prices and death-rates, but only the proportional changes in them.

the death-rate from phthisis.   It may be stated further that the price of potatoes per cwt. in the ten years 1864–73 averaged 53d. ; in the ten years 1894–1903, it averaged 40d.   These are the means of the extreme values given in the Annual Reports of the Registrar-General for Ireland.

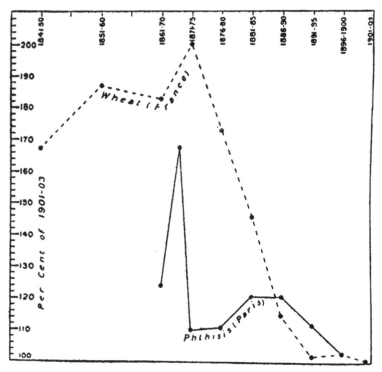

FIG. 21.—Proportional Death-rates from Phthisis in Paris, 1861–69 to 1901–02,
and Price of Wheat, 1841–50 to 1901–02

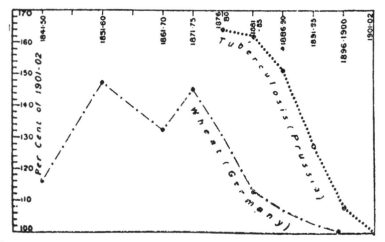

FIG. 22.—Proportional Death-rates from Tuberculosis in Prussia, 1877–80 to
1901–02, and Price of Wheat, 1841–50 to 1901–02

Fig. 21 shows the course of the phthisis curve for Paris and the wheat curve for France.   As already stated, it is probable that in Paris the phthisis rate has declined little, if at all.   Even if we accept the official figures of declining phthisis, no correspondence is visible between the official figures of variation of phthisis rate

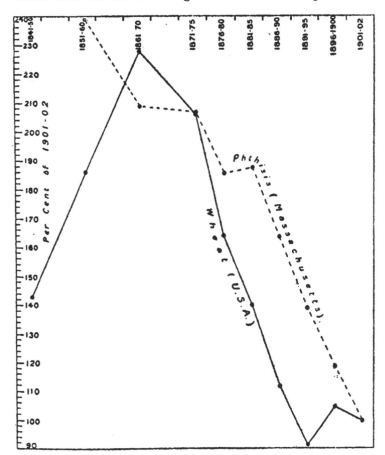

FIG. 23.—Proportional Death-rates from Phthisis in Massachusetts, 1851–55 to 1901–02, and Price of Wheat, 1841–50 to 1901–02

and price of wheat.   The proportional phthisis rate increased from 111 in 1876–80 to 121 in 1881–85, while the proportional price of wheat fell from 173 to 146.   Between 1891–95 and 1901–02 the price of wheat has been almost stationary, and the recorded death-rate has fallen from 112 to 100.

As will be seen in Fig. 22, the form in which figures are available compels comparison between Germany and Prussia, and also the substitution of tuberculosis for phthisis. Between 1876–80 and 1886–90, tuberculosis declined only from 164 in 1876–80 and 162 in 1881–85 to 151, while wheat declined from 130 to 107; while between 1886–90 and the present time, the decline of wheat has only been from 107 to 100, that of tuberculosis from 151 in 1886–90 and 128 in 1891–95 to 100.

In the United States, where the margin of wages is great, and where the price of wheat cannot be of such vital importance, the two curves are fairly correspondent up to 1890, but then diverge widely : a rise of wheat from 91 to 100 since 1891–95 having been associated with a fall in phthisis from 139 to 100 in 1891–95, and 119 in 1895–1900.

The data given above for the course of phthisis and of wheat prices are connected by the following coefficients of correlation:[1]—

Price of Wheat and Phthisis Death-rates

	Period of Observation.	Coefficient of Correlation.
England and Wales . .	1866–1902	+ ·90
Scotland	1868–1902	+ ·87
Ireland	1866–1902	– ·80
Prussia	1877–1901	+ ·55
Paris	1866–1902	+ ·31

Expressed in words these figures summarise the preceding tables and curves by showing a close co-variation between phthisis rates and wheat prices in England and Scotland ; moderate and poor co-variation in Prussia and France respectively ; and considerable inverse co-variation in Ireland.

TOTAL COST OF FOOD

The data for a review of total cost of food in certain countries from 1877 are furnished in Government Blue Books (1903, pp. 215 and 224). " Index numbers " are employed in the following table based on the retail prices collected by the Labour Department of the Board of Trade, of bread, flour, potatoes, beef, mutton, bacon, butter, tea and sugar ; value being attached

[1] The sense in which this term is used is stated in the Note on p. 295.

to each of these articles in accordance with the annual amounts spent by households in the purchase of the various articles.

TABLE LI

Relative Figures for Total Cost of Food and Phthisis

	Total Cost of Food.		Phthisis in			Tuberculosis in Prussia.
	United Kingdom.	Germany.	England and Wales.	Scotland.	Ireland.	
1877–80 .	135	112	166	157	93	165
1881–85 .	126	105	149	144	97	163
1886–90 .	102	99	134	128	99	145
1891–95 .	98	103	119	120	99	121
1896–1900.	94	99	108	114	99	104
1901 . .	100	100	100	100	100	100

(The cost of food and the phthisis death-rates respectively in 1901 are stated as 100 ; the other figures being given in proportion to the values for 1901)

The same values are also shown in Figs. 24 and 25.

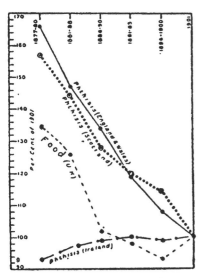

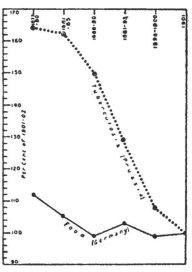

FIG. 24.—Proportional Death-rates from Phthisis in England and Wales, Scotland, and Ireland, and Cost of Food in the United Kingdom, 1877–80 to 1901

FIG. 25.—Proportional Death-rates from Tuberculosis in Prussia, and Cost of Food in Germany, 1877–80 to 1901

It will be noted that in and since 1886–90, the price of food has remained almost stationary ; during the same period the phthisis death-rate in England has fallen in the proportion of 134 to 100, and of Scotland in the proportion of 128 to 100.   In Ireland a rise of phthisis has been accompanied by a marked decrease in the cost of food, though Ireland has experienced the same cheapening of food as Great Britain.

In Germany (Fig. 25) between 1877 and 1886 the death-rate from tuberculosis in Prussia was stationary, while the total cost of food fell from 115 to 95, or from 112 to 105 in the consecutive periods 1877–80 and 1881–85.   On the other hand, in the period 1886–90, in which the cost of food was as low as in 1901, the death-rate from tuberculosis was 50 per cent. higher.

The correlation coefficients which connect these data are as follows :—

Total Cost of Food and Phthisis Death-rates

	Period of Observation.	Coefficient of Correlation.
England and Wales . .	1877–1901	+ ·90
Scotland	1877–1901	+ ·88
Ireland	1877–1901	– ·49
Germany	1877–1901	+ ·42

These figures show close co-variation between the phthisis rate and the total cost of food in England and Wales and in Scotland, poor co-variation in Germany, and some inverse co-variation in Ireland.

TOTAL COST OF LIVING

The figures enabling the relationship between total cost of living and the phthisis death-rate to be stated, are derived from the second Fiscal Blue Book (Memoranda, etc., Second Series).   They refer to workmen's expenditure in London and large towns in Great Britain, the relative price in 1900 being in each case stated as 100. The proportional costs in 1881–85 and in 1900 respectively were : for food 133 and 100, for rent 89 and 100, for clothing 105 and 100, for fuel and clothing together 75 and 100 ; and for all the

above four chief items of workmen's expenditure 116 and 100.[1]
The cost of living in the United Kingdom has therefore declined
considerably, as compared with what it was in 1881.

Fig. 26 shows the course of the phthisis death-rate, and the
total cost of living in England and Wales.

The total cost of living in England has been fairly uniform
during the last fifteen years; during approximately the same
period the phthisis death-rate has declined in the proportion
of 134 to 100.

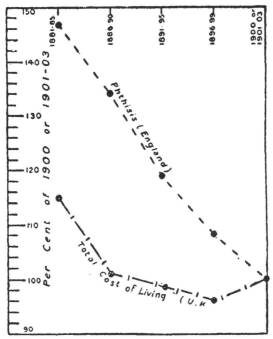

FIG. 26.—Proportional Death-rates from Phthisis in England,
and Total Cost of Living, 1881–85 to 1901–03

There are independent reasons for believing that in Ireland
the prices of total food, clothing, fuel, and rent have varied in
the same directions and approximately to the same extent as
in Great Britain; and on this assumption the coefficient of
correlation has been calculated for Ireland as well as for England
and Scotland.

[1] The proportional weights adopted in giving the data in Fig. 26 have been :
food, 7 ; rent, 2 ; clothing, 2 ; fuel and light, 1, of a total expenditure on these
items of 12.

Thus when to cost of food is added that of clothing and fuel and rent, which in importance are second only to the cost of food, the direct co-variation with the phthisis rate becomes less marked in Great Britain and some inverse co-variation continues to be shown in the experience of Ireland.

Total Cost of Living and Phthisis Death-rates

	Period of Observation.	Coefficient of Correlation.
England and Wales . .	1880–1903	+ ·76
Scotland	1880–1902	+ ·76
Ireland	1880–1903	− ·24

WAGES

It may be suggested that the lack of correspondence between cost of living and death-rate from phthisis may be due to the disturbing effect of changes in wages. Unfortunately, exact comparison of wages can only be made from official data for workmen engaged in skilled trades and for agricultural labourers. It is probable, however, that these wages give some clue to the corresponding wages of other workmen.

Table LII. compares the recent experience of different countries.

TABLE LII

Comparison of Rates of Wages in Skilled Trades

	United Kingdom.	France.	Germany.	United States.
Number of quotations of wages on which the following results are based	470	248	184	141
	s. d.	*s. d.*	*s. d.*	*s. d.*
Mean weekly wages for { 1. Capital cities . . .	42 0	36 0	24 0	75 0
15 skilled trades { 2. Other cities and towns .	36 0	22 10	22 6	69 4
Percentage comparison { 1. Capital cities . . .	100	86	57	179
(United Kingdom = 100) { 2. Other cities and towns .	100	63	63	193

British money wages are the highest in Europe, and the margin over the cost of living is probably the greatest in Europe.

The Board of Trade's Report gives the following *comparison of average family incomes* :—

United Kingdom.	France.	Germany.	United States.
100	83	69	123

The preceding official data are confirmed by facts independently collected by Dr. Shadwell (1905, vol. ii. pp. 81 and 91). He gives the following ratios for wages of unskilled labourers in the three countries :—

England.	Germany.	United States.
100	79	143

and he believes that these figures more nearly represent the actual state of matters than those in Table LII., which give the ratios for skilled workmen as 100, 57, and 179 in the capitals, and 100, 63, and 193 in other towns.

The only comparison of wages practicable between different parts of the United Kingdom is for agricultural labourers. The data for this comparison are derived from an important report by Mr. Wilson Fox, C.B. (Cd. 2376, p. 5). He gives the following table :—

TABLE LIII

Average Earnings per Week (including the Value of all Allowances in Kind) of Able-bodied Male Adult Ordinary Agricultural Labourers

	1902.	1898.	Percentage Increase between 1898 and 1902.
	s. d.	*s. d.*	
England . . .	17 5	16 9	4·0
Wales	17 7	16 6	6·6
Scotland . . .	19 5	18 2	6·9
Ireland. . . .	10 9	10 2	5·7

On p. 5 of the same report Mr. Fox remarks : " There is no doubt that the position of a farm labourer in Ireland is not so good as in other parts of the United Kingdom, but it may be added that he gets his house and fuel cheaper, and frequently has the opportunity of renting land on which he grows potatoes and keeps pigs, goats, and poultry."

This report enables a comparison to be made for agricultural labourers over a long series of years in the three parts of the

16

United Kingdom. The following table illustrates the course of wages on certain sample farms between 1850 and 1903. The rates of wages are expressed in percentages, the year 1900 being taken to represent 100 :—

TABLE LIV

	1850.	1860.	1870.	1880.	1890.	1900.	1903.
England and Wales (69 farms) .	64	76	82	91	90	100	101
Scotland (6 farms) . . .	50	60	71	85	91	100	103
Ireland (10 farms) . . .	56	63	71	81	90	100	101

Mr. Wilson Fox, in answer to an inquiry, kindly writes me the following statement (May 16, 1906) : " As stated on p. 220 of the Report " (*On the Wages, etc., of Agricultural Labourers in the United Kingdom*), " the employers who furnished these records were asked if the allowances in kind, given in addition to cash wages, had varied during the period of years for which wages were quoted, and you will see from the notes appended to the various records that on the whole there was very little variation, the tendency being to increase the extras as well as the rates of wages. It seems safe to assume, therefore, that there has been no diminution in the social well-being of farm labourers in Ireland, and that the steady rise in wages shown on p. 137 is not overstated."

TABLE LV

Ratio of Average Rates of Wages in Different Countries (exclusive in all Cases of Agriculture) (Cd. 1761, p. 275).   Wages in 1900 = 100

Years.	United Kingdom.	France.	Germany.	United States.
	Principal Groups of Trades.	Mean of Skilled Trades.	Groups of Principal Trades under Imperial Insurance Scheme.	Average of all Trades.
1881–85 . .	83·4	86·9	...	90·5
1886–90 . .	84·6	...	80·9	93·3
1891–95 . .	89·4	...	84·9	95·8
1896–99 . .	91·7	96·0 (1896)	92·7	96·0
1900 . . .	100·0	100·0	100·0	100·0

Comparing the past with the present, there has been great increase of wages all round (Tables LIII. and LV.).

The greatest increase has been in Germany, the least in the United States. The above ratios indicate the course of wages in each country, not the absolute amounts. Germany, which shows the greatest increase of wages, still pays its workmen a lower average wage than that in other countries. Unfortunately, the comparison for Germany does not extend back beyond 1886. Between 1886–90 and 1891–95 the death-rate from tuberculosis fell 15 per cent., while wages rose 5 per cent.

In Norway between 1885 and 1900, wages have increased in different industries from 24 to 53 per cent. Its phthisis death-rate meanwhile has not decreased.

Thus in Germany and in Ireland wages lower than the British are associated with a higher phthisis rate, while in the United States much higher wages are associated with a much higher phthisis rate. In Great Britain and the United States rise of wages has accompanied decrease of phthisis ; in France no such correspondence has appeared; and in Ireland and Norway considerable increase of wages has been associated with some increase of, or with a stationary death-rate from, phthisis.

Amounts of Food Consumed

Without entering into the figures which are given in detail elsewhere (1906, p. 343), it may be said that no uniform correspondence is to be found between the figures of food consumption per head of population and those of phthisis. England with the lowest phthisis rate has by far the highest consumption of meat, though not of other foods ; and Belgium, with substantially the same phthisis rate and the same decrease as England in the period under examination, consumes less meat than any country except Ireland, and less than half the amount consumed in England. France, with a large and steadily increasing consumption of meat and of other foods, has, judging by Paris, the largest phthisis death-rate, with no certain evidence of improvement.

Pauperism

Hitherto we have dealt with the experience of various

countries in regard to the positive elements of well-being. It remains to see to what extent these results can be checked by figures expressing the absence of well-being. Owing to the different methods of relieving poverty, we can only examine the figures relating to poverty in the countries of the United Kingdom, using for this purpose the poor-law returns. Before doing so, it is desirable to realise what figures of pauperism really indicate. Pauperism is officially-relieved poverty ; and poverty itself, while most often due to absence of means, may also arise from the unskilful, careless, or mischievous use of means, from thriftlessness, sloth, or intemperance. The conditions which accompany poverty, such as protracted exposure to infection, insufficient nutrition, and ignorance, work in a vicious circle with the conditions that cause it, till it is difficult or impossible to distinguish those elements of poverty representing destitution, and relievable by the provision of ampler means, from those which are of an origin independent of material supplies, and which would persist even in a community free from economic deficiencies. Poverty therefore is itself a most complex phenomenon, not to be remedied by any single set of measures ; and figures of actual poverty, even if they could be had, would not in themselves suffice to estimate the causes from which the poverty arose nor the steps which would be necessary to remove them. In fact, however, we have not figures of poverty, but only of pauperism, *i.e.* of State-relieved poverty. The amount of pauperism depends obviously, not alone on the extent of poverty, but also on the test or standard by which the scale of relief is determined ; and a given amount of poverty will beyond doubt yield very different figures of pauperism at various epochs and in various districts according to the scale of relief which happens to be applied. These considerations need to be remembered when an attempt is made to bring the complex phenomena of pauperism into relation with experience as to phthisis. It will be seen, shortly, that in the United Kingdom during the period under observation there has been a correspondence between the variations of phthisis and those of pauperism so marked as to justify the use of the figures of total pauperism as approximate indexes of the total amounts of phthisis, when the actual phthisis figures cannot be had. This does not mean that the variations in pauperism explain the variations in the death-rate from phthisis. Within the bundle of phenomena which constitute pauperism such an explanation may be found ; but until we ascertain which individual element or elements of the bundle contain the explanation, to explain the figures of phthisis by

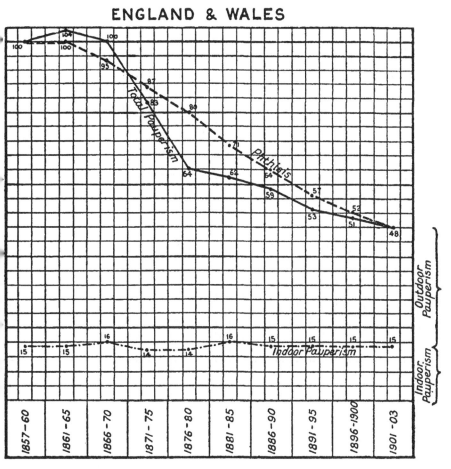

FIG. 27.—England and Wales. Showing the relative Changes in the Number of Indoor and of Total Paupers and in the Deaths from Phthisis per 100,000 of Population from 1857–60 to 1901–03

those of pauperism is for any practical purpose to explain a complex *ignotum* by a yet more complex *ignotius*.

In considering the experience of Great Britain it must be

remembered that about 1870 there was a vigorous and largely
successful movement for insisting on the "house-test" for relief ;
and the sudden drop of total pauperism about this date and
during the subsequent decade arose largely from this cause.

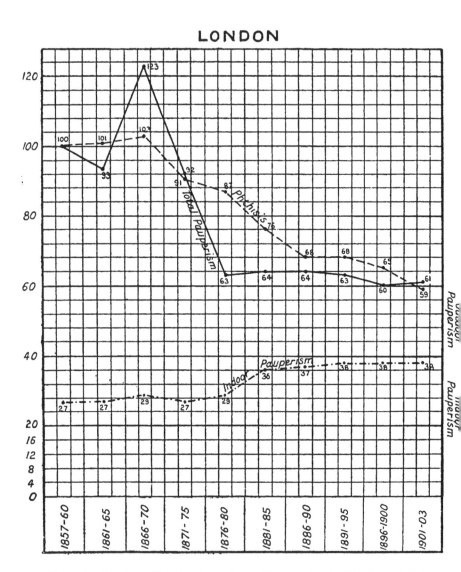

FIG. 28.—London. Showing the relative Changes in the Number of Indoor
and of Total Paupers and in the Deaths from Phthisis per 100,000 of Population from 1857–60 to 1901–03

Simultaneously there was great improvement in the workhouse accommodation, particularly in its infirmary department. The experience of Ireland has been even more striking, because in the opposite direction to that of England and Scotland. In

SCOTLAND

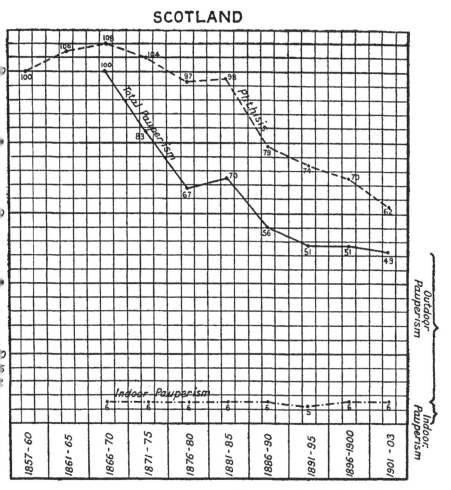

FIG. 29.—Scotland. Showing the relative Changes in the Number of Indoor and of Total Paupers and in the Deaths from Phthisis per 100,000 of Population from 1857–60 to 1901–03

Ireland, as shown in Fig. 30, a rigid system in which indoor, *i.e.* institutional, relief was almost alone given, has been superseded by a largely outdoor, *i.e.* domestic, system. As in the England

IRELAND

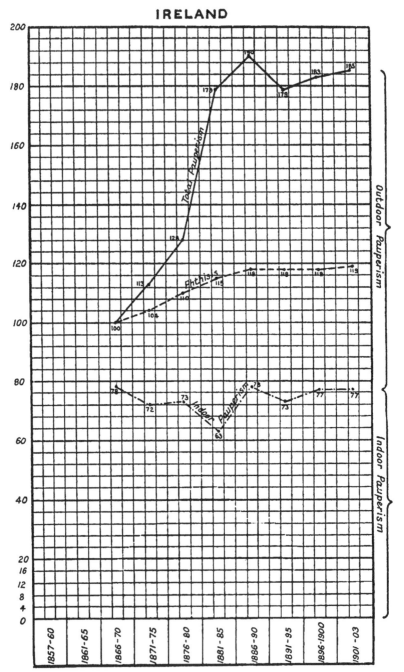

FIG. 30.—Ireland. Showing the relative Changes in the Number of Indoor and of Total Paupers and in the Deaths from Phthisis per 100,000 of Population from 1857–60 to 1901–03

of former times, this has been associated with a great increase of official pauperism ; and apart from the facts which independently make it improbable that this increase of official pauperism was due to increase of privation in this very poor country, such a sweeping change in administration must have produced an increased number of paupers for a given amount of destitution.

Unfortunately there are no figures of pauperism for foreign countries suitable for comparison with our own ; and it is therefore desirable to examine those of the United Kingdom with some minuteness. The course of pauperism in each country of the United Kingdom and in London is shown in Figs. 27 to 30. In order to compare the curve of total pauperism in each instance with the corresponding curve of the phthisis death-rate, the curves of total pauperism and of phthisis have been reduced to the same scale by stating the experience for the earliest period in each instance as 100, and the subsequent rates in their proportion to this.

It will be seen that if allowance be made for the reduction in the relief figures introduced about 1870 by the more rigid insistence on the " house-test," there is a correspondence between the curves of phthisis and of total pauperism. The following table shows the corresponding percentage declines of each for the whole period and for its constituent quinquennia :—

TABLE LVI.—ENGLAND AND WALES

Percentage Declines of Rates of Phthisis and of Pauperism

	1866-70 to 1901-03.	1866-70 to 1871-75.	1871-75 to 1876-80.	1876-80 to 1881-85.	1881-85 to 1886-90.	1886-90 to 1891-95.	1891-95 to 1896-1900.	1896-1900 to 1901-03.
Phthisis Death-rate.	49·8	9·4	8·1	10·2	10·3	10·9	9·6	6·8
Total Pauperism-rate	52·3	17·7	22·1	3·7	4·2	9·5	5·4	6·0

The total decreases for the entire period—49·8 per cent. for phthisis and 52·3 per cent. for pauperism—are surprisingly close. Individual quinquennia show some discrepancies ; but as phthisis has a long course and may have a still longer period of latency, and as any administrative influence is likely to operate slowly, a close quantitative relation between the figures for short periods cannot be expected.

The correspondence in London and Scotland when allowance has been made for changes in administration, though not so close as in England and Wales, is nevertheless close.

In Ireland, if we make the necessary allowance for the great increase of outdoor relief due to administrative causes shown in Fig. 30, and compare the subsequent curve of pauperism with that of phthisis, a close correspondence is seen. It would be unsafe to assume on historical grounds alone that the lack of exact parallelism between the earlier parts of the curves of phthisis and pauperism is due merely or mainly to administrative change. There is, however, independent evidence of the fact. It has already been shown (p. 241) that the economic condition of Ireland has not become worse, and that so far as can be measured by the tests already given it has improved. Agricultural labourers in 1881 formed 46·0 and in 1901 44·3 per cent. of the total male population of Ireland over 10 years of age ; and between 1870 and 1900 the wages of these labourers had increased 42 per cent. Food has become cheaper, rents are low, overcrowding has declined, and is less marked than in Scotland (p. 227). It is clear that poverty has been growing less in Ireland during the period of observation, and that the increase of pauperism has therefore been due to altered administration and not to increase of destitution.

The figures of pauperism and of phthisis for the entire period are connected by the following correlation coefficients :—

Correlation between Total Pauperism and Phthisis

	Period.	Coefficient of Correlation.
England and Wales . .	1866–1903	+ ·89
Scotland	1868–1902	+ ·90
Ireland	1866–1902	+ ·83

These figures summarise a close co-variation in each of these countries between phthisis death-rate and total pauperism. This result is what would be expected from the pathology of the disease. However minutely pauperism is analysed, each element which is disclosed is such as would favour an increased phthisis rate.   In each of these countries, therefore, the figures of pauperism confirm the *a priori* expectation that pauperism contains enough phthisiogenetic influences to make its figures vary closely with the figures of phthisis.

CHAPTER XXXIII

TUBERCULOSIS IN COMMUNITIES OF VARYING SANITARY EDUCATION AND SANATORIUM PROVISION

KOCH teaches on *a priori* grounds that direct infection has a preponderating influence on the prevalence of phthisis ; and the facts here reviewed will be found to lead by another road to the same conclusion. In a passage quoted by Dr. Bulstrode (1903, ii. p. 208), Koch says : " The fact that tuberculosis has considerably diminished in almost all civilised States of late is attributable to the circumstances that knowledge of the contagious character of tuberculosis has been more and more widely disseminated, and that caution in intercourse with consumptives has increased more and more in consequence."

This statement, so far as I am aware, has not been supported by evidence, and it is by no means a consequence of Koch's discovery that tuberculosis is infectious. Before such a statement can be accepted, it must be shown, not only that caution in intercourse with consumptives has increased, but also that the increase of this caution occurred at a period and to an extent warranting the inference. Prior to 1884 when Koch's discovery of the tubercle bacillus was first fully set out, suspicion of infectivity had no notable influence on medical or public action. Had Koch's contention on this point been correct, the chief

TABLE LVII

Percentage Decline in Phthisis Death-rate

	1871–75.	1876–80.	1881–85.	1886–90.	1891–95.	1896–1900.	1901–04.
England and Wales . .	9·4	8·1	10·2	10·3	10·9	9·6	6·8
Scotland . . .	3·5	7·2	8·0	10·9	6·3	4·5	13·1 (1901–02)

reduction of phthisis should have occurred since 1884. In Germany this has been so : in Great Britain it is otherwise.

Table LVII. gives the quinquennial percentage decline of the phthisis rate before and since 1885 in England and Wales and in Scotland (the last period is two years).

The rate of decline was substantially as great before as since the infectivity of phthisis became generally known to the medical profession. In recent years the rate of decline has diminished. In Scotland the rate of decline has been more irregular.

The figures of other countries are interesting in the same connection.

TABLE LVIII

Percentage Decline of the Death-rate from Phthisis or Tuberculosis between

	1881–85 and 1886–90.	1886–90 and 1891–95.	1891–95 and 1896–1900.	1896–1900 and 1901–02 or 1903 or 1904.
Switzerland . . .	2	8	3	$1\frac{1}{2}$
Prussia	7	15	16	7
Paris	0	5	7	3

In several of these countries a slackening of the rate of decline of the phthisis death-rate is noticeable in recent years. It will not be contended by the anti-contagionist that education and consequent precautions have caused this diminution in the rate of decline. Neither, on the other hand, is it possible to show that the extremely limited action taken on directly preventive lines has so far impressed itself on national statistics. As the matter stands, there is no evidence of a causal connection sufficiently large to be traceable between the decline of the phthisis death-rates and the progress of education in hygienic matters.

Similarly, no practical result can have followed from the amount of voluntary or compulsory notification of phthisis which has occurred in England. This is by no means because notification has no useful part in the prevention of tuberculosis, but because it is useless without the administrative mechanism which is necessary for turning it to account for the welfare both of the community and of the patient. No valid conclusions as to the utility of notification could be drawn from the experience of towns which are not so equipped, or which have been so only for a short term of years ; and in view of the important part which notification should play in a properly arranged mechanism for the control of tuberculosis, the error of attempting to draw such conclusions is more than an academical fault, and is much to be deprecated.

Nor conversely can it be imagined that similar educative influences have been entirely absent from Ireland and Norway, in which an increase, or from France in which probably no decline, of phthisis has occurred. The action taken in consequence of knowledge of the infectiousness of phthisis has doubtless varied greatly in different countries and in different parts of the same country. In Germany alone can treatment in special sanatoria have any claim to the decline which has occurred, as the use of these elsewhere has until a few years ago been on a very small scale compared with the total amount of disease. Sanatorium treatment, furthermore, has, with the same exception, been employed chiefly for well-to-do patients who from the public

TABLE LIX.—SANATORIA IN GERMANY

Year Opened.	Public.	Private.	Prussia.
	Number of Beds.	Number of Beds.	Tuberculosis Death-rate per 1000.
1854	...	300	...
1873	...	120	...
1875	...	80	...
1876	...	114	...
1881	...	100	307
1885	...	12	311
1887	...	100	290
1889	...	205	279
1892	94	...	248
1893	103	...	248
1894	...	275	237
1895	196	...	231
1896	195	...	217
1897	504	...	214
1898	958	135	197
1899	590	119	202
1900	817	...	205
1901	794	66	196
1902	811	...	...

health standpoint need it least.   Even in Germany the sanatorium treatment of phthisis was, as will be seen in Table LIX., on a very small scale until after 1892, when the first popular sanatoria were opened (Santoliquido, 1903) ; and these institutions cannot have played more than an insignificant part in the great decline of the death-rate from tuberculosis which took place between 1886–89 and 1890–93.   Of the great value of sanatoria in the treatment of phthisis there can be no doubt, nor of their even greater educational value ; but their main utility lies in the future.

CHAPTER XXXIV

THE GENERAL RELATIONSHIP OF INSTITUTIONAL SEGREGATION TO TUBERCULOSIS AND CERTAIN OTHER INFECTIOUS DISEASES

WE have seen that both general improvement in communal health and each individual measure which tends to produce it must work powerfully towards the reduction of tuberculosis, but that nevertheless the disease has varied in communal experience in a quite irregular relation to each and all of these important influences. In the words of Sir William Broadbent (1905, p. 118) :—

> Supposing that the best possible sanitation, the best possible food, and the best possible conditions of life, were an adequate protection against phthisis, we ought to have no such thing amongst the better classes. But it does get there somehow.

In Norway, Ireland, France, and Austria, the same influences of improved general health, well-being, and sanitary education have operated as in Great Britain, Germany, Belgium, and the United States, side by side with widely different variations in the respective death-rates in these countries from tuberculosis. Similar discrepancies have been seen when other elements of sanitary environment have been compared with the variations of the disease.

It will next be seen that the only constant correspondence between the variations in the prevalence of tuberculosis and in any element of sanitary environment consists in the relation to tuberculosis of the institutional segregation of patients.

Whether for good or harm, the segregation of infective patients is likely to influence the spread of tuberculosis. The operation of this measure on tuberculosis follows obviously from the infectious character of the disease; and it will be convenient here to recall what has been described on this subject in Part I. The vast majority of pathologists and hygienists are agreed that the chief source of infection in human tuberculosis is the tuberculous human patient. Whether he is more infectious at early or at later stages has not been ascertained definitely; but in cases of pulmonary tuberculosis it may be assumed safely that the infectivity varies with the amount of the sputum. There is no evidence that with advancing disease the patient becomes less able to disseminate infection ; on the contrary, in advanced cases the patient is less able to control its hygienic disposal. The period of latency of the disease appears to be very variable. Small doses of infection lead to immediate limitation of the disease, which may be followed after a long interval by invasion of other parts of the body from the localised tuberculous lesion. Pending such an explosion the lesion may be utterly unrecognisable by clinical symptoms. Experimentally, statistically, and clinically, it has been shown that " the disease as a rule advances not by a continuous progress, but by a series of successive invasions separated by variable intervals. After each invasion, or, as it has been termed, eruption of tuberculosis, there is a temporary self-limitation of the disease." The earlier invasions may date years back. During the patient's life they may be wholly unsuspected or evidenced only by the recollections of an earlier attack of pleurisy or hæmoptysis, often many years prior to the diagnosed tuberculosis ; and this earlier attack may itself be a secondary result of a still earlier disease in the bronchial or mesenteric glands.

The infection of tuberculosis, in short, is often acquired without at the time causing any recognisable illness in the infected person. Most acute infections, as for instance that of scarlet fever, are either followed by a recognised attack of the disease within a few days, or the person escapes entirely. The infection of tuberculosis, while it appears to require a much larger dose or more protracted exposure before evident disease is produced, may, on the contrary, be saved up within the infected person for years, and be discovered only after lapse of time and change of circumstances have destroyed the chance of tracing its origin. The infection which may be spread by an individual patient, or even by a whole group of patients within the practice of a single physician, may thus be wholly or partially concealed, and give rise to a mistaken estimate of the infectivity of the

17

disease.   No better evidence of this fact can be needed than
the historical circumstance that for many centuries the existence
of any infectivity at all escaped recognition, and indeed did not
become accepted doctrine until it had been demonstrated by
actual experiment on animals.   But though commonly unknown
by the patient and his family, and commonly unrecognisable
even to the physician in charge of the infecting case, the com-
municated infection remains within the body of the community
as a standing danger.   In the proportion in which such latent
infections come ultimately to fruition as disease they are bound
to appear in the actual experience of the community ; and it
is necessary to turn to that experience for sure and unspeculative
guidance in seeking to master the disease.

It is evident that institutional segregation is different
qualitatively from domestic segregation.   The average home,
both in its bedrooms and its living rooms, has far less special
accommodation per head, and a far lower standard of precautions against infection, than the average institution.   Two
persons and often three may occupy the same bed in the
home ; never more than one in the hospital.   In institutions,
and by reason of the abundance of gratuitous labour, notably in
workhouse infirmaries in this country, the average standard of
cleanliness is far higher than in most homes.   Spittoons and
spit-cups are provided and cleaned, washing of body and bed-
linen is not spared, and the floors, etc., of each room are kept
scrubbed and kept free from dust.   In private houses, the
crowding of furniture, the presence of mats and carpets, and
the exigencies of life in the families of the poor, do not encourage
and sometimes do not even permit of such frequent and persistent cleanings.   It follows that the inmates of the home,
including children of the most susceptible age, must be far
more exposed to infection when the patient remains at home
than are the inmates of an institution to which he is transferred.

It remains to see how far the institutional segregation of
infective patients which is secured in institutions in general
has in actual fact served to control the spread of the disease.
Before turning to the facts of communal experience by which
these theoretical anticipations are confirmed, a hypothetical case
suggested by Sir Hugh Beevor (1905) may serve to illustrate the
order of magnitude of the influence under consideration.

Let it be supposed that no influence was operating to control the prevalence of consumption except that of institutional segregation. In Brighton 20 per cent. of the total consumptives are segregated in its workhouse infirmary, and for the purpose of this calculation this proportion may be supposed to hold good for England and Wales. The examples given on p. 274 suggest that one-third of a year may be taken as the average stay of each patient, and Sir Hugh Beevor in common with others apparently would put the total period of infectivity at three years. If these figures hold good for England and Wales, it follows that just over 2 per cent. of the total infection of phthisis is prevented from spreading outside institutions. On this supposition, and if personal infection were the sole means of communicating the disease, the death-rate from phthisis ought to have declined in each year to the extent of the segregation, namely, 2 per cent. A reference to Table LVII. shows that from 1871 to the present time the decline year by year in the death-rate from phthisis has been usually under 2 per cent. The calculation, although interesting and suggestive, does not, of course, give any accurate measure of the institutional segregation of phthisis, nor even of its practical effect. Other influences besides segregation have been operating, some to restrain and some to promote the spread of the disease ; the extent of segregation may have been more or less than has been assumed ; its quality must undoubtedly have varied from place to place ; and when figures such as those of a single town are considered, the order of magnitude of which is vastly less than those of the whole country, the result is influenced by migration as previously indicated. The calculation shows, however, that the influence of segregation in institutions, as practised in England, has an order of magnitude fully sufficing to explain by itself the decrease of phthisis which has been secured, and it illustrates aptly the far-reaching result which may be hoped for from the withdrawal of infection from the community even to an extent which on careless inspection may appear to be too slight to have exercised an appreciable effect.

A brief statement of the history of typhus fever in Ireland and of leprosy in Norway throws some side-light on the influence of segregation in two other infectious diseases, one very acute and the other very chronic in its course. These diseases, like tuberculosis, have in the past been associated very closely with

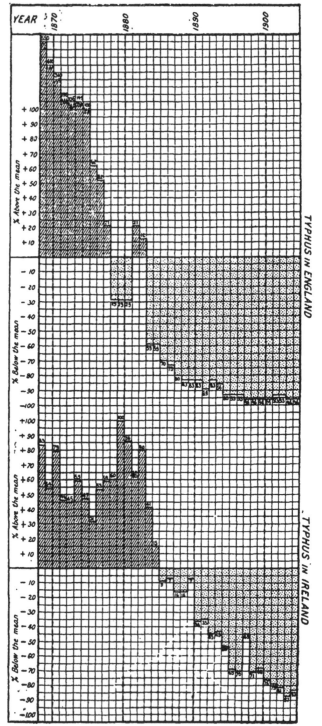

FIG. 31.—Comparison of the Changes in the Death-rates from Typhus and from percentage deviations from the average

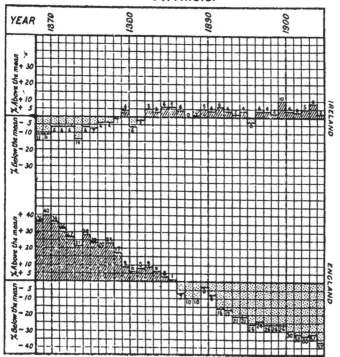

Phthisis in Ireland and in England and Wales, as shown in each country by death-rate for the entire period.

unwholesome conditions of life, and the history of their decline is instructive in its bearing on the problem of tuberculosis.

TYPHUS IN IRELAND.—The history of typhus in Ireland is closely wrapped up with that of want and famine. Famine has caused rapid spread of typhus, in the main because it has increased enormously the wanderings of vagrants from one part of Ireland to another, and to other countries. The disease began to abate when fever hospitals were generally provided, and when the families of infectious patients became relatively immobilised by the provision of poor-law relief. Fig. 31 displays the course of the death-rate from typhus and from phthisis in Ireland and in England since 1868. It will be seen that typhus has declined greatly in both countries ; in England it has approached extinction, and in Ireland it is following, though more slowly, in the same direction.

Phthisis, on the other hand, though it has declined greatly in England, in Ireland has not only not declined, but has even shown some increase. In the light of these national experiences, it can scarcely be maintained that diminution of domestic over-crowding and improvement in housing, — which have been regarded as the predominant factors in the decline of both diseases, —can have produced for typhus a diminution in both countries, and for phthisis a diminution in one country and none in the other. The detailed facts given in Chapters XXX.–XXXII. show that in both countries there has been marked diminution of overcrowding, improvement in housing, and cheapening of the means of living along with increase of wages. These facts justify the inference that some *differentia* between the two countries exists for phthisis, which does not exist for typhus fever ; and the history of the two diseases in Ireland and in England fits in with this inference. In Ireland the chief mass of sickness, especially of phthisis, is treated domestically (see pp. 280 and 282 for details, and especially p. 284 for the facts bearing on the quality of institutional treatment in Ireland). This is not the case in regard to typhus fever. By means of fever hospitals and by preventing the wanderings of the poor, the dissemination of typhus has been greatly diminished; and Ireland has secured a decrease of typhus, as has also England by similar means. In both countries, doubtless, diminished domestic overcrowding and clearing of crowded courts and other dwellings has helped in producing the result; but the detailed experience of Ireland [1] clearly indicates that the immobilisation of infection has been the chief operative factor.

LEPROSY IN NORWAY.—The history of leprosy forms an interesting chapter in the history of disease, more particularly so in its bearing on the history of tuberculosis. Both diseases are caused by bacilli producing granulomatous tissue changes; in both there may be a long period of latency before the signs of disease appear; and in both the disease is commonly protracted and intermittent in its progress. Both likewise are diseases to which the designation "sub-infectious" has been applied, though the name is misleading, and is no more applicable to them than to syphilis, in which similar phenomena of long latency of symptoms, and of protracted and intermittent course are seen, and in which, furthermore, hereditary predisposition is not known to occur. The further interest attaches to leprosy, that acute differences of opinion exist as to the cause of its partial or complete disappearance from England and some other countries, which recall the similar differences of opinion as to the cause of the great decline of tuberculosis in certain countries during the last forty years.

The history of the disappearance of leprosy has been associated with the existence on a very considerable scale of leper asylums in the countries from which the disease has disappeared. In mediæval England such lazar houses were numerous, and although complete segregation of all patients was never secured, there doubtless was segregation of a large percentage of the total cases during a considerable part of their illness. Here again the resemblance to what has been happening in the case of tuberculosis, as will be shown shortly, is striking. There is no intrinsic difficulty in accepting it as fact that in leprosy,—in which, as in tuberculosis, infection occurs chiefly after protracted infection of an intimate character, — the isolation of lepers must, if carried out to a sufficient extent, have served to bring about a steady decline and eventual disappearance of this disease. This conclusion is confirmed by the experience of Norway, which amounts almost to a check experiment. In this country until

[1] Further details of the history of typhus in Ireland are given in an address by the author on "Poverty and Disease as illustrated by the Course of Typhus Fever and Phthisis in Ireland" (*Journal of the Royal Society of Medicine*, Dec. 1908).

far on in the nineteenth century there were leper asylums. As Dr. Vandyke Carter put it, there never prevailed in Norway " the same systematic and rigorous opposition to the leprous pest as was aroused in Europe generally." During the first half of the nineteenth century leprosy was increasing in Norway. Thus the yearly average number of fresh cases of leprosy ascertained and

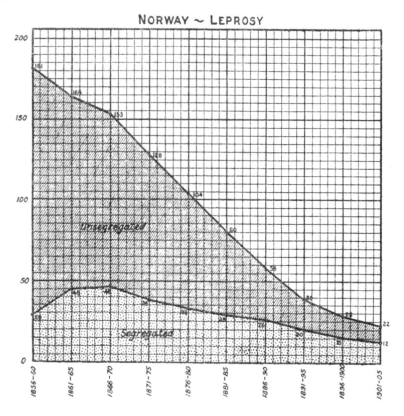

NORWAY ~ LEPROSY

FIG. 32.—Norway. Number of Total Lepers and of Lepers in Asylums per 100.000 of population, 1856-60 to 1901-05

registered in 1840-45 was 43, in 1846-50 it was 124, in 1851-55 it was 219, in 1855-60 it was 233, and in 1861-65 it was 225. Even allowing for the possibility of increasing accuracy of registration, it is clear that there was no decline in this disease. In 1856 notification of cases by medical men became compulsory, and for all years onwards the official statistics state the total number of known cases of the disease and the number segregated in asylums. The diagram on preceding page shows these facts for quinquennial periods. It will be observed that the steady pursuit of an intelligent policy of segregation of leprous patients,—almost entirely without compulsion,[1]—has been associated with a steady and continuous decline of the prevalence of leprosy. At no time has there been total segregation of all known cases. Of the total cases about 16 per cent. were segregated in 1856–60, 27 per cent. in the next period, 30 per cent. in 1871–75, 32 per cent. in 1876–80, then 36 and 46 per cent. in the two next periods, the proportion of segregation in the three most recent quinquennial periods being about 52 per cent. of the total known cases. In the light of our knowledge that leprosy is a communicable disease, of its history in other countries, and of the close correlation between the phenomena of segregation and diminution of disease (which is expressed by a coefficient of correlation of ·95 for the entire period), it is reasonable to give the chief place to segregation as the means by which the diminution of disease has been secured.

[1] Some indirect compulsion has been exercised by refusing non-institutional relief.

CHAPTER XXXV

TUBERCULOSIS IN COMMUNITIES WITH VARYING AMOUNTS OF INSTITUTIONAL SEGREGATION

THE exact measure of institutional segregation of phthisis is the ratio stating how many of the total days of sickness (number of patients and number of days of sickness) is passed in institutions. This ratio and the equivalents for it which have to be used in practice may for convenience be called the *segregation ratio*. The need for equivalents for the ratio as stated above arises from the fact that we are dealing with actual recorded experience, and the statistical material has to be taken from the records as they happen to exist. These records appear in very various forms in different communities. In existing circumstances of notification they can never state directly the number of days of tuberculous sickness, and only exceptionally for comparatively small communities can they state the number of such days passed in institutions. It becomes necessary therefore to select other figures which vary approximately with the total days of tuberculous sickness and the total days of tuberculous sickness passed in institutions. Such figures may represent them respectively on quite different scales; but so long as comparison is made only between segregation ratios, in which the substituted figures represent similar phenomena, the particular scale on which they represent the phenomenon of institutional segregation is of no consequence. From the records in various countries we can learn either how many of the total deaths from all causes and from tuberculosis or from phthisis occur in institutions, or how many of the total paupers are indoor paupers, or how many cases of tuberculosis or phthisis are treated in institutions, and how many deaths from these diseases occur in the whole community for each case treated in an institution.

From what has been said, it will be seen that these figures

measure with approximate accuracy the ratio which states how many of total days of tuberculous sickness are passed in institutions. Thus, for instance, in the absence of change of type of disease and of material change in efficiency of treatment, the number of deaths from tuberculosis is an approximate measure of the number of cases, and so is the number of deaths from all causes for short periods during which the relation of the death-rate for phthisis to that for all causes does not vary markedly.

The fraction of total deaths in the population occurring in institutions is by far the most direct measure of the amount of sickness, and Table LX., calculated from the census returns, shows for England and Wales how preponderantly public institutions are occupied by the sick and not the healthy. Deaths are taken at the average for 1891-95 and 1901-03 respectively, the difference between these and the deaths for 1891 and 1901 being immaterial for the present purpose.

TABLE LX

Per 100,000 of Total Population and per 100 Deaths in Total Population there were in

	Workhouses including Workhouse Infirmaries and Schools.		Hospitals.		Lunatic Asylums.		Total Institutions.	
	Inmates per 100,000 Total Population.	Deaths per 100 Deaths in Total Population.	Inmates per 100,000 Total Population.	Deaths per 100 Deaths in Total Population.	Inmates per 100,000 Total Population.	Deaths per 100 Deaths in Total Population.	Inmates per 100,000 Total Population.	Deaths per 100 Deaths in Total Population.
1891 . .	630	7·1	95	3·5	276	1·1	1001	11·7
1901 . .	641	8·1	120	5·5	280	1·5	1041	15·1

The fraction of deaths in the total population occurring in public institutions was accordingly fifteen times as large as the fraction of the total population which was housed in these institutions.

Apart from figures of mortality, the nearest approach to a satisfactory index of tuberculosis is probably to be found in the number of the pauper population. It is the last part of the population to be reached by ameliorating influences tending to control tuberculosis, and would therefore be expected to have a higher sickness rate than the general population, and to yield figures of which the variations will correspond with some accuracy to the variations in prevalence of tuberculosis. We have seen that this theoretical expectation has been verified, at least for the United Kingdom, in the close co-variation of the numbers of paupers and of deaths from tuberculosis respectively over a long period ; and the numbers of paupers relieved during the periods here in question do therefore actually represent on some scale those of total cases of tuberculosis during the corresponding periods.

In using these indirect measures of institutional treatment of tuberculosis and of its prevalence, it must be remembered that they are indirect and approximate. Thus, for instance, figures for institutional treatment usually give the number of cases and not days of treatment, and while they tell how many people were segregated in institutions, do not show the average duration, still less the quality of the treatment. Any of these indirect forms of segregation ratio has therefore to be verified wherever possible by the application to the same community and period of one or more other forms of the ratio, and checked where practicable by a special examination of sample constituent communities whose figures are included in the total. This has been done so far as the information obtainable has allowed. It will be seen that the results obtained by applying different ratios to the experience of the same country and period are usually, though not invariably, in good agreement ; and where this is not the case, fortunately other data have been available to explain the discrepancy and enable a more correct segregation ratio to be formed.

Where, again, the segregation ratio—the proportion of sick days spent by consumptives in institutions—is expressed as the proportion of total paupers who receive indoor relief, it is assumed that the number of days of sickness is the same in each class. This assumption is probably incorrect ; but to such extent as consumptives admitted to indoor relief are, in fact, treated longer than the average of other paupers, the error would be to exhibit the extent of segregation as being less than it really is, and for the present purpose the figures may therefore be used with safety.

As has been pointed out previously, the phthisis rates with which these ratios should be compared are not those for the same but for a somewhat later period, the interval representing the time taken for the effect of segregation to show itself. For the present purpose this comparison can in any sufficiently long series of years be made with the phthisis figures of the same year, not because the phthisis is affected immediately by simultaneous changes in other phenomena, but because the numerical difference between closely consecutive phthisis figures in the present material happens to be small.

The countries in which the fullest records of experience have been obtained in regard to institutional segregation are England and Wales, Scotland, and Ireland. It is not always realised how large a proportion of the total population is at any one time in public institutions; and, without quoting the actual figures, Table LXI. shows to the nearest whole number the number of total population at the censuses of 1891 and 1901 to every one inmate of a public institution.

TABLE LXI

For every Inmate of a Public Institution the Total Population of the Country was

	England and Wales.	Scotland.	Ireland.
1891	99	164	82
1901	96	137	69

The figures available for England and Wales and for London permit a statement of the fraction of total deaths in the population occurring in institutions, which, as we have seen, is one of the measures of the amount of institutional segregation. Tables LXII. and LXIII. give these figures, together with those of the death-rate from phthisis for a considerable period. They show that the decrease in phthisis was accompanied by a large and steady increase in institutional segregation measured by the fraction of total deaths occurring in institutions; and the rate at which these changes occurred is shown more conveniently in Figs.

33 and 34, in which the rate of change of the phthisis death-rate is shown by the side of the rate of change of the segregation ratio, the curve for the segregation ratio being inverted as shown on the left-hand scale.

TABLE LXII.—ENGLAND AND WALES

Percentage of Total Deaths in Public Institutions

Years.	Workhouses and Workhouse Infirmaries.	Hospitals.	Lunatic Asylums.	Total Institutions.	Death-rate per 1000 of Population from Phthisis.
1869–70 . .	5·7	1·9	0·7	8·3	2·45 (1866–70)
1871–75 . .	...	...	...	8·8	2·22
1876–80 . .	6·3	2·4	0·9	9·6	2·04
1881–85 . .	6·6	2·9	1·0	10·5	1·83
1886–90 . .	6·7	3·4	1·1	11·2	1·64
1891–95 . .	7·2	3·9	1·1	12·2	1·46
1896–1900 . .	7·7	4·6	1·4	13·7	1·32
1901–03 . .	8·5	5·9	1·8	16·2	1·23

TABLE LXIII.—LONDON

Percentage of Total Deaths in Public Institutions

Years.	Workhouses and Workhouse Infirmaries.	Public, Lunatic, and Imbecile Asylums.	M. A. B. Hospitals.	Other Hospitals.	Total Institutions.	Death-rate per 1000 of Population from Phthisis.
1852–55 . .	9·6	0·7	...	...	16·7	...
1856–60 . .	9·0	0·6	...	...	16·3	...
1861–65 . .	9·0	0·4	...	...	16·2	2·80
1866–70 . .	9·1	0·5	...	...	16·3	2·86
1871–75 . .	9·8	0·5	...	...	17·3	2·51
1876–80 . .	11·3	0·4	...	...	18·6	2·40
1881–85 . .	12·3	0·4	...	...	20·5	2·11
1886–90 . .	11·8	1·9	0·7	8·7	23·1	1·88
1891–95 . .	13·3	2·0	2·0	9·4	26·7	1·87
1896–1900 . .	14·8	2·1	2·1	10·2	29·2	1·80
1901–03 . .	17·7	2·8	2·2	12·2	34·7	1·65 (1901–04)

Thus in England and Wales, in the period 1866–1903, segregation measured by the fraction of total deaths occurring in institutions has approximately doubled, and the death-rate from phthisis has approximately halved ; in London segregation has not quite doubled and the phthisis death-rate is rather more than half. The closeness of numerical correspondence may be and probably is accidental, for, as pointed out above, close numerical concordance is not to be expected in the courses of complex associated phenomena operating among other complex influences. The data show, however, not only a very close

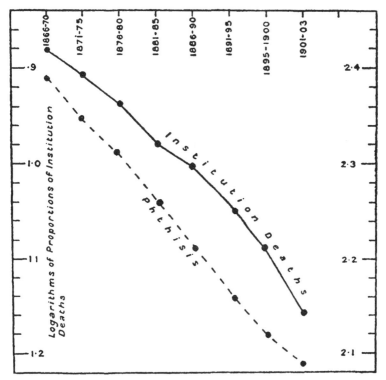

FIG. 33.—England and Wales. Logarithmic Curves showing Rates of Change in the Phthisis Death-rate and in the Proportion of Institutional to Total Deaths from all Causes

correspondence between the increase of total institutional segregation measured by the ratio in question and the decrease of phthisis, but an even more striking similarity in the rates at which these changes have occurred. The experience is summarised in the high correlation coefficients of ·91 for England and Wales (1878–1903) and ·90 for London (1866–1904).

The experience so far as it is available of the chief individual classes of institutions exhibits the manner in which this result has been obtained.

Workhouse infirmaries have been the most important agency

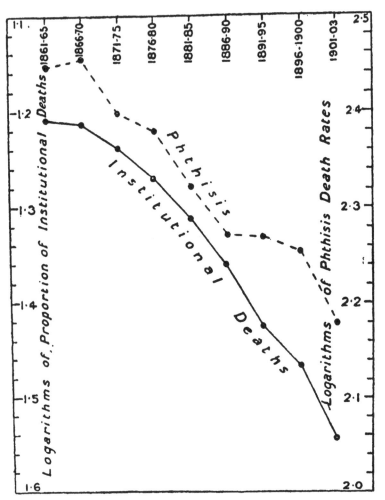

FIG. 34.—London.   Logarithmic Curves showing Rates of Change in the Phthisis Death-rate and in the Proportion of Institutional to Total Deaths from all Causes

in segregation.   These institutions are used to a much greater extent for tuberculosis than in the earlier history of poor-law administrations.   Figs. 27 and 28, expressing the data of Tables

LXV. and LXVI., have shown the general reduction which has occurred in total pauperism side by side with the steady maintenance of indoor relief at a stationary level in England and Wales, and an actual increase of indoor relief in London. In 1848–49 over 60 out of every 1000 inhabitants of England and Wales were paupers as against 20 in 1902–03. The whole of the reduction was in persons receiving outdoor relief, and the number of indoor paupers remained stationary at from 7 to 8 per 1000 of population. Thus of the total pauper population, who, as we have seen, are the most subject to disease of all kinds and notably to tuberculosis, the segregation in workhouses in 1848–49 amounted to about one-eighth, and was increased by 1902–03 to over one-third. The fact expressed in these figures is explained by Mr. Fleming, who speaks of the " great change in the character of workhouse inmates during recent years. . . . The able-bodied inmates are gone and the sick inmates have come " (1902–03, p. 84). When the frequency of tuberculosis is remembered, these figures and this fact become equivalent to the statement that, as has been seen already for the total institutions for England and Wales, there has been during a period of vast reduction in tuberculosis also a vast increase in the extent of segregation of tuberculous patients in workhouse infirmaries.

As a matter of practical importance, individual inquiry has been made among 27 Boards of Guardians in London and 85 of the chief provincial towns, to ascertain the extent to which workhouse infirmaries treat consumptives in separate wards. In 12 of the metropolitan infirmaries out of the 27, consumptives were treated wholly in the same wards as other patients, and in only 9 were they treated entirely in separate wards. Out of the 85 provincial infirmaries only 23 treated consumptives wholly and 13 partially in separate wards. It appears therefore that, although separate treatment is not rare, the more common practice is to treat consumptives in general wards. Incidentally it may be observed that taken in context with the general reduction in the prevalence of phthisis, this fact is very striking evidence of the superiority of segregation in infirmaries over what is practicable at home, and agrees well with the general considerations to which attention was drawn on p. 258. It must be remarked further that, although these results show great good to have arisen without the use of separate wards, it is obviously

18

desirable to have consumptive patients treated separately when it can be arranged.

Figures are not available in most cases to express the duration of stay of consumptives in workhouse infirmaries. For all diseases the average number of days' stay for each patient in certain provincial infirmaries in 1897 was: Salford, 97; Leeds, 95; Croydon, 86; Birmingham, 74; West Derby, 60; Kensington, 48. From the nature of the disease the stay of consumptives was probably longer on the average; thus in Kensington in 1897 all patients had an average stay of 48 days, consumptives of 144 days in 1898 and 95 in 1902. In Sheffield in 1904 the average stay of each phthisical patient was 311 days, and in Brighton 221 days. While therefore the segregation of each patient must have extended over a large portion of the period of his illness, there is considerable variation in the period of segregation in different towns. The existence of this variation indicates that while increased segregation in institutions has been followed by decrease in phthisis in various towns and countries, the decrease caused by institutional segregation must have varied at least according to the differences in average duration of treatment and according to any other variations in the efficiency of the segregation.

After workhouse infirmaries, the most important institutions for segregation of tuberculosis are lunatic asylums. The percentage of lunatics treated with relatives and others was 18·4 in 1859, and fell to 5·5 in 1902. The death-rate from tuberculosis in borough and county asylums in 1901 was 15·8 per cent. of the inmates, or over ten times as great as in the general population. Of these tuberculous lunatics the majority were tuberculous on admission, according to the results of Dr. Mott (1905). Subject therefore to such allowance as may be required by the fact that lunatics seldom expectorate,[1] the segregation of each tuberculous lunatic has been equivalent to the withdrawal from the community of ten ordinary tuberculous persons. The proportion of lunatics in asylums to the total population in 1902 was over 0·3 per cent., and their segregation must therefore be taken to have been equivalent to the withdrawal of say 3 per cent. of normal population or the same amount of average

---

[1] They are often dirty in their habits, and large numbers of tubercle bacilli must be passed in the fæces.

infection from the community. The average stay of each patient is about five years, or far longer than in any other great class of institutions. When the considerable increase in the extent to which lunatics are now lodged in asylums is considered, it is evident therefore that during the period of decline of tuberculosis a large, sustained and increasing segregation of tuberculous patients has taken place in these institutions.

The disproportion between accommodation and need in the case of special hospitals is too great for them to have had a large effect on the total amount of tuberculosis. In the past considerable numbers of consumptives were treated in general hospitals, but the returns of most of them show an increasing unwillingness to admit such patients. Thus in the Royal Infirmary (general hospital) of Glasgow the proportion of total deaths due to phthisis has fallen from 16·9 per cent. to 4 per cent. With this decrease of treatment of phthisis in general hospitals has been associated the great increase of its treatment in workhouse infirmaries.

The experience of large towns has been similar to those of the whole country. For the reasons described on p. 207, the experience of small towns into and out of which there is much migration is, like the experience of separate quarters of large towns, of very doubtful value. In certain towns the segregation

TABLE LXIV

	Brighton.		Sheffield.		Salford.	
	Phthisis Death-rate.	Proportion Per Cent. of Total Deaths from Phthisis in Institutions.	Phthisis Death-rate.	Proportion Per Cent. of Total Deaths from Phthisis in Institutions.	Phthisis Death-rate.	Proportion Per Cent. of Total Deaths from Phthisis in Institutions.
1866–70 .	2·95	9·6	...	...	...	...
1871–75⎫ 1876–80⎭ .	2·47	11·7	... 2·23	... 6·3	... ...	... ...
1881–85⎫ 1886–90⎭ .	1·93	14·3	1·90 1·70	7·9 10·3	... 2·36	... 14·4[1]
1891–95 ⎫ 1896–1900⎭ .	1·63	15·8	1·51 1·35	14·3 20·0	1·94 1·78	19·2 23·5
1901–04 .	1·40	20·2	1·25[2]	26·1[2]	1·82	27·6

[1] 1884–90. [2] 1901–05.

ratio has been obtained in the more direct form of the part of
the total deaths from phthisis which occurred in institutions.
Of the total deaths in London from phthisis, 31·4 per cent. in
1889 and 33·5 per cent. in 1904 occurred in workhouses, workhouse infirmaries, and sick asylums ; in Sheffield the proportion in
workhouse infirmaries and sick asylums was in 1876–80 only 6·3
per cent., and it rose in 1901–05 to 26·1 per cent. ; in Salford in
1884–90 it was 14·4 per cent., rising to 27·6 per cent. in 1901–04;
in Brighton it was 9·6 in 1866–70, rising to 20·2 per cent. in
1901–04.   The course of these figures is set out in Table LXIV.
by the side of the phthisis death-rate for the towns in question,
and, as was seen in the country as a whole, and for institutions
as a whole, there is shown constant increase of segregation in
workhouse infirmaries accompanying constant decrease of
phthisis.

Coefficients of correlation summarising this correspondence
for a long series of single years work out at ·67 for Salford
from 1884 to 1904, and ·80 for Sheffield from 1876 to
1905.

Summarising all this experience, it will be seen that in England
and Wales a large and continuously increasing amount of institutional segregation of phthisis, measured by the fraction of
the total mortality occurring in institutions, has been accompanied for nearly forty years by a large and continuous decrease
of the disease, and that throughout the entire period each of
these changes has gone on at much the same rate as the other.
The same association appears when segregation is measured
in the more direct form of the fraction of deaths from phthisis
in the whole community occurring in institutions as seen in
the experience of certain large towns.

These results may now be compared with those obtained by
regarding segregation as measured by either the fraction of
total pauperism which is treated in institutions, or the ratio
in which the number of paupers treated in workhouses and
workhouse infirmaries stands to the total number of deaths
from phthisis in the community.   The results obtained in either
of these ways confirm the conclusion obtained by the use of the
other measures of segregation.

Table LXV. is a summary in quinquennial periods of the
data for this comparison for the individual years from 1866 to

TABLE LXV.—ENGLAND AND WALES

	Number per 100,000 of Population of			Segregation Ratio. For every 100 Indoor Paupers there were the following Number of	
	Deaths from Phthisis.	Indoor Paupers.	Total Paupers.	Deaths from Phthisis.	Total Paupers.
1866–70 . .	245	726	4652	34	641
1871–75 . .	222	662	3828	31	578
1876–80 . .	204	668	2982	31	446
1881–85 . .	183	730	2870	25	393
1886–90 . .	164	709	2749	23	388
1891–95 . .	146	687	2489	21	362
1896–1900 .	132	692	2356	19	340
1901–03 . .	123	688	2218	18	322

1903. A clearer view of the total result is given in Table LXVI., which shows for England and Wales, and also for London, the respective percentages which the phthisis death-rate and the segregation ratio in question of 1901–03 are of the corresponding figures of 1866–70.

TABLE LXVI

In	Phthisis Death-rate for 1901–03 as Per Cent. of Phthisis Death-rate for 1866–70.	Ratio $\frac{\text{Indoor}}{\text{Total}}$ Pauperism for 1901–03 as Per Cent. of same Ratio for 1866–70.	Ratio $\frac{\text{Indoor Pauperism}}{\text{Total Phthisis Deaths}}$ for 1901–03 as Per Cent. of same Ratio for 1866–70.
England and Wales .	50	50	53
London . . .	58	38	44

This experience for the entire series of individual years is expressed by a coefficient of correlation of − ·94 between segregation measured by the fraction of pauper population treated in institutions and the phthisis death-rate.

The rate at which segregation, measured by comparison of indoor and total pauperism, has varied is shown in context with the rates of variation of the death-rate from phthisis in Fig. 35.

Each of these results is closely similar to that obtained by the previous measures of segregation. In the whole country segregation, measured in any of the ways, has approximately doubled, while the death-rate from phthisis has been halved.

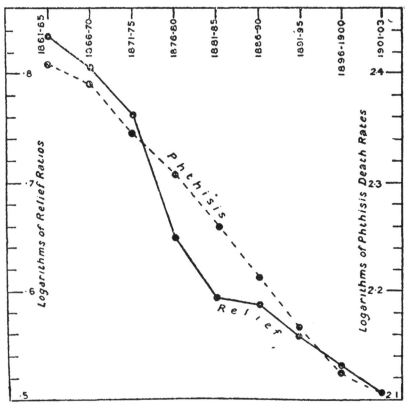

FIG. 35.—England and Wales. Logarithmic Curves of Phthisis Death-rates and of Ratio of Indoor to Total Paupers, 1861–65 to 1901–03

In London exactly the same has happened; measured by the fraction of the pauper population treated in institutions, the amount of segregation has more than doubled.

No figures are available for Scotland or Ireland by which segregation can be expressed in terms of institutional deaths. Measured by the other ratios, the data for Scotland are given in Tables LXVII. and LXVIII., and in Fig. 36.

TABLE LXVII.—SCOTLAND

| | Number per 100,000 of Population of | | | Segregation Ratio. | |
| | | | | For every 100 Indoor Paupers there were the following Number of | |
	Deaths from Phthisis.	Indoor Paupers.	Total Paupers.	Deaths from Phthisis.	Total Paupers.
1866–70 . . .	259	253	3896	102	1540
1871–75 . . .	248	224	3210	111	1433
1876–80 . . .	230	235	2597	98	1105
1881–85 . . .	211	236	2742	89	1162
1886–90 . . .	188	224	2168	84	968
1891–95 . . .	176	212	1978	83	933
1896–1900 . .	168	227	2085	74	919
1901–03 . . .	147	242	1922	61	794

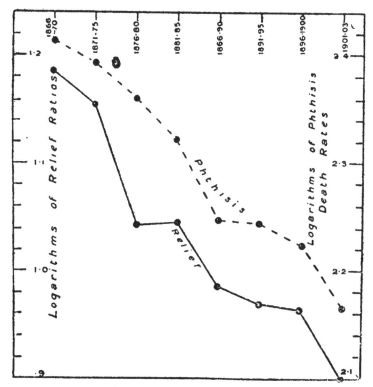

FIG. 36.—Scotland. Logarithmic Curves of Phthisis Death-rates and of Ratio of Indoor to Total Paupers, 1861–65 to 1901–03

In Scotland as in England the facts for the two terminal periods as given in the following table bring out more clearly the relationship between the different factors.

TABLE LXVIII.—SCOTLAND

Phthisis Death-rate for 1901–03 as Per Cent. of Phthisis Death-rate for 1866–70.	Ratio $\frac{\text{Indoor}}{\text{Total}}$ Pauperism for 1901–03 as Per Cent. of same Ratio for 1866–70.	Ratio $\frac{\text{Indoor Pauperism}}{\text{Total Phthisis Deaths}}$ for 1901–03 as Per Cent. of same Ratio for 1866–70.
56	52	60

As in the experience of London, the proportionate extent of segregation appears to have been somewhat larger when measured by the ratio of indoor to total paupers than when measured by the more direct ratio of indoor paupers to total deaths from phthisis in the whole community. On both measures, however, these data show very close correspondence between increased segregation and decrease of the death-rate from phthisis; and in the more direct segregation ratio, given in the 3rd column approximately, the same numerical closeness appears between the increase of segregation and the decrease of the phthisis death-rate as was seen in the experience of England and Wales and of London; a decrease of the phthisis death-rate of about 56 per cent. having been associated in Scotland with an increase of about 60 per cent. in institutional segregation. As with England and Wales, the rates at which segregation has increased throughout the entire period have been much the same as the rates at which the death-rate from phthisis have declined. The experience is summarised by a coefficient of correlation of − ·91 between segregation, expressed as the fraction of total pauperism treated in institutions, and the phthisis death-rate.

The data for Ireland are given in Tables LXIX. and LXX.

In Ireland a decrease in the amount of institutional segregation has been accompanied by an increase in the death-rate from phthisis; and measured by the more direct segregation ratio, there is again numerical identity between the extent

TABLE LXIX.—IRELAND

	Number per 100,000 of Population of			Segregation Ratio. For every 100 Indoor Paupers there were the following Number of	
	Deaths from Phthisis.	Indoor Paupers.	Total Paupers.	Deaths from Phthisis.	Total Paupers.
1866–70 . . .	182	963	1233	19	128
1871–75 . . .	190	882	1389	22	158
1876–80 . . .	200	903	1569	22	174
1881–85 . . .	208	1019	2198	20	215
1886–90 . . .	213	954	2332	22	244
1891–95 . . .	214	906	2204	24	243
1896–1900 . .	213	944	2244	23	237
1901–03 . . .	215	947	2272	23	240

TABLE LXX.—IRELAND

Phthisis Death-rate for 1901–03 as Per Cent. of Phthisis Death-rate for 1866–70.	Ratio $\dfrac{\text{Indoor}}{\text{Total}}$ Pauperism for 1901–03 as Per Cent. of same Ratio for 1866–70.	Ratio $\dfrac{\text{Indoor Pauperism}}{\text{Total Phthisis Deaths}}$ for 1901–03 as Per Cent. of same Ratio for 1866–70.
118	186	121

to which the death-rate from phthisis has increased and the extent to which institutional segregation has decreased. In two respects, however, the experience of Ireland appears to differ from that of England and Wales and of Scotland. The absolute amount of segregation, although steadily decreasing, has nevertheless, so far as gross figures are concerned, been greater than in England and far greater than in Scotland, while the phthisis death-rate has not only increased but has from 1881–85 onwards been higher than in England and from 1886–90 onwards than in Scotland. Moreover, the rates at which the apparent extent of segregation has changed in Ireland during the period in question show much less numerical concordance with the corresponding changes in the phthisis death-rate than has been seen in the experience of England and Wales and of Scotland. Each of these discrepancies is merely one of quantity and not of kind, and leaves segregation and the death-rate from phthisis varying universally as in England and in Scotland. Their explanation throws a light on the practical working of institutional segregation.

Theoretically the discordance might be due to one or more of three causes. The concordance in England and in Scotland might have been mere coincidence. This explanation, as will be seen shortly, is inadmissible because the comparison of institutional segregation with phthisis in a considerable number of other countries shows similar concordance. Presuming therefore that institutional segregation tends to reduce phthisis, it might be that in Ireland the influence of factors tending to increase phthisis has been greater than in either of the other countries. To some extent this has probably been the case ; but although it might assist in explaining the greater prevalence of phthisis at the present time in Ireland than in England or Scotland, it has no bearing on the increase in Ireland itself, unless Ireland at the present time is in a worse economic and sanitary condition than in the past, which, as already seen, is not the case. An examination of the demographical and administrative conditions of the country gives, however, independent and direct explanation of the lower specific result produced by institutional segregation in Ireland. It has been seen already that the population of Ireland contains a smaller proportion than either England or Scotland of persons at the ages specially liable to die from phthisis, and a higher proportion of persons at the ages when pauperism mostly occurs. Apart, therefore, from any question of specific efficiency, the specific result of pauper segregation must have been lower in Ireland than in England or in Scotland. This apparent reduction of specific result of segregation in workhouses is the greater because, as is shown in the Reports of the Irish Local Government Board, many artisans and labourers when sick, in the absence of other medical institutions, resort to the workhouse infirmary for all classes of diseases ; and their cases, which would include a much lower proportion of tuberculosis than occurs among paupers, swell the figures of apparent segregation. So much is clear as to the specific result of what appears as segregation in Irish experience, apart from any question of its specific efficiency. There is, however, unanimous and conclusive evidence that the quality of the segregation is notably inferior in Ireland to that given in England or in Scotland. The extent of institutional segregation is greater in Dublin than in the rest of Ireland, the indoor paupers in the Unions of North and South Dublin numbering 94 per 1000 in 1903, as compared with 80 per 1000 in the rest of Ireland. The average stay of each pauper in workhouses in North and South Dublin is 70 days, in the rest of Ireland 39 days. Clearly therefore the institutional segregation of phthisis may be taken to be more extensive in Dublin than in the rest of Ireland. Yet Sir Charles Cameron (*Ann. Rep.* 1904, p. 31) says concerning Dublin :—

" The hospitals rarely keep consumptives whose cases are hopeless, to the termination of their disease by death. If such cases were retained in hospital, it would prevent the circulation of much tuberculous infective matter."

This statement is confirmed by the data contained in a return, kindly supplied by Mr. J. E. Devlin of the Irish Local Government Board, which has enabled me to calculate the average duration of residence of phthisical patients in the Dublin workhouses. It is shown in the following table, in comparison with similar returns for English workhouses.

TABLE LXXI

Average Residence (in Days) of all Phthisical Patients in Workhouses, to Time of Discharge or Death (not including Patients still in the Institution)

Institution.	Days.	Based on Experience of the Undermentioned Number of Patients who have	
		Left the Institution.	Died in the Institution.
North and South Dublin Workhouses, 1904–05	53	272	156
Brighton Infirmary, 1897–1905 . .	175	165	181
Kensington Infirmary, 1888 . .	144	107	68
,, ,, 1902 . .	95	151	112
Sheffield (Firvale) Infirmary, 1904 . .	311	...	...

The above return relates to North and South Dublin, which in 1903 had a population of 379,666.

It will be noted that, unlike the experience of Kensington Infirmary (see p. 274), the institutional residence of consumptive patients in the Dublin workhouse is less than that of all patients in the aggregate.

In addition to the necessarily low specific effect of segregation in Ireland due to the constitution of the population, to the much shorter duration of average residence in workhouse infirmaries in Ireland than in England or in Scotland, and to the very imperfect conditions of Irish workhouses which diminish the efficiency of segregation, the great increase in outdoor relief must have exerted a powerful influence in promoting the prevalence of tuberculosis, owing to its inevitable effect in increasing domestic at the expense of institutional treatment, and to its effect in continuing an enormous number of domestic foci of tuberculous infection such as are invariably implicated in the average home treatment of phthisis among the poor.

On these grounds the lower specific value of institutional segregation in Ireland need not be taken into further consideration.[1]

The experience of the United Kingdom will now be compared with that of foreign countries, and it will be seen that the inquiry is carried into a larger number than was used in examining the other factors of phthisis. This course is desirable in regard to segregation and was unnecessary for the other factors, because each of the factors discussed earlier in this paper showed failure to maintain co-variation between the factor and the phthisis death-rate in one or more of the countries examined. This failure does not appear when segregation is tested over the

---

[1] Comparisons have been freely made in this inquiry between the condition of different countries at a given period as regards food, housing, etc. ; but the necessity of caution in making a similar comparison between different countries as regards segregation has been emphasised. The reason for this is obvious. Such factors as a given amount of food, of house accommodation, wages, etc., mean much the same in any country, and can with approximate accuracy be compared with the corresponding phthisis death-rates in each country. It is otherwise with segregation until we can obtain more accurate measures of its duration and its character as well as of the number of segregated persons. Administrative variations like those shown in the experience of Ireland are enormous ; and country can only be compared with country so far as the general trend of observation goes. Each country needs separate study as to the contents of any institutional segregation which its statistics show.

same countries, and it is therefore necessary to extend the inquiry over a wider area in order to make sure that the continued concordance was not fortuitous.

The death-rate from phthisis in Norway (1904, p. 30) was—

1881-90.	1891-1900.	1901-02.
141	189	192 per 100,000 of Population [1]

In 1902, of the total deaths in Norway 5·9 per cent. occurred in hospitals and lunatic asylums. The average duration of treatment of all the patients treated in hospitals in 1902 was 35 days. It is evident, therefore, that there is comparatively little institutional treatment of sickness in Norway as a whole, together with increasing phthisis. Separate hospital statistics could not be obtained for Christiania, but facilities for hospital treatment are doubtless more extensive than in the rest of Norway, and there has been considerable fall in its phthisis rate.

No Swedish statistics for the entire country are obtainable.

TABLE LXXII

Death-rate per 100,000 of Population from Phthisis

	1861-70.	1871-80.	1881-90.	1891-1900.
All Swedish towns together . .	306	324	300	270
Stockholm	433	406	346	292
Gottenburg	279	326	322	303
All other towns	195	299	277	256

Stockholm is the only town of Sweden showing any marked decline in its phthisis rate. The detailed statistics show, both in small and large towns, either insignificant declines, or a stationary phthisis rate. There are few hospitals in Sweden, as shown by the following extract from the report to the Paris Congress on Tuberculosis (1905, p. 205) :—

" Notwithstanding the excellent general organisation of Swedish hospitals, only a small number of consumptives can be treated in them, owing to the fact that the great majority of the hospitals were organised only for the case of acute diseases. The official figures for 1890–1900 show that only about 1500 tuberculous patients have been treated each year in all the provincial hospitals of the kingdom, while the number of

[1] See footnote on p. 213.

patients suffering from tuberculosis is about 60,000 (1905, p. 4)."

Stockholm is better furnished with hospitals than the other towns, and it alone shows any decline of phthisis, though its death-rate is still very high.[1]

As regards Denmark, statistics are obtainable only for Copenhagen. These have been kindly furnished by Dr. E. M. Hoff.

TABLE LXXIII.—COPENHAGEN

Phthisis and Hospital Treatment

Years.	Phthisis Death-rate per 100,000 of Population.	Percentage of the Total Deaths from Phthisis which occurred in Hospitals.	Cases of Phthisis treated in Hospitals Per Cent. of Total Deaths from Phthisis in the Population.
1860–64 . . .	307	...	...
1865–69 . . .	297	...	...
1870–74 . . .	342	...	...
1875–79 . . .	314	...	...
1880–84 . . .	289	30	77
1885–89 . . .	251	27	88
1890–94 . . .	205	25	83
1895–99 . . .	183	28	80
1900–04 . . .	149		147

Evidently there is, as Dr. Hoff states, a large amount of institutional treatment of phthisis in Copenhagen ; and he adds that the average number of days' treatment for each patient has in recent years increased much more rapidly than the number of patients. More recently, further particulars have been published (1905, p. 7). It is stated that—

" Notwithstanding the enormous increase of accommodation required, owing to the growth of the town and new ideas concerning phthisis, up to the present all requests for admission have been satisfied ; and no consumptive desiring to be admitted has hitherto been refused owing to lack of room."

In 1895, on an average 40 beds in the municipal hospitals were always · occupied by consumptives (deaths from phthisis

---

[1] R. Koch quotes Carlsson's statement that 410 cases of pulmonary phthisis are being cared for in the hospitals of Stockholm, " no small number for a city of 300,000 inhabitants " (*Lancet*, 26, v. 1906, p. 1450. Nobel Lecture on " How the Fight against Tuberculosis now stands ").

in that year in Copenhagen, 661) ; in 1904, the number of beds thus always occupied was 270, not including the Sanatorium of Boserup (deaths from phthisis in Copenhagen in 1904 were 632). The mean duration of treatment of three successive series of cases of phthisis, in years 1890–1904, was as follows :—

TABLE LXXIV.—COPENHAGEN

	Mean Duration of Stay in Hospital in Days.	Mean Duration of Stay (Days) in Hospital of Patients	
		Dying in the Hospital.	Leaving the Hospital.
Series I. . .	40	42	40
„ II. . .	107	112	105
„ III. . .	107	98	110

The reduction of phthisis in Copenhagen, therefore, has been associated with a large amount of institutional treatment of the disease in general hospitals. The co-variation of the phthisis death-rate for Copenhagen during the period of 1880–1904 and of

TABLE LXXV

Years.	Prussia.			Berlin.		
	Rate per 100,000 of Population of		For every 100 Deaths from Tuberculosis the Number of Patients with Tuberculosis treated in Hospital was	Rate per 100,000 of Population of		For every 100 Deaths from Tuberculosis the Number of Patients with Tuberculosis treated in Hospital was
	Deaths from Tuberculosis.	Cases of Tuberculosis treated in General Hospitals.		Deaths from Tuberculosis.	Cases of Tuberculosis treated in General Hospitals.	
1877–80 . .	319	43	14	337	231	69
1881–85 . .	311	53	17	332	255	77
1886–90 . .	291	65	23	294	282	96
1891–95 . .	248	77	31	244[1]	291[1]	119
1896–1900 .	212	91	43	213	313	147
1901–02 . .	192	124	64	210	284	136

[1] Returns for 1891 missing.

the deaths from phthisis which occurred in the hospitals of Copenhagen is summarised in a correlation coefficient of ·57. When segregation is measured for the same period by the proportion of cases of phthisis treated in hospitals to total deaths from this disease, the coefficient of correlation with the phthisis death-rate is ·68.   These figures (Table LXXV.) express a fair co-variation between segregation as measured above and the phthisis death-rate.

Table LXXV. shows that, while in the whole of Prussia the number of cases of tuberculosis treated in general hospitals has increased from 14 for every 100 deaths from this disease in 1877–80 to 64 per 100 deaths in 1901–02, the death-rate from tuberculosis has declined from 3·19 to 1·92 per 1000.   Similarly in Berlin the number of cases treated in Berlin has increased from 69 per 100 deaths from this disease in 1877–80 to 136 per 100 deaths in 1901–02.

There is reason for believing that the duration of treatment as well as the number of hospital patients has increased.   It will be noted (Table LXXV.) that the proportion of cases treated in hospital was greater throughout in Berlin than in Prussia. Collateral evidence shows that the duration of treatment of each patient has been shorter in Berlin than in Prussia.   Approximately while Berlin had 153 beds (for all patients in its general hospitals) for every 100 in Prussia, it had 241 patients for every 100 in Prussia, for equal populations.

The above experience is summarised in correlation coefficients between the annual returns of segregation and of phthisis or tuberculosis death-rates of ·95 for Berlin and ·93 for Prussia, showing close co-variation of the two phenomena.

It will be remembered that the general hospitals indicated above are not sanatoria.   The limited operation of the latter has already been described on p. 254.

In Brussels the death-rate from tuberculosis has declined from 3·21 per 1000 in 1886–90 to 1·97 in 1901–03.   In the two great hospitals of Brussels (St. Jean and St. Pierre) the number of deaths from tuberculosis to every 100 in the whole city was 12·2 in 1886–90, 15·6 in 1891–95, 17·3 in 1896–1900, and 38·9 in 1901–03.   I am unable to obtain further information as to the character and duration of the hospital segregation of consumptive patients in Brussels, but the experience of Brussels appears to fit in with that of Copenhagen and of English towns. The correlation coefficient between the annual segregation ratios from 1888 to 1903 and the corresponding phthisis death-rates in Brussels is ·76.

In 1902, 4828, *i.e.* 41 per cent. of the total deaths from tuberculosis of the lungs and larynx in Paris occurred in its public hospitals. The average duration of stay in hospital of all patients admitted to its general hospitals was only 23·6 days in 1901 (Dr. J. Bertillon). The institutional treatment of phthisis in Paris is very short, and can have but little effect in preventing infection. We have already seen that in Paris there is probably no considerable decline of the death-rate from phthisis, and that it remains much higher than that of any other city for which statistics have been obtained.

There is among the medical profession of Paris an impression that the Paris hospitals are a focus for tuberculous infection. Thus, M. Mesurier states that the hospital attendants " suffer cruelly from contagion in the wards, two-thirds of them becoming tuberculous (1905, p. 9)." He states also (1905, p. 16) that the hospitals contain 30 to 40 per cent. of consumptives. On the other hand, Dr. S. Bernheim, Vice-President of the Société Internationale de la Tuberculose (1905, p. 173), states :—

" The Paris hospitals scarcely suffice for patients suffering from acute diseases, and can only, in view of their number, exceptionally admit consumptives. Furthermore, all the hospitals in our large centres of population, were they restricted to the treatment of tuberculosis, would not suffice for a tenth part of the consumptive poor of these towns."

The two statements here quoted can be partially reconciled by the fact that Paris hospitals are generally so overcrowded that consumptives make a very short stay in them.

Dr. Bernheim, in a later paragraph, says :—

" A consumptive never improves in our hospitals. We can allow the death in one of our beds of a consumptive with cavities ; and, on the contrary, the curable consumptive has his fever increased in the presence of patients with serious lesions ; and, in the inevitable overcrowding, rapidly passes beyond the first stage of the disease, and on leaving the hospital has no further prospect of recovery. In this sombre statement I leave out of consideration the contamination of the hospital ;

and do not wish to speak of the unhappy typhoid patient who often leaves the hospital with consumption which he has acquired there."

On the whole, it may be said that in balancing the possibilities of infection in Paris homes and hospitals, it is doubtful on which side the dangers are greatest. These hospitals, with a few exceptions, cannot under recent conditions be regarded as institutions tending to reduce total infection. As a whole, neither the extent of accommodation nor the average length of treatment is comparable with what is found in other countries. This, coupled with the uncertainty of the death returns, would make it unsafe to include the French statistics, even if they were available, in the consideration of the problem.

In the cities of the United States a considerable and increasing proportion of cases of phthisis are institutionally treated. In Cincinnati, in 1885, 18·6 per cent., and in 1902–04, 34·6 per cent., of the total deaths from phthisis occurred in its public institutions. In San Francisco, in 1885–87, 30 per cent., and in 1902–04, 38 per cent., of the total deaths from phthisis occurred in its public institutions. In New York, in 1884, the death-rate from phthisis was 3·86, in 1903 it was 2·40 per 1000 of population. In 1882-84, 22·0 per cent., and in 1901–03, 26·0 per cent., of the total deaths *from all causes* occurred in public institutions. Dr. Hermann Biggs writes me that he cannot give separately the number of deaths from phthisis in the public hospitals of New York ; but he states that a census of tuberculous patients in the public institutions in the boroughs of Manhattan and the Bronx has been taken twice a year for a series of years, and that the number of beds available for phthisis has greatly increased. At the present time there are 2100 to 2200 beds, chiefly for the care of advanced cases. Fifteen years ago the number specially devoted to this purpose was scarcely more than a quarter of this number, certainly not in excess of one-third. He adds that in little more than a year they will probably have over 3000 beds for tuberculous patients : though even this number is insufficient. The number of deaths from phthisis in Manhattan and the Bronx in 1903 was 5250. This implies— assuming the above beds to be always occupied—that every advanced case of phthisis in the city has had in recent years an opportunity of being segregated in a hospital during 21 weeks. Doubtless a smaller number, representing the poorest and therefore the most dangerous part of the phthisical population, were segregated for a correspondingly greater part of the year.

During the years 1881–1903 the coefficient of correlation between the phthisis death-rate and the proportion of deaths occurring in public institutions was ·75. This figure in itself shows a well-marked co-variation of the phenomena in question. Its significance is the more notable when it is considered in connection with the amount of overcrowding in New York.

CHAPTER XXXVI

THE RELATIVE INFLUENCE OF INSTITUTIONAL SEGRE-
GATION AND OF OTHER MEASURES FOR THE CON-
TROL OF TUBERCULOSIS

THE results disclosed by Chapters XXVIII. to XXXIII. may be said to have added nothing of practical value to the knowledge described in Part I. of this volume. They indicate the probability that tuberculosis is affected to a greater or less extent by general sanitary conditions, town life and over-crowding, and the various elements of well-being ; but the probability disclosed in this way is not so strong as that result-ing from the facts given in Part I., which indeed place the con-nection beyond doubt. Neither line of investigation, however, has succeeded in measuring the respective extent of influence exerted by the important factors in question.

The experience of institutional segregation differs from that of the other factors of the death-rate from tuberculosis, both because the nature of its influence on the prevalence of the disease cannot be inferred with certainty from the facts given in Part I., and because not only the nature but the relative extent of this influence is demonstrated clearly from the statis-tical results. On theoretical grounds it has long been recognised that the institutional segregation of patients suffering from an infectious disease may influence its prevalence in two ways. It may restrain the disease by segregating foci of infection from the general population, or it may spread it by exposing to infection from these foci persons in or about the institutions not suffering from the disease in question. With tuberculosis it has till recently been a moot point whether these theoretical results actually appear in practice, and which of them is the more important. The records of segregation analysed in the pre-ceding pages give a decided answer to this question. Each group of records shows, not as a matter of hypothesis or theory, but as the teaching of actual experience, which gives the final touchstone for final conclusions and action, that with no more precautions than are taken in well-conducted general infirmaries the increase of institutional segregation has been associated with reduction of tuberculosis in the community affected by it ; and that the segregation of a decreased proportion of the total bulk of tuberculosis has been associated with an increase of the disease. The scale of the observations and the number of communities examined is so large as to eliminate the chance that this correspondence has been due to mere coincidence ; and it follows that these associations of segregation, with the prevalence of tuberculosis, have not been accidental, but have occurred because segregation has had an influence on the disease, and because it has done more to restrain infection than to spread it.

By comparing the several experiences of the communities examined, we have been able to obtain information as to the relative importance of institutional segregation and of the other factors of the death-rate from tuberculosis. We have examined the records of a large number of communities exhibiting the respective variations of the several factors affecting the death-rate from tuberculosis side by side with the variations of this death-rate. Each of these factors was thus tested in the actual experience of many large communities over the same period of history. In the series of communities subjected to this test, institutional segregation was the only factor of which the variation was always associated with a variation in the prevalence of tuberculosis in a constant relative direction. It would not have been surprising had the influence of institutional segregation been masked by that of opposing factors, as has been seen (p. 221) to have occurred in many countries with the important influence of urbanisation ; or contrariwise, it would not have been surprising if more than one influence had varied with the prevalence of tuberculosis in a constant relation. In either case the question as to which influence had predominated in affecting the prevalence of tuberculosis would have been left open. In fact, however, no influence except that of institutional segregation has appeared in actual experience in a constant relation to the amount of tuberculosis, and it must therefore be accepted as having been the predominant influence.

The administrative consequences flowing from this result are obvious in principle from what has been stated previously, and further reference in detail is made to them in Part III. (p. 394).

Some general reflections may be permitted as to the method by which the result has been obtained. It has involved necessarily much repetition of inquiries concerning the factors of the prevalence of tuberculosis as the experience of each country came under review ; in many of these experiences questions subordinate to the main issue have had to be asked and answered by further reference to communal experience in order that doubts arising in the course of the investigation might be eliminated. The presentation of the argument would have been far simpler and easier if the number of these reiterations had been reduced and the doubts ignored ; but the results would have been inconclusive and intellectually dishonest. Those who have read this section attentively may have found some or all of it tedious and wearisome ; the collection, calculation, and above all the conspective criticism of its data has certainly been far more tedious and wearisome. Such, however, is the condition upon which alone the records of communities large enough to be worth studying by this macroscopic method will consent to give up their secrets.

The experience which these records contain is not arranged in the orderly sequence of a text-book, but is intermingled in an almost endless intricacy. The chief difficulty in handling it lies in arriving at the assurance that the material examined is sufficient for the purpose in view. The temptation to stop short of what is necessary for sound conclusions does not lie mainly in the reluctance to continue the protracted labour of accumulating, arranging, and comparing data ; nor to persons of elementary scientific honesty does it consist in the fear that continued investigation may upset conclusions previously reached ; but rather in the fact that many of those whom the solution most concerns may decline to follow the more detailed argument associated with protracted investigation, when it becomes as intricate as it has to become if the results of the investigation are to be trustworthy. Such investigations are apt to be judged by summaries which are often imperfect, misleading, or even inaccurate ; and the work is subjected not to the welcome criticism which is based on equal labour, but to random and often irrelevant conjectures, hypotheses, and speculations.

Although the continued search for the full truth may, as indicated above, even obstruct its recognition, no part of the search can be omitted with safety. The attempt to find a royal road to truth and to express it as a whole by suppressing essential parts, leads too often to indolent work and slovenly thought ; and this in the public health service is not to be tolerated. We are not engaged in academic labours, of which the prize shall go to the winner, and it is at the choice of each man to neglect his preparation. The servant of public health is working on the lives of men, and should be laying the foundations of national prosperity and happiness. He belongs to an order of sanitary priests, and if he forms or announces conclusions without having used fully and faithfully the material at his disposal, he belies his vocation and abuses his trust. " The day is short, and the work is much, and the labourers are slothful, and the reward is great, and the master of the house presses."

NOTE ON CORRELATION COEFFICIENTS

The coefficient of correlation between two columns of figures is a number, never greater than unity, which expresses the closeness with which deviations of figures in one column from their mean value follow deviations in the corresponding figures of another column from their mean.   In the case of perfect direct correlation, *i.e.* when all corresponding deviations from mean values vary in the same sense of excess or deficiency and bear the same ratio to each other, the coefficient is 1 ; in the case of perfect inverse correlation, where the senses of variation in corresponding pairs of figures are opposite and the ratio of their magnitudes is the same, it is –1 ; and it may have any intermediate values according to the nature of the case.   The closer the coefficient is to ± 1, the nearer is the approach to constant co-variation of the pairs of figures ; and where no influences but those represented by the figures are operating, a high correlation coefficient on a sufficient number of figures is the numerical expression of strong inductive evidence that there is some connection—whether causal or otherwise is a matter for subsequent discussion—between the phenomena represented by the two groups of figures.   In practice it is rare for two groups of phenomena to be free from disturbing influences ; and the correlation-coefficient measures therefore for practical purposes the influence of one group of phenomena on the other to such extent as it predominates over or is assisted by the other influences in operation.   Within certain limits the manner in which the deviations are measured may vary according to the circumstances of the case. The effect of any such variation would, however, only be to alter the final result by a relatively small amount ; and coefficients of correlation, computed on any single system, represent the closeness of relations between such curves as appear in Part II. far more distinctly than any general impression that can be derived from mere inspection of the curves. The usual form taken for this coefficient is the ratio of the arithmetical mean of the products of corresponding deviations in each group of figures from the arithmetical means of the values in the respective groups to the product of the square roots of the arithmetical means of the sums of these deviations squared ; that is to say

$$\frac{\frac{1}{n}\Sigma(xy)}{\sqrt{\left(\Sigma\frac{x^2}{n}\right)}\sqrt{\left(\Sigma\frac{y^2}{n}\right)}},$$

where x and y are the deviations from the arithmetical means of the respective series.

Without discussing the precise mathematical reasons for the selection of this form of coefficient and the processes by which its validity is demonstrated, it is worth while to verify the fact that, by whatever mathematical considerations the coefficient in question may have been obtained, it is a quantity of which the magnitude must always depend on the closeness with which the phenomena to which it refers stand in some relation to each other. This may be seen very shortly. It can be shown by simple algebra, and is here assumed to have been proved, that this fraction can never be greater than 1. If the two groups of phenomena were unconnected by any causal link whatever, that is to say, if there was no reason why a deviation x_n of any figure in one group from the arithmetical mean of that group should be accompanied by a deviation $\pm y_n$ of dependent magnitude and constant relative direction in the corresponding figure of the other groups, then in any long series of pairs the deviation of figures in each group from the arithmetical mean would be as often positive as negative, and their values would be distributed evenly on each side of the mean. Hence the products of the pairs of deviations (xy) of which the sum (Σxy) forms the numerator of the fraction will be as often positive as negative, and when added together with their proper signs will exactly balance each other, and the sum will be 0. In other words, when there is absolutely no causal link between the phenomena, this correlation coefficient will become 0. If there is any causal link, then to such extent as they are governed by the causal relation the figures expressing the phenomena will always deviate from their respective arithmetical means in a common direction or always in opposite directions ; the members of every pair of corresponding deviations will in every case be either both greater or both less than the arithmetical mean of their respective groups (i.e. always $+x$ and $+y$ or always $-x$ and $-y$), or else in every case one will be greater and the other less (i.e. always $\pm x$ and $\mp y$). Therefore the products of which the sum enters into the numerator will either always be positive or always be negative, and the sum total of the products will accordingly be either a positive or a negative quantity of which the magnitude will depend on the number of terms to be added. It follows therefore that the more the co-variant terms, the larger will be the numerator ; and as the whole coefficient can never exceed ± 1, the closeness with which its value approaches ± 1 will be a measure of the closeness with which the phenomena under examination are connected by cause directly or inversely.

PART III

MEASURES FOR THE REDUCTION AND ANNIHILATION OF TUBERCULOSIS

CHAPTER XXXVII

GENERAL NATURE OF PREVENTIVE MEASURES:
INDIRECT MEASURES

IN Part I. and Part II. of this volume we have discussed in full the causation of phthisis, and the factors which have produced the decline already secured in the death-rate from this disease. It has been seen that, on the one hand, an infective agent, the tubercle bacillus, is the essential agent in causation, and that, on the other hand, various influences other than infection favour or inhibit the spread of the disease. If our review of the factors of past decline of phthisis is correct, the diminution of infection outweighs in importance the diminution of the conditions favouring infection, though historically the two have been acting in combination in most countries. To remove infection most completely we must have the earliest diagnosis of disease. The early recognition of an infectious disease is therefore the first step in preventive measures against it. The cases recognised thus early must then be notified to those whose duty it is to inaugurate and ensure the execution of measures against further spread of infection, and to discover its source in the notified case. This must be some other case of the same disease, either human or animal ; and the detection of the source, when practicable, will enable wider measures to be taken against infection ; while at the same time the removal or improvement of the conditions, which in the instance in question have favoured infection, will aid in preventing the occurrence of further cases. Around the notified case centre our further preventive measures, which are none the less preventive in character because they consist largely in the most effective treatment of the patient himself. Wherever practicable, the sanatorium treatment of the patient at an early stage will be secured, with a view to his cure and to his being trained in the details of the hygienic life which offers

him the best prospect of recovery and of efficiency after returning home. Should recovery not be secured, the hospital
treatment of the patient, especially if he is poor and cannot
secure good nursing at home, is indicated at a later stage ; and
if he recovers but partially, the conditions for modified work
under favourable conditions need careful consideration. All
these and many allied problems require to be studied, and
some attempt at stating the principles of action is made in the
following chapters. In this chapter we may now consider in
outline the indirect measures against phthisis, which in the
aggregate are very important in its prevention.

INDIRECT MEASURES AGAINST PHTHISIS.—*The Teaching of the
Laws of Health.*—Of these measures the most important of all
is the inculcation of the laws of health. Hygiene should be
one of the most important subjects in the curriculum of every
scholar in the higher classes of our elementary schools, and
every teacher should be thoroughly competent to teach it.
In a paper read before a Conference of Medical Officers of Health
in 1890, I pointed out that as the entire school population
passed through the higher standards in our elementary schools,
we had here the means of systematically teaching the science of
health to at least six-sevenths of the entire population of the
next generation; but that for this purpose " it was necessary that
teachers competent to teach the subject should be provided."
The same opinions have been frequently expressed ; and it is
satisfactory to find it stated in a circular issued by the Board
of Education in November 1907 that that Board " are urging
the necessity of giving special instruction in the principles of
hygiene to all students in every type of training college, so that
they may be able to deal profitably with this subject in the
schools." With such teaching in schools and the correlative
practice of school hgyiene, each school will gradually become
an example of the application of the laws of health, and the
homes of the people will quickly benefit also.

Fresh Air and Cleanliness.—In such a scheme of teaching
hygiene the importance of an abundance of fresh air, of strict
cleanliness of person and environment, and particularly of avoidance of dust, will be emphasised ; and thus something will be
done towards securing three great conditions for the prevention of
phthisis. The importance of nasal breathing will also be taught,

as a means of filtering the incoming air, and of preventing the formation of adenoids, which are a favourite nidus for tubercle bacilli. If, as appears to be the case, artificial feeding with the ordinary bottle-teat, and particularly the constant use of the " dummy-teat," favour the production of adenoids, an additional reason is furnished for the abolition of the latter and the encouragement of breast-feeding of babies. The dangers of dust illustrate the need for having school-drill and all gymnastic exercises on dustless floors and in an atmosphere which approximates to that of the external air.

Ill-nutrition and Fatigue.—Defective nutrition may favour tuberculosis, either by allowing latent foci to come into activity or by favouring new infection. Over-fatigue is a contributory influence similar to ill-nutrition, in which the toxic effect of the products of fatigue replaces the effect of inanition ; and in context with over-fatigue, it is convenient to group the ordinary occupational disadvantages which combine with over-fatigue to lower the inhibitory powers of the workers, favouring catarrhs, and rousing into activity foci of infection, which may have remained latent in the bronchial or other lymphatic glands for many years (pp. 74 and 137). In the poor the two often unhappily coincide. If food is carefully chosen, even the very poor seldom suffer from dangerous mal-nutrition ; but if bread and tea alone take the place of porridge, cheese, herrings, with bread and other very cheap but highly nutritious foods, mal-nutrition opens the way to a dangerous extent to invading tubercle bacilli. Over-fatigue probably causes a much larger number of attacks of tuberculosis than mal-nutrition, and much of the excess of pulmonary tuberculosis among men as compared with women is due probably to this. It is not suggested that there is not abundant infection in the workshops ; nor that the dust of workshops is not largely responsible for the result under consideration. If a reliable test for the limits of physiological fatigue were applicable, which would eliminate the element of personality in the testing, and would enable work to be given in accordance with individual fitness, much avoidable disease might be prevented. At present we are without any such test, capable of being used in practical life.

Alcoholism.—Alcoholism, like excessive fatigue, loads the circulation with toxic matter, diminishes the normal phagocytic action of the body cells, and makes the individual more prone to every form of infection, and especially to tuberculosis. As already seen, alcoholic indulgence, when it involves the frequenting of public - houses, implies increased risk of infection by tuberculosis (pp. 159 and 181; and it is scarcely practicable in most instances of phthisis among the intemperate to distinguish between the two factors. It is fairly clear, however, that even among those classes of intemperate persons, who have not been exposed to convivial infection, an excessive death-rate from phthisis prevails.

Poverty.—There is no need to reconsider in detail the relation of poverty to phthisis, as Part II. is largely devoted to this problem. Poverty and tuberculosis are allied by the closest bonds, and nothing can be simpler or more certain than the statement that the removal of poverty would effect an enormous reduction of the death-rate from tuberculosis. It is, however, essential in order to secure clear conceptions of causation, to investigate; differentially in various communities the separate operation of overcrowding, ignorance, mal-nutrition, increased opportunities for infection, as constituent elements of poverty. This has been done in pp. 224 to 255, and the preceding remarks as to the teaching of hygiene, the removal of over-fatigue and mal-nutrition, the encouragement of alcoholic temperance, and of cleanliness, represent the practical issue of this investigation. There remains to be considered the influence of housing.

Housing Conditions.—Although the death-rate from phthisis is not proportional to the quality of the housing accommodation in compared communities (pp. 225 and 229), the death-rate from this disease in any given community is always higher among those badly than among those more favourably housed (p. 147). That improved housing is not the *main* influence determining the past decline in the death-rate from phthisis is shown by the evidence given on pp. 227 and 228. This does not imply that improved housing accommodation is not imperative in the public interest, but only that such improved accommodation has not been the *predominant* influence in causing the decline of the death-rate from phthisis.

Other things being equal, however, every improvement in conditions of housing will secure a diminution of tuberculosis. This applies both to structural and to functional conditions of housing ; to improvement in respect of light, air, and ventilation ; and to improvement in internal cleanliness of dwelling-rooms, and diminution of overcrowding. Dwellings to which light gains free access will always be kept cleaner than dark and sombre dwellings; sunlight has a special purifying action of its own (p. 53). But even more important than these important structural conditions is the manner of using the dwelling-rooms. The structural improvements owe a large share of their importance to the fact that they render internal cleanliness easier, and its absence more quickly detected. In many houses, unfortunately, bedrooms are overcrowded, while other rooms remain partially or completely unoccupied. The teaching of the laws of health, the reduction of the waste of money on alcoholic drinks, the elevation of the moral standard, must gradually diminish this variety of overcrowding. As already indicated, the best means for diminishing the risks of overcrowding is to secure the institutional treatment of the sick (pp. 149 and 224), especially of the tuberculous sick. This brings us back to the evil done by overcrowding in favouring the spread of infection ; in this chapter we are concerned with its action in lowering the resistance to infection ; and although this must be placed on a lower platform than the direct effect in spreading infection, every effort must be made persistently to spread out the sleeping accommodation of each family over all the rooms available for this purpose, and to insist on the increase of this accommodation as required. This latter problem is one of the most difficult in practical sanitation. To secure its complete solution involves a wider attack on the problems of poverty, and an increase of the family income in some instances, and in others a determined attempt to prevent the waste of the family resources in dissipation and gambling (see also p. 206).

CHAPTER XXXVIII

THE EARLY RECOGNITION OF PHTHISIS IN RELATION TO ITS PREVENTION

THE NEED FOR BETTER ORGANISATION OF MEDICAL TREATMENT.—For both its successful treatment and the complete prevention of spread of infection, phthisis must be recognised at an early stage. A very large proportion of cases, especially those occurring among wage-earners, are not diagnosed until some such serious symptom as pleurisy or hæmoptysis (spitting of blood) occurs. Even when pleurisy occurs, this acute disease is often treated without the phthisis which it commonly indicates being diagnosed. Under the present conditions of medical treatment immediate improvement in the expedition with which phthisis is diagnosed cannot be anticipated. For the working man can seldom afford to leave his work until actually disabled; and too often he cannot afford to pay a doctor's fee for treating a cough, which he may regard as of comparatively small importance. The provident system of medical attendance has not been generally successful in this country, and is not likely to become so in the absence of compulsory membership. Even when adopted, its full benefits have not been secured, in part owing to the absence of arrangements for consultations, where necessary, with physicians having special experience in chest ailments. My views on this point, which has a most important bearing on the prevention of tuberculosis, are set forth in the following remarks taken from a recent address (Sept. 1907).

Doctors have never been doing so much and such good work on behalf of the public as at present ; but this work is being done under conditions involving the petty worries of fee-collecting, the stress of competitive commercialism, the strain of work which for most doctors is excessive in order to secure a " living wage," and the " sweating " of the medical profession by hospitals, friendly societies, and similar organisations. The doctor earning his livelihood among the artisan and labouring classes not only has to do excessive work under harassing conditions without leisure, but he is in a large measure cut off from consultation with doctors having special knowledge in the very considerable proportion of complicated cases which come under his care. To the patient in the same classes the conditions are equally unsatisfactory. However willing he may be to pay the doctor's fee—which may be as low as 1s. 6d., or even 6d. —his limited means necessitate delay in obtaining medical aid until compelled by urgent symptoms, and necessitate dispensing with this aid at the earliest possible moment. He realises also the absence of skilled consultation in difficult cases, and that by attending at a hospital to which his employer has subscribed, or to which he in his workshop has given his penny a week, he may have an additional chance of being thoroughly overhauled, and of securing special skill. Even if the patient is a member of a club or provident dispensary, similar reflections apply under the present unco-ordinated conditions, in which facilities for skilled special consultations are not organised. Thus, in a large proportion of the total mass of sickness, the medical welfare of the public is not secured, partly because the rates of remuneration of club doctors and of doctors attending the poor are so scanty that only doctors of exceptional mental and physical capacity can afford time or energy to examine each patient thoroughly, and partly because medical consultations cannot be secured in difficult cases.

The following are some of the principal respects in which the present medical service frequently fails :—

1. *Diagnosis is belated.* This is inevitable for the largest proportion of the population, under circumstances which involve payment of a fee or seeking for a hospital letter and then waiting several hours in an out-patient department. The dangers of delaying diagnosis are too well known to need detailed consideration. . . . In chronic infectious diseases, like phthisis, the difficulty of obtaining early diagnosis is nearly as great as with acute infectious diseases, and in non-infectious diseases the normal condition among the masses of population, especially those who do not belong to clubs, is to shirk medical advice until it becomes relatively ineffective.

2. *Treatment is curtailed* and its efficiency diminished by similar considerations of expense.

3. When patients are treated under present circumstances in dispensaries and in out-patient departments, the *waste of time* involves a serious economic loss to the community.

4. There are no co-ordinated arrangements for *medical consultations* in all difficult cases.

5. *Valuable information as to the incidence of disease* is wasted under the present conditions of medical service.

6. There is *a great waste of information as to the existence of conditions conducing to disease*, which might promptly be removed under more systematised conditions of medical attendance. At the present time sanitary inspectors and health visitors are busily engaged in inspecting houses, without medical knowledge and with only haphazard and very occasional information of the conditions in the households of the poor, which the poor-law medical officer, the dispensary doctor, and the " 6d. doctor," know to be aiding the continuance of disease and preventing its banishment. The one set of officials, unless indefinitely multiplied, cannot properly locate the foci of mischief ; while poor-law and dispensary doctors and the doctors generally among the poor are in possession of information of urgent importance to the public health; information which, under present conditions of inco-ordination, is almost entirely lost. Overcrowding and dampness of the house occupied by a bronchitic or consumptive patient, the uncleanly and careless nursing of children, the numerous minor cases of food poisoning, are examples of conditions of direct importance to the public health ; and the present system must be regarded as both extravagant and inefficient, inasmuch as it fails to bring all available information concerning such conditions systematically and punctually to the knowledge of a properly organised system of preventive medicine. My meaning will be made clearer by giving a practical instance of co-ordination in further detail. It must be noted that the co-ordination required in the interests of the public health is not solely that between all medical practitioners, preventive and curative, but also between them and such officials as sanitary inspectors, health visitors, and nurses ; and the efficiency of co-ordination may be measured by the extent to which steps taken for the control of a single disease are

applied without cost to the direct control of general sanitary conditions.

The experience of Brighton in the notification of pulmonary tuberculosis is an instance of successful co-ordination of measures for the treatment and prevention of this disease with those for the entire public health control of the town. The Public Health Department of the town is the focus of all the measures—prophylactic, curative, and sanitary—which are taken in the treatment and the prevention of this disease. The officer who visits the notified case obtains full particulars of the sanitary condition of the patient's home and secures the necessary disinfection and sanitary improvements. He obtains information as to the health of other occupants of the house, and directs them into the avenues of medical relief, supplying hospital letters when a private doctor cannot be afforded. He arranges the removal of the patient to the sanatorium if the doctor considers this desirable, and there the patient is trained and treated, so that when discharged there is little risk of his continuing to infect others. It will be seen that under such an arrangement—an arrangement which would be improved under a system in which the doctor himself would to a large extent take the place of the inspector—one visit serves several ends, and automatically, and without expense, the information which it affords is distributed to the departments really concerned. By this co-ordinated arrangement an economy of time, energy, and money is secured, which would be impracticable if separate authorities administered the departments concerned. . . . Hospital reform, as a measure by itself, would not cure either the grievances of the public or of the medical profession. Even were all free dispensaries and all out-patient departments of hospitals abolished, the willingness and competence of patients to pay sufficient fees would not thereby be increased, nor would the ability of the general practitioner to do excessive work for insufficient pay.

Yet at the present time the coexistent but unco-ordinated systems have failed lamentably to provide what the health of the community requires—means for ensuring effectively the early recognition and proper treatment of all disease. I hope and believe that what has been done already towards securing this end is merely a phase in the evolution of the system which will attain it ultimately. The total expense under a co-ordinated system, worked with due economy, might or might not be greater than that entailed under the present inefficient and unco-ordinated system ; and it may be asked whether the increased cost can be justified economically. The economical justification, as I have already indicated, will be found in the decrease of sickness which must follow, with the corresponding decrease of poverty and inefficiency and invalidity ; in other words, the economical, like the medical, justification and commendation of a complete medical service consists in its being a branch of a general service of preventive medicine.

I see no reason to expect that such a medical service, whether partial or general, would tend to deprave any part of the community morally, any more than the system of free (that is rate-paid) education has tended to pauperise the parents of the children who benefit by it. There would be, I think, no difficulty in proving that each additional form of medical aid officially given up to the present time, so far from undermining self-help, has imposed new duties and responsibilities on the recipients of such help ; while in the aggregate these measures have been largely instrumental in securing the immense improvement in the public health already realised.

Some essential features of the medical service to which I look forward will be obvious from my previous observations. At present we have medical officers of health dealing with sanitation and the prevention of infection, poor-law medical officers dealing with sickness under the most adverse home circumstances, school doctors and nurses knowing nothing or next to nothing of the home conditions which baffle their work, factory surgeons out of touch with local public health administration, and a large body of private practitioners daily in touch with environmental evils that they cannot remove. The picture which this mere enumeration calls up of work which overlaps in some directions and leaves serious gaps in other directions, and which in both instances means an enormous waste of knowledge of enormous value to the public health, shows that systematic co-ordination is indispensable to medical as well as to economical efficiency. The considerations previously advanced indicate that on all grounds the extended medical service must be primarily a preventive service. It must be a medical service for the general community and not merely for its sick members, and must call into activity every individual and collective means for the preservation of health as well as for the cure of disease. Information of preventive value must no longer be allowed to run as at present into culs-de-sac, but must be utilised to the full extent for the public welfare. This can only be effected when preventive medicine is regarded as a whole, and the many fragmentary portions of it—now unconnected and relatively inefficient—are no longer allowed to continue relatively impotent ; and when every branch of curative medicine is included in its scope.

THE REMOVAL OF IGNORANCE.—Next in importance to the removal of all hindrances to early treatment comes teaching the public the significance of the early symptoms of tuberculosis. This will doubtless be done in connection with the instruction in hygiene in the higher classes of elementary and other schools. Such facts as the following if thoroughly realised would go far towards annihilating this disease.

1. Consumption is curable, in the majority of instances, if treated at an early stage.

2. Every cough not yielding to ordinary treatment within a limited period, indicates the necessity for (a) thoroughly examining the patient's chest, and (b) examining the patient's expectoration for tubercle bacilli.

3. Every case of pleurisy must be regarded as likely to be followed by consumption, failing persistent attention to a hygienic life.

And there is no reason why this knowledge should not be impressed upon every boy and girl before leaving school, as well as upon those who have already left school. At the same time it should be made plain that scrofulous glands, abscess of bones, and some deformities of the spine are due to tuberculosis.

On the part of doctors practising among the masses of the population much more needs to be done to ensure the early recognition of tuberculosis. More time needs to be spent in ascertaining the antecedents of each patient, his exposures to infection, and the method of onset of the symptoms from which he is at present suffering.

DIAGNOSIS BY HISTORY.—Symptoms otherwise obscure are often at once elucidated when an accurate history is obtained from the patient. The occurrence of languor and lassitude, of occasional " bad colds " or " bronchitis," of a persistent cough for some weeks, of indigestion and " anæmia,"—one or more, or all of them at different times—may indicate merely passing sickness, or may form the early symptoms of phthisis ; and the significance of these symptoms can often be discovered by obtaining an accurate domestic and personal history from the patient.

The diagnosis by history,—aided by such symptoms as the above,—is in reality a diagnosis of

THE SO-CALLED PRÆ-TUBERCULOUS STAGE.—Reference to the schemes on pp. 64–70 and 75–77 shows that there is strong reason for believing that in many cases of phthisis years of primary latency have elapsed between the reception of the tubercle bacilli with the formation of the first nodule of disease, and the first recognisable symptom of disease. In some cases, doubtless, resistance is steadily and increasingly lowered by the reception of further doses of infective material. In other cases, active tuberculosis is due probably to the quickening of the long latent primary foci. This stage of primary latency cannot correctly be called a præ-tuberculous stage, as infective nodules are already present; but it is known under this name, and in it no clinical evidence of tuberculosis is found. It is in this stage that the greatest good can be done.

The patient can be suspected of being tuberculous, and action taken accordingly. Given a complete system of notification of phthisis, or a system fairly complete among the classes whose children attend public elementary schools, it is possible to pay special attention to the children of notified cases. This is already done to a considerable extent, but action on these lines is capable of wide extension. In Brighton the notified cases, chiefly parents, are removed to the Borough Sanatorium for a month's treatment and education in the management of their illness ; and hospital tickets are pressed on any members of the family who show the least sign of failing health, and who cannot afford a private doctor. Scholars from such families should receive special preference in any scheme for providing country holidays. They are already given special preference in the provision of free breakfasts and dinners for the poor in connection with elementary schools. Extensions of action on these and allied lines, combined with the more frequent medical inspection of children from tuberculous families than of other children, will gradually ensure the early diagnosis and the preventive treatment of the members of suspected families.

LOSS OF WEIGHT.—In persons of tuberculous family history periodical weighing is one of the best means of ensuring the early recognition and treatment of disease. The weight should be taken and recorded at least four times a year—once a month if there is any reason for anxiety. If along with loss of weight, or in children failure to increase in weight, the patient's temperature is apt to rise for apparently small reasons, the suspicion of tuberculosis is increased.

TUBERCULIN TESTING, ETC.—Of means for the early detection of tuberculosis, other than physical examinations and the testing of the sputum, the use of tuberculin is the best known. The value of this test in the detection of bovine tuberculosis is well established; though, as Sir .J. MacFadyean has pointed out—(1) an animal may not react for some considerable period after infection ; (2) a distinct reaction may be unobtainable in some advanced cases of tuberculosis ; and (3) in a considerable number of cases a second reaction is not possible for some days or weeks after the first. It appears therefore that the reaction when it occurs is trustworthy, but that a negative result is less reliable. Although there are differences of opinion on the point, its general use as a means of diagnosis of disease in man is to be deprecated, in view of the possibility mentioned by Dr. J. E. Squire that it seemed to him to " cause an increased activity in the tuberculous focus."

CALMETTE'S OPHTHALMIC METHOD.—A local method of using tuberculin as a means of diagnosis has been described recently by Calmette, which may prove to be valuable. He places inside the eyelid one drop of an aqueous solution of a precipitate obtained by adding 95 per cent. alcohol to tuberculin. If conjunctivitis develops within twenty-four hours, it is stated to be proof positive that the patient is suffering from tuberculosis ; no inflammatory reaction seems to occur in other than tuberculous patients. If more detailed investigation shows that this method of employing the tuberculin product is harmless and free from fallacy, it promises to be very valuable in the diagnosis of obscure complaints which may be tuberculous. If it should lead to the general adoption of an earlier treatment of tuberculosis than has hitherto been secured, it will be an immense boon.

OTHER SPECIAL MEANS OF RECOGNITION.—The Röntgen ray photograph of a chest in which there is an early tuberculous focus sometimes shows a shadow at the affected part. This is by no means a certain means of diagnosis, and cases have been described by Theodore Williams and others in which the physical signs (by percussion, auscultation, etc.) revealed evidence of disease not shown by the Röntgen rays. In fact, no special means of diagnosis will supersede the necessity for

(a) careful physical examination of the patient, and

(b) bacteriological examination of his sputum for tubercle bacilli.

PHYSICAL EXAMINATION.—In cases in which there is cough with or without expectoration, in which the patient has repeated " bad colds," or in which even without these symptoms a patient with a tuberculous family history suffers from indigestion, anæmia, or languor, a thorough examination of the chest by a competent doctor is indicated. Such an examination will frequently detect the presence of lung disease, either before there is expectoration or before tubercle bacilli can be found in it.

The occurrence of jerky breathing or of feeble inspiration is suspicious. A scattered fine sibilus, often heard only on deep inspiration or expiration, was emphasised by Sir William Broadbent as important. When the physical signs are more marked and there is dulness and crepitation after coughing, the diagnosis is relatively easy, and the disease is scarcely at its earliest stage.

EXAMINATION OF SPUTUM.—Very commonly the disease is first recognised when tubercle bacilli are found in the expectoration. This cannot be regarded as satisfactory, for the occurrence of expectoration and the presence of tubercle bacilli in it mean that the encapsulation of the tubercle nodule by the surrounding tissues has ceased to be effective, and *closed* has been transformed into *open* tuberculosis; non-infectious into infectious disease. For weeks, months, or even years in very slight cases the tubercle bacilli may not find their way out of the body.

Thus Allbutt quotes Turban as failing to find tubercle bacilli in the sputum in the first stage in 59·8 per cent. of 408 cases.

And yet in actual public health experience of the notification of phthisis, surprise is frequently expressed by doctors when sputum sent by them for examination at the public health laboratory shows tubercle bacilli. It is clear therefore that the possibilities of early diagnosis of phthisis are not realised in a notable proportion of cases. It must be added, furthermore, that each year a considerable number of specimens of thick purulent expectoration are sent for official examination, from patients who have been treated—usually for bronchitis—for months before this step towards complete diagnosis is taken. I append a copy of the form of certificate of results of examination of sputa which is in use in my own office.

PUBLIC HEALTH OFFICES,

TOWN HALL,

_____190___

Dear Sir,

     I beg to inform you that the specimen of sputum from

_____

*of*_____

*has been examined, and tubercle bacilli were*_____

_____

_____

Yours faithfully,

_____

Dr. _____   *Medical Officer of Health.*

NOTE.—The failure to find the tubercle bacillus does not, of course, prove that the patient from whom the specimen was taken is not suffering from pulmonary phthisis.

Tubercle bacilli can sometimes only be found after repeated examinations.

The early morning expectoration should preferably be sent for examination.

The patient's address should be given when each specimen is sent.

CHAPTER XXXIX

THE MEDICAL PRACTITIONER IN RELATION TO PREVENTIVE MEASURES AGAINST PHTHISIS[1]

THE PATIENT MUST NOT BE KEPT IN IGNORANCE.—When the presence of phthisis has been ascertained, the first duty of the doctor is to inform his patient. Anxious relatives will occasionally urge him not to do so, but the cases in which he is justified in withholding the information in my opinion are few ; and both relatives and the patient can with intelligent explanation be made to understand that it is in the latter's interest to secure intelligent co-operation between him and the doctor. Phthisis is an eminently curable disease. Its cure is hastened and rendered more certain if the patient is convinced of the necessity for and the wisdom of adopting the prescribed measures, — both the treatment in the more limited sense of the word, and the treatment which consists in care as to sputum, thus diminishing the danger of re-infection.

WHAT DANGER IS THERE OF INFECTION IN PHTHISIS ?— The relative infrequency of infection of hospital nurses by tuberculosis is important from the medical practitioner's standpoint, as a study of it supplies him with the main indications for safeguarding the health of the relatives and attendants of his own consumptive patients. He is already aware that the channels of infection are limited. The following scheme sets forth the main dangers. This scheme does not pretend to be logical or exhaustive, but it serves to draw attention to some of the more important points :—

[1] A large part of this chapter has already been published in an Introductory Address given by the author at the Mount Vernon Hospital for Consumption, on " The Relation of the Medical Practitioner to Preventive Measures against Tuberculosis," *Lancet*, January 30, 1904, p. 282.

I. The infection.
1. Dose.
2. Cumulative dosage.
3. Closeness of contact.
4. Lack or absence of precautions.
5. Defective ventilation and cleansing of rooms.

II. Receptivity.
1. Inherited.
2. Acquired.
1. Exhaustion from nursing, etc.
2. Depressing emotions.
3. Insufficient nutrition.
4. Defective ventilation and cleansing of rooms.

In hospitals, long before the communicability of phthisis was recognised, expectoration was received into spittoons and large dosage of infection was thus prevented. Similarly hospital wards have usually been well ventilated and kept scrupulously clean, all surfaces both of walls and floors being washable. Again, hospital nurses are not so long on duty as wives or other relatives, the contact between them and the patient is less intimate as well as less prolonged than that of home nurses, they have periodical holidays, are well fed, and are not subjected to the same extent to the influence of depressing emotions or of insanitary house conditions. They are better trained in regard to the washing of hands and other personal precautions. In view of the above circumstances, the difference between the infectivity characterising phthisis in hospital and in private practice is easily understood.

I can imagine no better means of converting those who underrate the infectivity of tuberculosis than the task of administering the notification of this disease in a large town, of interviewing some 300 patients each year, of examining over 200 patients who are yearly treated for a month or more each in a borough sanatorium with a view to train them so as to diminish the probability of their continuing sources of infection, of obtaining the family and personal histories of each of these, and tracing, as one gradually comes to do, links of infection, which, although individually they may not be conclusive, when connected together become as convincing as any evidence can ever be regarding a communicable disease of chronic course.

DUTY OF THE DOCTOR TO THE PATIENT AND TO THE PATIENT'S FAMILY.—The first duty of the family practitioner in relation to a case of phthisis obviously is to do his best for the patient. Incidentally his position by implication involves that he is, at least partially, the guardian of the health of the patient's family. Happily, the interests of both patient and relatives are identical, and the measures most conducive to the patient's recovery will also give the maximum protection to the other occupants of the same house.

Having (1) made an early diagnosis of the disease, and (2) acquainted the patient and his relatives with the nature of the disease, the further indications for the doctor are : (3) to investigate and, if possible, ascertain the most likely source of the patient's infection ; (4) to treat the patient (under this head will come not only dietetic and medicinal treatment, but the question of sanatorium treatment and the control of the general hygiene of the patient) ; (5) to train the patient to control his cough, as far as practicable to cough and to expectorate only when means are available for preventing the dissemination of infective matter, to train him to live in the open air, to eat heartily, and to attend to every detail of personal hygiene ; and (6) to protect the attendants on the patient from infection, from over-fatigue, from impaired nutrition, carefully training them on the same lines as the patient himself, whose recovery depends largely on the state of their health.

INVESTIGATION OF SOURCES OF INFECTION.—The investigation of possible sources of infection may appear to be somewhat remote from the duties of the family practitioner, and yet success in the treatment of the patient may be wrapped up in the fulfilment of this indication.   The three most common sources of infection are : (1) domestic, (2) occupational, and (3) public-houses.   So far as domestic infection is concerned, in well-to-do families the medical adviser will have the opportunity of investigating possible unrecognised sources of infection in the same household.   In poorer houses this is not so.   The patient is treated as a club patient or at the dispensary or hospital. Domestic sources of infection cannot then be recognised by the medical attendant.   Even if he sees the patient at home he has no time to investigate the case fully.   It has been my frequent lot in visiting phthisical homes to find other unrecognised patients suffering from chronic tuberculous disease and innocently spreading more acute tuberculous disease to husband or wife or children.

If infection can be shown with some degree of probability to have been acquired in a dusty workshop or shop, an indication for treatment is at once obtained.   Even if the occupation

cannot be altered, the conditions of the workshop may be favourably changed, and if the medical officer of health and the
practitioner come into touch at this point the conditions of the
workshop can be improved and the patient's chances of recovery
increased without the slightest risk to the patient's pecuniary
welfare. At this point, however, we trench on the question of
notification of the case to the medical officer of health, and the
action which would follow such notification (p. 338).

If the patient is alcoholic, to insist on a change in his
habits in this respect, given that the patient's confidence
can be secured and that he is open to conviction, is the
best means not only of preparing him intelligently to carry out
his instructions and of enabling him to recover the resistance to disease which has been lowered by alcoholic indulgence, but also of stopping those visits to the public-house
which, as Dr. J. Niven has indicated, are a frequent means of
infection.

RELATIVE MAGNITUDE OF THE RISKS OF EXTERNAL AND
AUTO-INFECTION.—It may be urged that once phthisis is started
its subsequent course is determined not by external but by
internal infection, and that consequently the detection of the
sources of infection or even of other cases of phthisis in the
same house is not important from the private practitioner's
standpoint. This point is one of real importance. In the
card of precautionary instructions, of which a copy is given
on p. 324, the following sentence occurs : " The patient himself
is the greatest gainer by the above precautions, as his recovery
is retarded and frequently prevented by renewed infection
derived from his own expectoration."

Is the prevention of auto-infection by expectoration, which
has been already ejected from the mouth, important ? It is
well known that tubercle travels from one part of the body
to another by the lymphatics or blood vessels. It is also agreed
that healthy persons are infected chiefly by inhalation or ingestion of infective dust or by direct infection by minute particles
of ejected sputum. The patient is perhaps not likely to be
re-infected directly by the spray of his own sputum, but may
if this becomes dry ; and he may receive more massive re-infection if no precautions are taken to prevent the inhalation,
as dust, of desiccated sputum, or the swallowing of his own

sputum. I am unaware of any exact facts as to whether such re-infection is an important factor in the downward progress of the consumptive when considered in comparison with the auto-infection caused by the cross-inhalation of infective mucus into other bronchioles than those first affected; but whether the danger be greater or less, the swallowing of sputum should be prohibited, and experience shows that the improvement of the consumptive is greatest in those cases in which there is the most rigid care to prevent re-infection by dust, whether because in this way re-infection by the tubercle bacillus or because secondary infection by other micro-organisms is prevented. I attach much importance to the value of these precautions in preventing danger to others than the patient. Self-interest is a potent motive for beneficence.

THE EFFECT OF SWALLOWED TUBERCULOUS EXPECTORATION. —The occurrence of self-re-infection by swallowing expectoration is well established. Various statistics give the proportion of cases in which intestinal ulcers are found after death from phthisis, as from one-fourth to three-fourths or more of the total cases. The coincidence between tuberculosis of lungs and intestines might be due to the intestinal ulcer having been the primary seat of disease; but that this is not the correct explanation is indicated by the fact that intestinal ulceration is a late phenomenon in phthisis. The intestinal disease must therefore in most instances be due to spread of tuberculosis from other parts of the body, or to the swallowing of large quantities of tuberculous expectoration. That the last is most usually the explanation is shown by the fact that intestinal ulcers are much more rarely found where the lung is not implicated, and very rarely in general tuberculosis. Experimental observations point to the same conclusion. Cornet records that out of over 3000 animals on whom he experimented otherwise than by feeding, only in about eight cases were tuberculous foci found in the intestine and in isolated mesenteric glands. The extreme frequency of intestinal ulceration in young children and in the insane, who nearly always swallow their expectoration, points to the same conclusion.

On the other hand, instances occur in which prolonged swallowing is not followed by intestinal ulceration. It is likely, also, that in a certain number of instances of such ulceration infection has been received from the blood current, and not by the direct contact of tuberculous expectoration.

The evidence points clearly to the importance of the doctor warning his patient against swallowing his sputum. Some French physicians have gone so far as to advise washing out the mouth with a mild antiseptic after each attack of coughing ; but this does not appear to be necessary or likely to be carried out even if recommended.

THE DOCTOR IN RELATION TO DISINFECTION.—Assuming that a doctor is called in to a case of phthisis, and that up to that time no precautionary measures have been taken, his duty is not fulfilled by insisting on the adoption of all the measures enjoined in such a set of " precautionary instructions " as those given on p. 324. Infection has been repeatedly shown to cling to the lower part of the wall and to the floor of the consumptive's room. It also hangs about his pockets, bed-hangings, etc. If the doctor is to do the best for his patient he must rid him of old infective material. And he cannot in the majority of instances do this alone. He must in the interest of his patient call in the aid of the medical officer of health, who can arrange for efficient disinfection of the room and its belongings. Then, with a rigid system of cleanliness, re-infection of the room and repetition of danger from this source to patient and relatives can be greatly diminished.

THE DOCTOR IN RELATION TO NOTIFICATION.— Such an intimation of desire for disinfection is almost tantamount to a voluntary notification of the case to the medical officer of health ; and this voluntary notification can in the case of private patients be made only with the consent of the patient or his guardians. There are other reasons why such a voluntary notification is desirable.

1. The medical officer of health will probably be in a better position than the practitioner to detect the possible source of infection and thus to minimise any likelihood of continuance of infection when the patient resumes his occupation, etc.

2. The medical officer of health can not only enable the patient to " start fair," as indicated above, but he can do much to remove any insanitary conditions of home, workshop, or shop tending to retard recovery. It may be urged that sanitary authorities already have the power to abate overcrowding

and to insist on the cleansing and ventilation of houses, work-shops, etc. But sanitary officials are neither omniscient nor omnipresent, and their work is most productive of good when directed especially to houses in which the presence of a case of phthisis renders overcrowding, uncleanliness, and other insanitary conditions supremely dangerous. Without an army of inspectors it is impossible completely to control overcrowding and dirtiness of houses, and the notification of this disease gives valuable additional leverage in securing the abolition of minor insanitary conditions, the continuance of which is detri-mental to the consumptive.

3. The most conscientious and indefatigable doctor can usually only ensure the carrying out of a portion of the measures which I have ventured to bring within the range of his legiti-mate duties. He may do so if his patient is wealthy and intelli-gent. He certainly cannot if his patient belongs to the working classes, who contribute the vast majority of the cases of phthisis. Between these two extremes are patients in whose behalf a varying degree of intervention on the part of the local authority is required. There is no wish on the part of such authorities or their officers to interfere, but only to help. If proper steps for preventing indiscriminate expectoration, for destroying any infective material already deposited by the patient, and for tracing possible connections with other cases of phthisis, have been taken, the less the intervention of any one between the medical man and his patient the better. But in actual practice most phthisical patients have medical men in attendance only at intervals, and for a short portion of their total illness. Visits of an educational character are certainly needed in the intervals of professional attendance, if not also while the latter is in opera-tion. In actual experience in Brighton, although a considerable number of cases of phthisis have been notified in private as well as in dispensary and hospital practice, no appreciable friction has been caused by my visit or those of my assistants, and a large amount of carelessness as to the disposal of sputum has been thus stopped.

THE DOCTOR IN RELATION TO SANATORIUM TREATMENT.—A further duty to his consumptive patient devolves on the family practitioner. He has to decide whether he can secure for his patient the best medical and hygienic treatment at home, or whether a temporary stay in a well-organised sanatorium is needed. These points are more fully discussed in Chapter XL. As a rule, it may be said that both educationally and therapeutically the patient is benefited, and his relatives are freer from danger of infection if such a course of sanatorium treatment and teaching has been secured.

In the preceding remarks the ideal position of the medical practitioner in relation to tuberculosis has been indicated. Therapeutical measures are in the widest sense measures of prophylaxis, and the aid of measures of public and private hygiene is as indispensable to cure as are therapeutical measures. But the doctor in the majority of cases—*i.e.* those of the working classes—can scarcely be said to be the " family " doctor. Even in the higher social strata his efforts at prophylaxis may be hampered by prudential and other considerations, and he cannot undertake those wider inquiries which are required in order most completely to stop the sources of infection. Clearly, then, everything indicates the necessity of co-operation between doctor and medical officer of health, and the more complete this co-operation the greater is the benefit to the consumptive patient and to every member of the public.

CHAPTER XL

THE CONSUMPTIVE PATIENT IN RELATION TO PREVENTIVE MEASURES AGAINST PHTHISIS

ASSUMING that the patient has consulted a doctor who is imbued with the ideal view of his duties suggested in the last chapter, the duty of the patient is clear, though it necessitates a steady persistence in well-doing, which implies moral courage and perseverance as well as intelligent acceptance of the duties involved.

The patient will have handed to him a set of instructions, of which the following may be taken as an example. They will be amplified and explained more fully by the doctor. It may be added that in Brighton these cards are printed by the Corporation without any official headings or names, in order that every doctor may distribute them to his own patients.

The instructions are as follows :—

PRECAUTIONS FOR CONSUMPTIVE PERSONS

Consumption is, to a limited extent, an infectious disease. It is spread chiefly by inhaling the expectoration (spit) of patients which has been allowed to become dry and float about the room as dust, or by directly inhaling the spray which may be produced when a patient coughs.

Do not spit except into receptacles, the contents of which are to be destroyed before they become dry. If this simple precaution is taken, there is practically no danger of infection. The breath of consumptive persons is free from infection, except when coughing.

The following detailed rules will be found useful, both to the consumptive and to his friends :—

1. Expectoration indoors should be received into small paper bags and *burnt* immediately ; or into a receptacle which is emptied down the drain daily and then washed with boiling water.

2. Expectoration out of doors should be received into a suitable bottle, to be afterwards washed out with *boiling water*. If a paper handkerchief is used, this must at once be placed in a waterproof bag, the contents subsequently burnt and the bag washed daily.

3. Ordinary handkerchiefs, if ever used for expectoration, should be *put into boiling water before they have time to become dry* ; or into a solution of a disinfectant, as directed by the doctor.

4. *Wet* cleansing of rooms, particularly of bedrooms occupied by sick persons, should be substituted for " dusting " and " sweeping."

5. *Sunlight* and *fresh air* are the greatest enemies of infection. Every patient should sleep with his bedroom window *open* top and bottom, a screen being arranged, if necessary, to prevent direct draught.

6. The patient should, whenever practicable, occupy a separate bedroom. *Children should never sleep in the same bedroom* as the patient.

N.B.—The patient *himself* is the *greatest gainer* by the above precautions, as his recovery is retarded and frequently prevented by renewed infection derived from his own expectoration.

7. Persons in good health have little reason to fear the infection of consumption. *Over-fatigue, intemperance, bad air, dusty occupations, and dirty rooms favour consumption.*

Cure and Prevention are inseparable.—The first point needing to be grasped by the patient thoroughly is that measures for the cure of and measures for the prevention of consumption are to a large extent identical. Certain drugs have their value in treating consumption ; cod-liver oil is equally valuable in treating it and in preventing its development ; most other remedial measures used in the treatment of consumption would be still more effective if employed in preventing it.

The essential points in the treatment of consumption are—

(1) the prevention of further infection ;

(2) the prevention of the inhalation of dust of any kind ;

(3) the improvement of nutrition of the patient ;

(4) regulated rest until the disease has become entirely quiescent.

The first of the above points has been discussed on p. 319. The patient, as well as those about him, gains by observance of the precautionary measures as to coughing and the disposal of sputum. By avoiding the swallowing of sputum, he also minimises the chance of secondary intestinal infection.

The prevention of the inhalation of dust is an essential point in the treatment as in the prevention of consumption. It has been already seen that this disease is most prevalent among those engaged in dusty occupations ; and one of the great gains in sanatorium treatment is that the patient breathes a relatively dustless and aseptic atmosphere.

Similarly with regard to mal-nutrition and over-fatigue, the probability of recovery from consumption and of successful resistance to its infection, other things being equal, are both increased by diminishing or removing their operation.

HOME TREATMENT.—These points being settled, we may consider in detail the part which the patient has to play in curing his disease and preventing its spread. In this chapter the matter will be considered from the standpoint of the treatment of the disease at home. The following are the main points :—

(1) There must be no spitting into handkerchiefs, nor should handkerchiefs with which the mouth has been wiped be placed under the pillow. The exact details as to the disposal of sputum are given in Chapter XLI.

(2) If linen handkerchiefs are used at all, they must not be allowed to get dry after being used, but placed in water to which some washing-soda has been added. It is best, however, to use paper handkerchiefs or rags which can be burned.

(3) During coughing the patient must always hold something in front of his mouth.

(4) A fire in the bedroom always helps ventilation, and is useful for burning rags, etc.

(5) Cups, knives, spoons, etc., must be placed in boiling water containing some washing-soda before being again used.

(6) There is no need to sprinkle the floor of the room with disinfectants. Washing with soap and water suffices.

(7) The floor should be uncarpeted except for a rug at the bedside. The best plan is to have the floor covered with linoleum, washing this daily. The floor should *never* be dry-

swept. All articles not washable should be wiped with a damp duster. Curtains and other hangings are best discarded.

(8) The walls should be periodically cleansed, especially the part between the floor-level and about a yard above the level of the bed. Four methods of cleansing and disinfection are commonly adopted ; the help of the officials of the Sanitary Authority can be obtained in carrying out one of these :

(a) The wall-paper if dirty should be stripped off and burnt.

(b) A solution of chlorinated soda may be brushed on the walls.

(c) Formalin spray (1-50) may be employed.

(d) The German method of rubbing down the wall with bread-crumbs, and then burning the crumbs, may be adopted.

(9) The patient's room should be carefully chosen, so as to be convenient for nursing, and to enable the patient to get into the garden whenever practicable.

(10) The ventilation of the room should be specially studied. As a rule, the window and the door should both be kept wide open, and generally—by means of screens or otherwise—this can be arranged without leaving the patient in a disagreeable current of air. If the bedroom has two windows, there is no difficulty in securing the perflation of air which is desirable. The question of open doors and windows must be decided in each case according to circumstances. Gradually the amount of fresh air should be increased ; and a sanatorium-treated patient will seldom wish to go back to the imperfect ventilation which passes muster in most households. On the other hand, nothing is gained by increasing the discomfort of a dying patient.

(11) The thoughtful patient will save his nurse as much trouble as possible. She must have a sufficiency of sleep, exercise, and rest, and must not take her meals in the bedroom. The patient must further protect her by always placing a hand-kerchief in front of his face when coughing.

THE PATIENT'S OCCUPATION.—The preceding scheme of action is concerned chiefly with the patient's home-life. It has to be borne in mind, however, that during a large part of his illness he is still following his occupation. Commonly, if a wage-earner, he has drifted from the more to the less laborious occupations, and from the ranks of the steady wage-earners to the ranks of the casual workers. But in a large proportion of cases, the patient for a year, or even for many years, keeps at his work in the factory, workshop, shop, or office. As a rule, it is better that he should do so, than that in consequence of vague advice " to get a lighter job in the open air " he should drift into a condition of unemployment, he and his family suffering in consequence from ill-nutrition. If there is a definite prospect of more suitable work, it should be taken ; but it is of little use, for instance, to advise a clerk to become a farm labourer or even a market gardener, unless he is unusually strong and the disease is very early.

Assuming that the patient must keep to his present indoor occupation, what advice should be given ? It should first of all be urged upon him to come into a sanatorium for a month to receive the short course of treatment and teaching which is described on p. 349. If he continues his occupation after a month thus well spent, he is much more likely to do so without danger to others, and with a prospect by careful living of pro-longed work, than would otherwise have been possible for him.

The further advice needed consists chiefly in the avoidance of over-fatigue and of the inhalation of dust, and the proper use of his spit-bottle. This can be used judiciously, so as not to attract attention. In his home-life the ex-patient has the opportunity of counteracting to a large extent the influence of an unfavourable occupation. He can sleep in the open air, take judicious rest, and in other ways, so far as his means permit, follow the régime, the principles of which he has learnt while in a sanatorium.

The Patient in relation to the Sanitary Authority.— If compulsory notification of phthisis is in force in the town in which the patient lives, the doctor in attendance is required to notify the patient's illness to the medical officer of health. If such notification is invited under a voluntary system, the patient has it within his choice to prevent such notification. By so doing he will be acting unwisely in his own as well as in the public interest. This somewhat bold statement needs perhaps elaboration and proof, which it is not difficult to supply. In the first place, it can be made clear that *the patient will suffer no disability by having his case notified*. Thus the statement that " as soon as they made known that a man was a victim to the disease they advertised him as a dangerous person, and the public would continue to believe that," ignores the fact that notifications are confidential, that the information does not pass beyond the householder, that so long as the patient takes reasonable precautions as to his sputum, there is no interference with his home-life or his occupation.

In the absence of grave mal-administration the notion that notification will involve any interference with a man's occupation may be banished as unfounded. At the same time, it is true that, quite irrespective of notification, the public have become much more alive to the possibilities of infection in phthisis, and have ofttimes taken exaggerated action concerning it. The best means for reducing such fears to their proper magnitude is to be able to reassure the public that every case of phthisis is notified and the proper precautions have been taken.

Secondly, the patient himself benefits from notification so far as both his domestic and industrial circumstances are concerned. (a) *Domestically* the patient has offered to him any disinfection that may be required in the interest of himself and his family. For the poor, sputum bottles and paper handkerchiefs are supplied. Under a well-organised system of notification, sanatorium treatment is offered (see p. 347). If any sanitary defects are found in the house, these are remedied. Damp walls, unventilated staircases, windows that do not open top and bottom, all militate against the patient's recovery, and may be remedied as the result of an official visit.

(b) *Industrially* the patient only benefits indirectly. No visits to patients are made at workshops or shops, in any town with the administration of which I am acquainted. To make such visits would be a foolish mistake. But, quite apart from the patient himself, workplaces are visited, and defects discovered and remedied, the remedy of which might otherwise have been greatly delayed. No Sanitary Authority possesses a sufficiently large staff immediately to discover all sanitary defects. Very few Sanitary Authorities have a staff of sanitary inspectors sufficiently large to enable them to visit each house and workplace in their district once annually. In the intervals of such visits conditions of overcrowding, dirtiness, and dustiness may long prevail. These conditions are much more dangerous where there is a case of phthisis than elsewhere. The notification of cases of this disease enables houses and workplaces in which such visits are particularly important to be visited at more frequent intervals, a great gain to the public health being thus secured.

Thirdly, the patient by allowing his case to be notified is contributing to the general health of the community. The notification of his case may lead not only to the removal of insanitary conditions favouring the spread of disease, but also to the discovery of other untreated cases in the same household; and by comparison with the official records may lead to the discovery of particular workplaces or of particular areas of a town in which phthisis is exceptionally rife.

CHAPTER XLI

THE PREVENTION OF INDISCRIMINATE EXPECTORATION

THE proper control of spitting and disposal of the sputum are probably the chief problems in the prevention of phthisis. They therefore deserve a special chapter, and by this means repetition of instructions can be avoided in other chapters. The closely allied question of instructions for coughing with proper safeguards is considered on p. 326.

As already seen, consumptive patients may discharge billions of tubercle bacilli daily in their expectoration (p. 104). This may be dangerous immediately while being scattered as fine spray; or after having become dried and pulverised, it may be subsequently suspended in the air and inhaled.

Indiscriminate spitting is much less dangerous in open places, for instance in a road, than in houses, public-houses, or other places of public resort, especially if these are dark and over-crowded. Dr. H. E. Annett (1902) collected by means of sterilised swabs 105 specimens of sputum deposited in the streets of Liverpool. Five of these were proved to contain virulent tubercle bacilli. Apart, however, from such actual deposits of expectoration, it is fairly certain that tubercle bacilli can seldom be found in the dust of streets in places protected from direct expectoration. The explanation of this is not far to seek. Notwithstanding the large amount of indiscriminate expectoration in streets, many factors tend to cause tubercle bacilli to perish within a limited period. When exposed in thin layers, direct sunlight kills them in a few minutes or hours and diffuse light in a few days. The cleansing of streets by rain or by road watering must have a very beneficial effect, both in washing the bacilli into the sewers and in preventing their dissemination as dust. At the same time expectoration in streets is an undoubted source of danger, especially when this expectoration is carried home on the skirts of ladies' dresses or on boots, etc.

How should the consumptive patient dispose of his sputum indoors and out of doors ?

INDOOR DISPOSAL OF SPUTUM.—The problem indoors is easily solved. A special spit-cup must be kept for the patient. If the amount of expectoration is not very great, it is a good plan to line this spit-cup with butter-paper, and then the daily expectoration can be easily emptied down a water-closet or slop-closet into the drain. A disinfectant is unnecessary in the spit-cup under ordinary circumstances ; but care must be exercised to ensure that the outsides of the cup are not fouled, and that flies are not allowed access to it. The spit-cup after being emptied should be washed out in boiling water containing some washing-soda, and subsequently washed again, before being used. If the expectoration is abundant and adheres to the sides of the spit-cup, it is convenient to render it less adhesive, and aid its removal from the spit-cup, by adding some soapy disinfectant to it before emptying it down the drain. If there is no water-closet system, the sputum should be burned, or if this is impracticable it should be boiled. In a sanatorium the spit-cups should be cleaned and sterilised with boiling soda solution, which may be done in a special apparatus heated by coal, gas, or steam. In this way the cleansing is effected with less trouble, and sterilisation is rendered certain. Floor-spittoons should never be tolerated. After expectoration, the patient's mouth is frequently soiled, and a paper handkerchief should be employed in wiping it. This should be at once burnt, or if this is impracticable it should be placed in the spit-cup. Japanese handkerchiefs suitable for this purpose are purchased by the Brighton Corporation at 5s. a thousand. These measure 14 inches square, and are cut into four before distribution. The patient should also be carefully trained to hold one of these handkerchiefs in front of the mouth while coughing.

OUTDOOR DISPOSAL OF SPUTUM.—A pocket spit-bottle is required for outdoor use. A very good and simple form consists of a wide-mouthed bottle, with a thick rubber stopper. It is easily cleansed, not easily broken, and of a convenient size for the pocket. Such spit-bottles can be obtained at 4d. to 5d. each when a gross are bought ; and both they and the Japanese handkerchiefs mentioned above are suitable for gratuitous distribution in public health administration. The spit-bottle can be cleansed thoroughly with boiling water containing some washing-soda.

It is well to carry the pocket spit-bottle in an indiarubber pouch or in a pocket having a detachable washable lining; and a similar bag should be used for soiled paper handkerchiefs.

THE DISPOSAL OF SPUTUM OF PATIENTS WITH ADVANCED DISEASE.—It is generally recognised that the danger of infection is greatest in advanced cases of phthisis. Objection has been taken to this view, because the sputum of early cases often contains multitudes of tubercle bacilli. Several points, however, need to be borne in mind: (a) Patients with early disease spend a large part of their day away from home, and much of the sputum they expectorate is deposited in the open. (b) Expectoration at this stage is much smaller in amount than at later stages. (c) The patient is not enfeebled by prolonged illness, and he still has the courage and strength to avoid fouling his handkerchief or his bed and body linen. There is a further reason why the sputum of advanced cases of disease is to be particularly feared when they are treated at home. The wife or other attendant is exhausted by prolonged nursing, and depressed by anxiety and sorrow, and is consequently much more liable to be open to infection than at an earlier period.

For these reasons a special importance attaches to the management of the sputum of patients with advanced disease.

Bedridden patients should never be allowed to keep a handkerchief under the pillow or in the bed. It should always be placed in a cleansable receptacle outside the bed. The patient's mouth must be covered with a paper handkerchief or rag while coughing, the mouth wiped with the same paper or rag after coughing, and the material where practicable at once burnt. The attendant's hands should be washed after performing these duties.

PUBLIC REGULATIONS AS TO SPITTING.—In recent years great advances have been made in the control of indiscriminate expectoration. In this country the Glamorgan County Council was the first to obtain the consent of the Secretary of State for the Home Department to a bye-law regulating spitting in public places. As originally drafted, the bye-law ran as follows :-

A person shall not spit on the floor of any public carriage, or of any church. chapel, public hall, waiting-room, schoolroom, theatre, or shop, whether admission thereto be obtained upon payment or not.

Any person offending against this bye-law shall be liable to a fine not exceeding £5.

The Home Office subsequently decided that the bye-law could not properly be made to apply to churches, chapels, schools, and shops, and the bye-law being amended in accordance with this decision came into operation. A considerable number of other Local Authorities have now adopted the same bye-law, the one commonly in force running as follows :—

No person shall spit on the floor, side, or wall of any public carriage, or of any public hall, public waiting-room, or place of public entertainment, whether admission thereto be obtained upon payment or not.

Any person who shall offend against this bye-law shall be liable for each offence to a fine not exceeding forty shillings.

Local Authorities owning tramways have also passed bye-laws forbidding expectoration in them, and prosecutions of persons offending against such bye-laws have been success'ul.

THE PREVENTION OF SPITTING IN PUBLIC-HOUSES, ETC.— In my local experience no difficulty has been experienced in securing the fixing on the walls of every bar of each public-house in the town of an enamelled iron tablet, size 6¾ × 4⅝ inches, having the following words on it :—

PREVENTION OF CONSUMPTION

YOU ARE

EARNESTLY REQUESTED

TO ABSTAIN FROM THE

DANGEROUS HABIT OF

SPITTING

The following correspondence took place before the tablets were exhibited, and it is reproduced here, as it may be useful to others :—

To the Sec., Licensed Victuallers' Association.
    ,,   Beer Sellers' Association.
    ,,   Brewers' Association.

DEAR SIR,—I enclose herewith a draft of a circular letter which it is proposed to send to each publican in the town.

It deals with a very important question, the importance of which with regard to the public health is becoming more and more realised.

The likelihood of securing compliance with the suggestions made in this circular letter would be greatly increased by your co-operation. Would it not be practicable for you to bring the question before your Association at their next meeting, with a recommendation that individual members of the Association should help in bringing about this desirable reform ?

If you have any suggestions to make as to improving the draft circular, 1 should be glad to receive them and to give them every consideration.— Yours faithfully,

MEDICAL OFFICER OF HEALTH

To the Proprietor or Tenant of
              Inn or Hotel.

DEAR SIR,—You will probably have learnt from the public press that it is now generally realised that consumption, which is the most fatal of all the infectious diseases, is spread by inhaling the dried spit or expectoration of patients suffering from this disease. It may not be so well known to you that the mortality from consumption among those engaged in public-houses is much heavier than that of the general public. Our national statistics show that if the deaths from consumption for the average of all men aged 25 to 65 engaged in various occupations be represented by 100, that of innkeepers and brewers is 140 to 148, and of male inn servants is 257.

This excess is doubtless due to the conditions to which those engaged in public-houses are exposed, among the chief of which is the frequent inhalation of dust derived from the expectoration of consumptives. This danger is greatly favoured by (a) the practice of indiscriminate spitting in the bars of public-houses, and (b) the common practice of allowing such spitting on the floor, sawdust being frequently provided for the purpose of receiving it. If expectoration on the floor is to be permitted, the spit should be washed up by means of a mop several times a day, before it has had time to become dry. Sweeping up of sawdust containing it is one of the surest methods of distributing a very dangerous infection to others as well as to the sweeper. The spit or expectoration is not a source of danger (unless directly inhaled when a patient is coughing) in the wet condition. Efforts should be therefore directed towards either *causing it to be immediately burnt in the fire*, or, failing this, *kept in a moist condition* until it can be destroyed.

It may be further remarked that expectoration indoors is very much more dangerous than expectoration out of doors. In the latter case its infectious properties are soon destroyed by sunlight. Hence, customers may fairly be asked to reserve their spitting for out of doors.

It is suggested that the accompanying tablet should be put up in the bar. Further supplies, which it is hoped will be displayed in every public room, may be obtained as desired. It is also strongly urged that no sawdust should be used on the floor, and that the sweeping of floors which may have been spat upon should be entirely discontinued, and daily mopping or washing substituted for it.

Spittoons have not been mentioned hitherto. If not carefully employed, they may increase the danger of infection. The floor around spittoons becomes soiled with spit; and, unless the spittoon contains water or other fluid and is carefully emptied daily and cleansed with actually boiling water, it is a possible source of danger.

I shall be glad to advise with you further on the subject if you think this desirable. If you have any suggestions to make as to practical means of carrying out the principle of prompt removal of the infection derived from dried spit, you will be conferring a public favour by communicating them to me.—I am, Sir, yours obediently,

MEDICAL OFFICER OF HEALTH

There is no difficulty in securing the exhibition of similar notices in each room of common lodging-houses, etc. Most railway companies now exhibit such notices in railway stations and in each compartment of railway carriages.

SHOULD EXPECTORATION IN STREETS BE FORBIDDEN?— When we remember the immense change which has taken place in our national habits as to spitting, it will be realised what progress has already been made in preventing the spread of infection by sputum. Not many decades since nearly every home was supplied with spittoons, and spitting into the fire or fireplace was common. Now spittoons are almost unknown except in public-houses and barbers' shops, and domestic spitting seldom occurs. If it does, the person finding it necessary to spit retires to a lavatory or water-closet. There is still much public nuisance from expectoration deposited on public pavements and roadways, and there must be carriage of infected material from such deposits by means of dress-skirts and boots into houses. It would not, however, be wise to ask for regulations forbidding outdoor expectoration, even though the operation of these was confined to towns, for such regulations would go beyond present public opinion, and would be systematically evaded. It would, however, be well to regulate outdoor expectoration, restricting it to certain defined parts of each street.

A bye-law to forbid outdoor expectoration, except over street gully-tanks, would do much to educate public opinion and keep the streets clean ; and a bye-law which, though less rigid than the above, would forbid outdoor expectoration except into the channel between the roadway and pathway would be beneficial. These bye-laws by calling attention to the need of frequent swilling of the street-channels would conduce to the public health, by the prevention of dust in general as well as in reference to tuberculosis.

CHAPTER XLII

THE NOTIFICATION OF PHTHISIS

U P to the present point we have considered preventive measures against phthisis chiefly in their relation to the patient and his doctor; slightly and incidentally, but viewed from the same standpoint, the relation of the public to the patient and his doctor. It is necessary that this wider aspect of preventive measures should now be more fully defined.

We need not fight over again the battle as to whether the conditions favouring infection or infection itself are the more important. Both are important, and no hygienist would be willing to content himself with removing insanitary areas, improving the ventilation, lighting, and cleanliness of houses, preventing industrial dust, and increasing the nutrition of the poor, without at the same time adopting measures against indiscriminate expectoration, or without, where practicable, removing advanced cases of phthisis from the midst of large families, in which they cannot be nursed suitably without risk to others.

The great advantage of having cases of phthisis notified is not only that each notification enables personal preventive measures to be taken against infection, but also that each case becomes the *point d'appui* for the detection of other hitherto unrecognised cases, and for the discovery and removal of insanitary circumstances and conditions either in domestic or industrial life. It converts the patient from a focus of infection into a focus of prevention.

OBJECTIONS TO NOTIFICATION OF CASES

It is perhaps somewhat belated to consider these, as very few now object to systems of voluntary notification and the action taken thereon, and there is an increasing volume of advocacy of compulsory notification of phthisis. It is, however, convenient to enumerate briefly the main objections which have been urged against notification, as their fallacy is not always recognised as clearly as it should be.

(1) It has been commonly urged that notification of cases is of relatively small value, because most of the cases—even in the absence of wilful concealment—will have been infectious for a long time before being notified, and that therefore attempts to destroy infective material derived from the patient can have only a partial and limited success. I can see no ground for this reasoning. It is agreed that risk of successful infection increases with increased dosage, and it is probable that advanced cases are usually more bacilliferous, or at least eject more bacilliferous sputum than early cases. It is evident, therefore, that at whatever stage precaution is taken, it must reduce the dose of infectious material and the risk of infection which varies with it. But this is really an understatement of the case. The healthy occupants of a tuberculous home may be compared to a city which is the subject of a protracted siege, in which the combined effects of arms, and starvation, and depressing emotions are at work. The inhabitants of such a city may escape with but little damage if the siege is raised at a comparatively early period; but they succumb if it is protracted. Similarly the healthy members of a tubercle-invaded household may be able to withstand infection if precautionary measures are begun as soon as the nature of the disease is detected and are continued thereafter; but they eventually fall victims to the cumulative infection if a fatalistic inertia is allowed to prevail, and no efficient precautions are taken.

(2) In the past some use has been made of the argument that as the tubercle bacillus enjoys a saprophytic existence apart from its human host, measures directed solely to preventing infection from the patient will be ineffective. The same line of answer as to the first objection holds in this case; and the objection involves the assumption, which should be unfounded in actual practice, that notification is not intended to be accompanied by measures of disinfection and cleansing directed against the bacillus in its exiguous saprophytic environment.

(3) The objection that equally efficient action against the defects found after notification can be taken apart from such notification, has already been answered (pp. 321 and 328).

(4) The risk of interference with the patient's occupation has been shown not to exist in practice (p. 329). On this point there has been confusion between the possible but unrealised evil effect of notification, and the independent fact that the public on their own initiative, and apart from notification, have occasionally had exaggerated fears as to the risks of working with consumptives.

THE IMPOSSIBLE MAGNITUDE OF THE TASK?—(5) It has been urged also that as phthisis is, unlike the infectious diseases now notifiable, a disease of protracted duration, the carrying out of official preventive measures is impracticable, and would, if attempted, involve a larger staff than is possessed by any local Sanitary Authority. This objection can be tested by an estimate of the number of cases of phthisis in an average population of 100,000 persons. This will be 380 on the basis of the data given in the table on p. 63. If we assume that there are five cases of active phthisis, each living a year of life in the community in which one annual death from that disease occurs, instead of three as assumed in the table, then there will be 633 cases among 100,000 persons. Many of these cases will need no visits from the medical officer of health or his assistant. To ensure a quarterly visit to 400 of them, about thirty visits would need to be made each week. The number of visits actually needed is much reduced by having consultations at the medical officer of health's office. By this means the cases not actually under a doctor can be kept under supervision with relatively little difficulty, especially when the medical officer of health is the medium through which sanatorium treatment is secured. In a larger population it is simply a question of additional help; but the above figures will show that the amount of help required is much less than has been stated.

LE SECRET MÉDICAL.—(6) The only valid objection is one which, in theory at least, presses hard against a voluntary system of notification. It is that, in the absence of a statutory obligation, the notifying doctor may be laying himself open to awkward consequences. This is a real difficulty, and must necessarily always limit the operation of voluntary notification of phthisis to patients of the poorer classes, and particularly to those treated in connection with the poor law or with public institutions. Among these patients I have found that visits

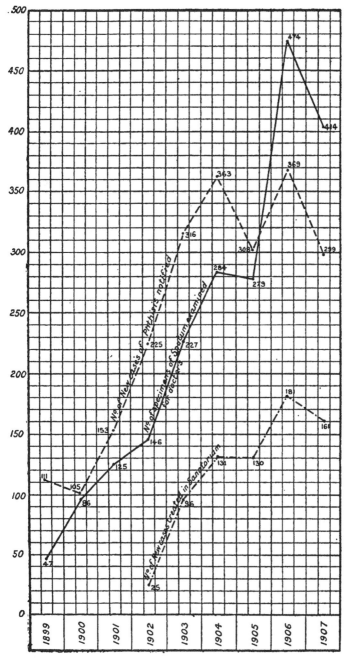

FIG. 37.—Brighton. Showing the parallelism between the number of Consumptive Patients treated in the Sanatorium, of cases of Consumption notified, and of Specimens of suspected Sputum examined

by the medical officer of health are not unwelcome, and that they are grateful for the help they receive in having their rooms cleansed and purified, etc. In our local experience in Brighton, we have secured in addition, under a voluntary system, the notification of a considerable proportion of cases of phthisis among persons above the wage-earning classes. This is owing partly to the fact that in a relatively small town personal influence counts to a greater extent, and partly to the provision of sanatorium treatment for the notified cases. This is shown clearly in the diagram on preceding page.

It will be noticed that specimens of sputum were more readily sent for examination by doctors when sanatorium accommodation became available. It may be added that in 1906, when the available beds at the sanatorium were increased from 10 to 25, a further marked increase of specimens of sputum occurred. The number of cases notified has, I think, approximated towards the maximum ; and, in the future, I look rather towards earlier notification of cases than to any great increase in their number.

In the light of an experience like the above, it is plain that voluntary notification may be practised on a large scale, and without involving any such risks as have been feared. My advice has always been, when consulted on the point by doctors, that they should not notify outside of hospital and dispensary practice, without first mentioning their intention to the patient. When the confidence of the inhabitants as well as of the family doctor has been gained, there is little difficulty in securing the notification of a large proportion of the total cases.

The advantages secured by notification are sufficiently indicated in the preceding pages and on pp. 321 and 328. Even with incomplete notification, a large mass of infection can be brought under control, and circumstances conducing to infection can be minimised.

THE GROWTH OF VOLUNTARY NOTIFICATION OF PHTHISIS.— Nothing is more remarkable in the history of English public health administration than the rapid conversion of the medical profession and of the public to the necessity for the notification of cases of phthisis. The tubercle bacillus was discovered by Koch in 1882, and Cornet's investigations into house-infection were published in 1886. Very soon after this, instructions began to be given to patients at several hospitals and dispensaries, defining the precautionary measures required. As early as 1887 and 1888, Dr. James Niven printed and distributed to every house in Oldham elementary directions for the prevention of infection. In 1892, Mr. C. E. Paget prepared for the North-Western Branch of the Society of Medical Officers of Health a memorandum of instructions in methods of prevention. At a meeting of the parent Society of Medical Officers of Health on August 4, 1893, the following resolutions were passed unanimously on the motion of the present writer :—

That the Society of Medical Officers of Health, while accepting the view that phthisis is an infective disease, in the prevention of which active hygienic measures should be taken, think it premature to recommend the compulsory notification of a chronic disease like phthisis. They are of opinion that it is incumbent on medical officers of health to take such steps as may secure—(a) the voluntary notification of cases of phthisis by medical officers of public institutions and such medical practitioners as agree that precautionary measures are desirable ; (b) the adoption of such precautionary measures, including the disinfection of rooms, as can be arranged in conjunction with the family practitioner. For this purpose the memorandum prepared by the North-Western Branch of the Society of Medical Officers of Health would give an excellent basis of action.

Towards the end of 1893 a scheme of notification recommended by Dr. Niven was adopted by the Oldham Medical Society, and by it urged, though unsuccessfully, on the Town Council. Had it not been for this failure, the voluntary notification of phthisis would, owing to Dr. Niven's pioneer action, have been much earlier adopted in this country than actually occurred. This scheme was published in the *Lancet* on November 18, 1893. In 1894 a voluntary system of notification of phthisis was begun in New York ; while from 1898 onwards the notification of cases of this disease was made obligatory on doctors in that city.

In England the voluntary notification of cases of phthisis was begun in January 1899 in Brighton, and in September 1899 in Manchester, and since then a considerable number of other towns have adopted it, with very varying success. In the following table the extent to which notification has succeeded is shown. In Sheffield compulsory notification of phthisis has been adopted under a special local Act, and its figures are compared with those of other towns in Table LXXVI. It will be noted that the number of cases notified is stated in terms of the total deaths from phthisis instead of in terms of population, in order to give a more accurate proportion between cases notified and total cases (which may be regarded as a constant multiple in each town of the number of deaths from phthisis).

TABLE LXXVI

Number of Cases of Phthisis notified in each Town to every 100 *Deaths from the same Disease*

	1894.	1895.	1896.	1897.	1898.	1899.	1900.	1901.	1902.	1903.	1904.	1905.	1906.
New York (compulsory notification from 1898) . .	94	112	167	201	173	153	137	175	197	211	251	265	...
Brighton (voluntary notification) .	...	...	...	...	...	61	61	93	128	174	209	179	202
Manchester (voluntary notification) .	...	...	...	...	...	38	138	118	112	113	109	142	126
Liverpool (voluntary notification) .	...	...	...	...	...	...	...	139	163	149	116	150	149
Sheffield (voluntary notification to 1904, compulsory notification from 1904) . . .	...	...	...	...	...	6	58	49	66	91	154	152	155

Under a voluntary system of notification in Brighton we have (December 1906) under observation and being visited at regular intervals 667 cases of phthisis, or about four times the annual number of deaths from this disease. In other towns than those named above the extent to which voluntary notification has succeeded varies greatly. In the Metropolitan boroughs dissatisfaction is generally expressed with the results of voluntary notification of phthisis, and the adoption of compulsory notification is being urged.

THE COMPULSORY NOTIFICATION OF PHTHISIS.—The risks of notification to the patient's pecuniary or social welfare have already been shown to be merely imaginary under a properly administered system. The information is confidential, and for an officer of a Local Authority to use it to the detriment of the patient would be likely to imply serious consequences to himself. I have never heard of any such instance of improper use of the information furnished by notification. The great advantage of compulsory notification is that it relieves the notifying doctor of any fear that he is improperly revealing confidential information. He is merely fulfilling his statutory obligation. This is a great gain, and usually must conduce to more complete and often to earlier notification of cases, and consequent earlier adoption of complete preventive measures. The experience of New York, however (Table LXXVI.), in which city the number of cases notified compulsorily was less for a couple of years than it had been under the previous system of voluntary notification appears to indicate that compulsion may occasionally carry with it some factor tending to depress the number of notifications. Sheffield under the guidance of Dr. Robertson was the first town to adopt the compulsory notification of phthisis, under a local Act, which came into force in January 1904. Sec. 45 of the Act dealing with this subject is as follows :—

SEC. 45, SHEFFIELD CORPORATION ACT, 1903

(1) (a) Every registered medical practitioner attending on or called in to visit any person within the City shall forthwith on becoming aware that such person is suffering from Tuberculosis of the Lung send to the Medical Officer of Health a certificate on a form to be supplied to him gratuitously by the Corporation, stating the name age sex and place of residence and employment or occupation (so far as can be reasonably ascertained) of the person so suffering and whether the case occurs in his private practice or in his practice as medical officer of any hospital public body friendly or other society or institution.

(b) Any such medical practitioner who fails to give such certificate shall be liable on summary conviction to a fine not exceeding forty shillings.

(c) The Corporation shall pay to every such medical practitioner for each certificate duly sent by him in accordance with this section a fee of two shillings and sixpence if the case occurs in his private practice and of one shilling if the case occurs in his practice as medical officer of any hospital public body friendly or other society or institution.

(d) A payment made to any medical practitioner in pursuance of this section shall not disqualify that practitioner from serving as a member of the Corporation or as a Guardian of a Union situate wholly or partly in the City or in any municipal or parochial office.

(2) (a) Where the Medical Officer of Health certifies that the cleansing and disinfecting of any building (including in that term any ship, vessel, boat, tent, shed, or similar structure used for human habitation) would tend to prevent or check Tuberculosis of the Lung the Town Clerk shall give notice in writing to the owner or occupier of such building that the

same or any part thereof will be cleansed and disinfected by the Corporation at the cost of the Corporation unless the owner or occupier of such building informs the Corporation within 24 hours from the receipt of the notice that he will cleanse and disinfect the building or the part thereof to the satisfaction of the Medical Officer of Health within the time to be fixed in the notice. If within 24 hours from the receipt of such notice the owner or occupier of such building has not informed the Corporation as aforesaid or if having so informed the Corporation he fails to have the building or the part thereof disinfected as aforesaid within the time fixed by the notice the building or the part thereof shall be cleansed and disinfected by the officers and at the cost of the Corporation under the superintendence of the Medical Officer of Health. Provided that any such building or part thereof may without any such notice being given as aforesaid but with the consent of the owner or occupier be cleansed and disinfected by the officers of and at the cost of the Corporation under the superintendence of the Medical Officer of Health.

(*b*) For the purpose of carrying into effect the provisions of this subsection the Corporation may by any officer authorised in that behalf who shall produce his authority in writing enter on any premises between the hours of ten o'clock in the forenoon and six o'clock in the afternoon.

(*c*) Every person who shall wilfully obstruct any duly authorised officer of the Corporation in carrying out the provision of this sub-section shall be liable to a penalty not exceeding forty shillings and if the offence is a continuing one to a daily penalty not exceeding twenty shillings.

(3) (*a*) The Medical Officer of Health generally empowered by the Corporation in that behalf may by notice in writing require the owner of any household or other articles books things bedding or clothing which have been exposed to the infection of Tuberculosis of the Lung to cause the same to be delivered over to an officer of the Corporation for removal for the purpose of disinfection and any person who fails to comply with such requirement shall be liable on summary conviction to a penalty not exceeding five pounds.

(*b*) Such articles books things bedding and clothing shall be disinfected by the Corporation and shall be brought back and delivered to the owner free of charge.

(4) If any person sustains any damage by reason of the exercise by the Corporation of any of the powers of sub-sections (2) and (3) of this section in relation to any matter as to which he is not himself in default full compensation shall be made to such person by the Corporation and the amount of compensation shall be recoverable in and in the case of dispute may be settled by a Petty Sessional Court.

(5) No provisions contained in any general or local Act of Parliament relating to infectious disease shall apply to Tuberculosis of the Lung or proceedings relating thereto under this section.

(6) All expenses incurred by the Corporation in carrying into effect the provisions of this section shall be chargeable on the District Fund and General District Rate.

(7) The Corporation shall cause to be given public notice of the effect of the provisions of this section by advertisement in the local newspapers

and by handbills and shall give formal notice thereof by registered post to every medical practitioner in the City and any other registered medical practitioner known to be in practice in the City and otherwise in such manner as the Corporation think sufficient and this section shall come into operation at such time not being less than one month after the first publication of such an advertisement as aforesaid as the Corporation may fix.

(8) The provisions of this section shall cease to be in force within the City at the expiration of seven years from the date of the passing of this Act unless they shall have been continued by Act of Parliament, or by Provisional Order made by the Local Government Board and confirmed by Parliament which Order the Local Government Board are hereby empowered to make in accordance with the provisions of the Public Health Act, 1875.

(9) The term " Medical Officer of Health " in this section shall mean the Medical Officer of Health for the time being of the City or any person duly authorised to act temporarily as Medical Officer of Health for the City.

The amount of notification hitherto secured under this local Act is, as shown in the preceding table, not materially more than in Manchester and Liverpool and less than in Brighton under systems of voluntary notification. It would, however, be unwise to base on these facts inferences as to the relative value of the voluntary and compulsory notifications of phthisis. Notification, whether voluntary or compulsory, is but a means to an end, and it may be that the circumstances of these communities including their arrangements for treating the notified patients differ so much as to render their statistics of notification almost incomparable. It has to be remembered in the first instance that Brighton has a population which is only one-fourth that of Sheffield, and from one-fifth to one-sixth of that of Manchester or Liverpool. This renders the personal supervision of notified cases by the medical officer of health relatively easy, and generally helps in smoothing the working of the system.

In the next place, no statistics are at present available as to the stage of disease at which cases of phthisis are notified. The third consideration is that

The success of notification, whether voluntary or compulsory, depends in the main on the extent to which a Local Authority and its officers can be helpful to the notified patients. And herein lies, I think, the success of successful voluntary notification.

Notification is the necessary channel through which the available help comes. Although it to some extent anticipates what is said in later chapters, the character of this help may be now summarised :—

(1) Paper handkerchiefs and pocket spit-bottles are provided whenever indicated.

(2) When the visits are made at the patient's home, every possible assistance is given in securing for the patient any help needed. The parochial authorities, the Charity Organisation Society, and other voluntary agencies are used as far as practicable. Where the patients are poor, out-patient letters for the local hospital or dispensary are given, in order that the patient may not be stinted of cod-liver oil and other remedies. Furthermore, if any other member of the same family appears to be failing in health and a doctor's fees cannot be afforded similar letters for the hospital or dispensary are given, the importance of early treatment of illness and of the maintenance of health being emphasised in every possible way.

(3) Sanatorium treatment is offered in all cases suitable for it, and in actual fact more than half of the total cases at present under observation in Brighton have spent at least four weeks in the Borough Sanatorium, and have there been taught the precautionary measures needed to prevent infection, and the personal régime indicated by their illness ; while at the same time their families have had a temporary holiday from the charge of the patient, the house has been disinfected, and the patient has returned with a knowledge of the means to avoid re-infecting it.

The chief reason for the success of voluntary notification of phthisis in Brighton has been the provision for the sanatorium treatment of notified cases. If the dates in the following table be compared with the curves in Fig. 37 the coincidence between the provision of increased sanatorium treatment and increased notification will be evident.

BRIGHTON

Voluntary notification of phthisis begun .   . Jan. 1899.
Four beds reserved at a sanatorium outside
    Brighton .   .   .   .   . May 1902.

Four beds opened for phthisis at the borough
    isolation hospital   .   .   .   . July 1902.

The number of beds for phthisis at the isolation
    hospital increased to ten   .   .   . Dec. 1902.

The number of beds for phthisis at the isolation
    hospital further increased to twenty-five . April 3, 1906.

At first the patients were admitted for only a month, the principle adopted being that of training the patients in personal hygiene, and in the general management of their illness, rather than of attempt at cure. The wisdom of this plan has been fully justified by experience. The majority of patients have been found to have extensive lung disease, often with cavitation, when admitted to the sanatorium. Such patients commonly have several years of life before them, but the experience of other sanatoria shows that prolonged treatment of many months, or even over a year, is necessary to ensure anything approaching to a cure even in cases in earlier stages of the disease. It is much more to the public interest to pass a large number of patients through the sanatorium and train them thoroughly in the hygienic requirements of their disease, than to treat a smaller number for a more protracted period. It is furthermore much more convenient for the patients, who often find it difficult or impossible to leave their families and work for longer than a month. Our experience is that advice as to the deposit and disposal of sputum given at home is commonly neglected ; and that it is very rarely neglected by patients who have been in the sanatorium. We welcome re-admissions to the sanatorium of patients whose health is again flagging. By this and other means, and by quarterly visits at the home of the patient, we keep in sympathetic relationship with the patients, and ensure the maintenance of precautionary measures against infection.

SHOULD THE NOTIFICATION OF PHTHISIS BE MADE GENERALLY COMPULSORY ?—The preceding facts and considerations will prepare the way to the conclusion that at present it would be inexpedient, unwise, and of relatively little use to advise the general adoption of compulsory notification of phthisis. Public opinion is not ripe for this step, and such notification would remain to a large extent a dead letter. Local Authorities are not ready to utilise the information thus received *to the benefit of the patient and of the public.* I place the two together, because they are substantially identical. It would, in my opinion, be premature for any community to adopt compulsory notification of phthisis which (*a*) does not possess a sufficient staff of skilled visitors, preferably medical men or women, to visit the notified cases ; and (*b*) does not possess sanatorium beds available for the treatment and training of consumptive patients. Under these circumstances compulsory notification can be made to work even in the present state of public opinion to the benefit of all concerned ; without such aid, I do not say that considerable good will not be done, but that the good done probably will not so far exceed that capable of being done under a voluntary system as to justify in most districts the addition at present of the element of compulsion.

CHAPTER XLIII

THE SANITARY AUTHORITY IN RELATION TO PREVENTIVE MEASURES AGAINST PHTHISIS

THE persons primarily concerned in the management of a tuberculous patient are the patient himself and his doctor. Happily preventive measures and curative measures overlap and to a large extent are identical. Hence when this fact is realised, the co-operation of patient and doctor in carrying out preventive measures may be confidently expected. Very often, however, it is not realised. Patients may be ignorant, careless, or indifferent. In the later stages of their illness they may be unable, unhelped, to adopt the necessary precautions. Many doctors furthermore are too busy to explain the necessary instructions as to precautionary measures ; and whatever the reason, these instructions are frequently found in actual official experience not to have been given until the visit of the medical officer of health or his assistant is made, or, when given, not to have been carried out. The intervention of the Sanitary Authority is necessary, under present conditions, to ensure preventive measures being taken to the extent required by the necessities of public health. Some parts of the duty of the Sanitary Authority in this connection have been already considered. Of these the first is to ensure the early diagnosis of the disease ; and for this purpose no Sanitary Authority can be regarded as fulfilling its duty which does not provide facilities for the

FREE BACTERIOLOGICAL EXAMINATION OF SPUTUM.—This is already being done in many towns, and should become universal. Further details on this point are given on pp. 52 and 314. Next comes the organisation of arrangements for the

NOTIFICATION OF CASES.—Whether this should be voluntary or compulsory will depend on local needs and possibilities, and on the considerations urged in Chapter XLII.

BYE-LAWS PROHIBITING INDISCRIMINATE EXPECTORATION form an important official means of preventing infection. The extent to which these are at present practicable is indicated on p. 334.

A case of phthisis having been notified, what action follows as the result of this notification ?

(a) COLLECTION OF NECESSARY INFORMATION.—The method to be employed depends on whether the patient desires sanatorium treatment, and whether this is available. In Brighton a very high proportion of the cases notified bring the notifications with them to the Town Hall, often with a letter from their doctor, applying for sanatorium treatment. The patient is then interviewed by the medical officer of health, and the full particulars indicated on the following inspection card are obtained. If the patient does not call at the Town Hall, the medical assistant of the medical officer of health visits him at home. Owing to patients being at work, or being unwilling at the first interview to give as full information as is required, a second or even a third visit is occasionally required before the complete history of each patient can be obtained. The information is written on a stiff four-paged inspection card 8×4 inches. The first page is as follows :—

NOTIFICATION OF PHTHISIS

Reg. No._____Sanatorium No._____

Name_____Age_____

Address_____ .. _ _   _____

Date of Notification _____Doctor_____

Recommended for Sanatorium by_____

Notes by Doctor_____

_____

_____

Date of Admission to_____

Date of Discharge from_____

Date of Change of Address_____

New Address_____

Dates of Visit_____

_____

_____

On the inside second and third pages information under the following headings is obtained :—

Duration and History of Illness_____

_____

_____

Places of Residence during Illness_____

_____

_____

Occupation and Workplaces during last 5 years_____

_____

_____

(a) Wages_____(b) Work regular_____

No. and Ages in same Family.	No. in 2nd Family.	History of Cough or Consumption among these.

Family History_____

_____

_____

Precautions :—

(1) Card_____(2) Handkerchiefs_____

(3) Pocket Spittoon_____

(4) Habits as to Spitting_____

_____

(5) Other Occupants of same Bedroom_____

_____

_____

(6) House_____

_____

_____

Habits as to Food and Drink_____

_____

Further Remarks_____

_____

_____

Likely Sources of Infection :—

(1) Same House_____   (4) Neighbour_____

(2) Companion_____   (5) Workmates_____

(3) Public-Houses_____   (6) Others_____

The fourth page deals with the sanitary condition of the home, especially as to cleanliness and crowding, space being left at the bottom for a summary of conclusions as to exposures to infection, which along with the statement of likely sources of infection at the bottom of p. 3 may lead to further inquiries and action.

Condition of Dwelling-house as to—

No. of available Dwelling Rooms_____

_____

Overcrowding_____

_____

Cleanliness
⎰ of Walls_____
⎪ of Ceilings_____
⎨ of Floors_____
⎱ of Bedding, etc._____

Dampness_____

Ventilation_____

Lighting, especially of Staircase _____

Size of Yard_____

Any Sanitary Defects_____

(*a*) Duration of each Case_____

(*b*) Latest Exposure to Infection before reputed date of onset_____

_____

(*c*) Duration of Exposure, etc._____

_____

(*d*) Previous Exposures_____

_____

The inquiry form may seem to be unnecessarily elaborate, but it is the result of long experience in the work ; and it has to be remembered that the information often accumulates gradually, as our acquaintance with the patient improves.

(*b*) GIVING OF INSTRUCTIONS.—At the first interview with the patient the card printed on p. 324 is given, and its contents are explained to him verbally.

At the same interview he is instructed in the methods of using paper handkerchiefs and a pocket spit-bottle.

(*c*) DISINFECTION.—The next step is to ensure cleansing or disinfection of the patient's room as required. The following directions, quoted from a circular prepared by Drs. Niven and Newman and myself in 1903 and issued by the National Association for the Prevention of Consumption, may be quoted at this point :—

The phlegm infects everything upon which it falls—handkerchiefs, books, papers, linen, floors, carpets, furniture, etc., and when dried and broken into dust is then readily inhaled by healthy persons.

On these facts rests the important question of disinfection. In endeavouring to prevent a consumptive person from spreading the disease, two sets of preventive measures are required :—1st. The removal or destruction of the infective matter disseminated by the patient's phlegm ; and, 2nd, the prevention of future dissemination. For the latter purpose the main object is not to permit any phlegm or discharge to become dry before being destroyed.   Before the consumptive person has learned the personal precautions which must be taken, and up to the time when he has been trained to carry them out carefully, he has probably distributed a considerable amount of infective matter.   This is especially liable to accumulate in a dangerous form at home, where the space is small, and light and ventilation are defective.   Infective particles will be found in greatest abundance on and near the floors, on ledges, and in room-hangings. But the personal clothing and bedclothes will also have become infected. Hence it is necessary to disinfect the floor, walls, and ceiling of the rooms occupied by the patient, as well as the furniture, carpet, bedclothes, etc.

If personal precautions are taken, the risk of infection is lessened, but it is impossible to prevent coughed-up minute drops of phlegm from being deposited in a room, and rooms should therefore be cleaned at least once in a month, the floors being scrubbed with soft soap, the furniture washed, the walls cleaned down with dough.   The ceiling should also be whitewashed every six months.

Disinfection of rooms which have been occupied by consumptive patients may be secured in various ways, but the following are the practical rules which must underlie any methods adopted :—

1. Gaseous disinfection of rooms, or " fumigation," as it is termed, by whatever method it is practised, is inefficient in such cases.
2. In order to remove and destroy the dried infective discharges, the disinfectant must be applied *directly to the infected surfaces* of the room.
3. The disinfectant may be applied by washing, brushing, or spraying.
4. Amongst other chemical solutions used for this purpose a solution of choride of lime (1 to 2 per cent.) has proved satisfactory and efficient.
5. In view of the well-established fact that the dust from dried discharges is infective, emphasis must be laid upon the importance of thorough and wet cleansing of infected rooms.
6. Bedding, carpets, curtains, wearing apparel, and all similar articles belonging to or used by the patient, which cannot be thoroughly washed, should be disinfected in an efficient steam disinfector.

In Brighton a formalin spray is used for disinfecting rooms. The preceding instructions when combined with direct precautions during the act of coughing suffice to prevent risk of infection.

(*d*) REMEDY OF SANITARY DEFECTS.—It is unnecessary to detail the means used for the remedy of overcrowding or other sanitary defects found in the consumptive's home, as in regard to these the usual procedure of sanitary administration will be pursued.   Notification has, however, secured their remedy earlier than would have been practicable under ordinary conditions (see also p. 321).

Nor for a similar reason is it necessary to detail measures

taken in regard to workplaces, for the removal of dust, the prevention of daily dust, and the limewashing of walls, etc. Notices against spitting in factories, workshops, etc., such as the one given on p. 334, are now exhibited fairly generally.

(e) EDUCATION OF THE PATIENT.—The great difficulty is to secure that the uneducated patient will adopt the simple precautions as to coughing and spitting which are needed to prevent infection. Most patients, whatever their class, are uneducated in this respect, but some patients acquire more easily than others the habit of taking the necessary precautions. My personal experience is that very few patients can be trusted to follow scrupulously the instructions as to coughing and spitting given on the card printed on p. 324, except in the light of the careful habits inculcated and the personal benefits received at a sanatorium. Hence I consider

(f) THE PROVISION OF SANATORIUM TRAINING AND TREATMENT as one of the most important duties of a Sanitary Authority in regard to phthisis. The details under this head are described in Chapter XLVIII.; but there is no difficulty in seeing that a medical officer of health or other official who goes with an offer of sanatorium treatment is in an infinitely better position for receiving a hearty welcome than when he merely asks questions which may be regarded as inquisitorial, and gives instructions which to the uninitiated may seem foolish.

(g) THE PROVISION OF MEDICAL TREATMENT FOR OTHER MEMBERS OF THE PATIENT'S FAMILY.—The welcome of the visitor is likely to be still more cordial when it is known that for suitable cases he has hospital or dispensary tickets, and can ensure continuous treatment not only for the patient, but also for other members of his household when this is indicated (see also pp. 318 and 348).

(h) REVISITS.—In some towns visits to consumptive patients are made monthly. In Brighton only a quarterly visit is made, and it is probable that more frequent visits would lead to friction. In order to prevent removal without the knowledge of the medical officer of health, notifications of change of address are paid for, thus ensuring in a certain proportion of cases prompt disinfection of the vacated rooms. With the same object, a fee of sixpence is paid to relieving officers who notify a case of phthisis, or who notify the removal of such a patient to the infirmary or elsewhere. The cleansing and disinfection of vacated rooms before they are occupied by another family is one of the most important measures in connection with the administrative control of tuberculosis.

(*i*) In connection with visits and revisits to the patient, the question of helping him in gaining his livelihood under the best conditions arises. The subject of the after-care of consumptives is discussed in Chapter XLVIII. There will doubtless be great future developments under this heading, but at present this matter is chiefly one for private enterprise and charity.

CHAPTER XLIV

EDUCATION AUTHORITIES AND TUBERCULOSIS

IN previous chapters stress has repeatedly been laid on the importance of teaching the laws of health (p. 302), and particularly on the necessity of having teachers taught these laws with special reference to the prevention of tuberculosis (p. 365). The necessity for teaching the patient the means of preventing the spread of the disease has been emphasised on pp. 318 and 332. The prevention of indiscriminate expectoration, which is discussed in Chapter XLI., bears on the same subject.

In all these particulars school authorities have duties which they cannot with propriety continue to ignore. This is true for all classes of schools, and not less true for secondary than for public elementary schools. The majority of children attend the latter, and the following remarks, produced from a paper on "The School in Relation to Tuberculosis," contributed by me to the International Congress on School Hygiene, August 1907, relate chiefly to them. It is convenient to reproduce here the remarks as to the amount of open and recognisable tuberculosis in schools, as well as those relating to its prevention.

Happily the Education Committees governing general elementary education in this country, although they have important specially delegated duties and have co-opted members, form part of the local Sanitary Authority, and there is every reason why they should actively co-operate to the fullest extent in securing the prevention of tuberculosis. The new machinery for the medical inspection of scholars will be an invaluable means to this end, especially in districts in which notification of cases of phthisis to the medical officer of health is in successful operation.

Elementary day - schools may be considered from the following standpoints :—(1) Whether tuberculosis is spread in them and to what extent ; (2) whether the conditions of life

and work in such schools tend to bring into activity latent
tuberculosis ; and (3) as important means for teaching and
training children so that we may obtain the aid of the next
generation in the rapid elimination of tuberculosis.

THE AMOUNT OF TUBERCULOSIS AT SCHOOL-AGES.—Before
we can arrive at any definite decision on the first point, it is
necessary to know how much tuberculosis there is among children
of school-age. So far as tuberculosis terminating fatally during
school-life is concerned, the figures of the Registrar-General's
reports enable this point to be settled with some approximation to accuracy for the age-periods 5 to 10 and 10 to 15,
which may be taken as practically coincident with school-ages.
Fig. 38 gives the death-rates from pulmonary and from all forms
of tuberculosis in the aggregate per million living at each age-
period in the decennium 1891–1900 (Decennial Supplement,
R.G., Dr. Tatham). The interval between the lower and higher
space in each column represents the death-rate from all forms
of tuberculosis, excluding pulmonary tuberculosis.

It will be noted that at ages under 5 pulmonary tuberculosis
only supplies about one-ninth ; at ages 5 to 10 less than one-
third ; and at ages 10 to 15 not much more than one-half
of the total registered mortality from tuberculosis. At higher
ages the proportion of pulmonary to total fatal tuberculosis
becomes greater.

It will be noted furthermore that at ages 5 to 15 the
death-rate from pulmonary and from all other forms of tuberculosis in the aggregate is lower than at any other age-period,
except at ages over 75. It is clear, therefore, that, as a
fatal disease, tuberculosis is relatively uncommon at school-
ages. Taking the ages 5 to 15 together, it is the registered
cause of death each year of only about seven out of every 10,000
children living, while pulmonary tuberculosis only supplies three
out of these seven.

As a means of spread of tuberculosis, pulmonary tuberculosis
is supreme, all other forms of tuberculosis being almost negligible
in this respect. How many cases of pulmonary tuberculosis
are there for every fatal case of this disease ? In adults the
proportion is usually given as three to one, though this is
probably too low (see p. 63). If we assume that there are
constantly as many as ten non-fatal cases for each annual death,

then three out of every thousand children at school-ages are suffering from pulmonary tuberculosis, on the basis of the figures of the last decennial period.

It does not follow that all these phthisical children are in attendance at elementary schools. Many of them doubtless will not be.

Compare this estimate with the actual results of examination

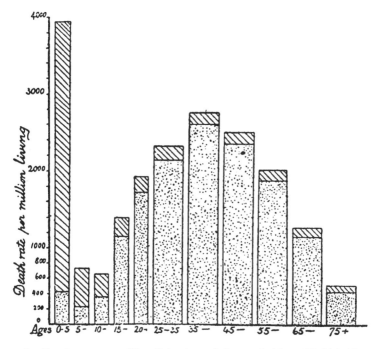

FIG. 38.—Death-rate per million living in each Age-period from Phthisis (dotted) and from other forms of Tuberculosis (lined)

of children in elementary schools. These are given more fully in a paper by Drs. Lecky and Horton of Brighton (1907). I need, therefore, only briefly summarise the results. They very exhaustively examined 806 children, of whom 491 were attending an elementary day-school, 241 in a parochial industrial school, and 74 in the workhouse. These children varied in age from 4 to 17. Only three cases of phthisis were found—one in the parochial school, one in the workhouse, and one in the elementary school. With these results may be compared the following, which are summarised in the same paper. At Dundee, Dr. A. P.

Low (1905) found no pulmonary tuberculosis in 517 children; at Dunfermline, Dr. Ash (1905) had a similar result in examining 1371 children. Dr. Mackenzie, in Edinburgh, found fourteen cases in 600 children; Professor Hay, in Aberdeen, three cases in 600 children; the Charity Organisation Society results, Edinburgh (Canongate schools), give nineteen cases in 1318 children. These results vary greatly, and it appears likely that there has been some confusion between bronchitis and phthisis in some of the observations, a very easy mistake unless a very careful examination is made.

Dr. Greenwood, at Blackburn, found 6·7 per cent. of phthisis in 1028 children referred to him, but these were children whose fitness for schools was already in question, and rather confirm the view, which is, I think, correct, that a child failing with phthisis usually does not remain in school long before his ill-health is recognised.

Omitting the above negative observations, and Dr. Greenwood's results, which represent a selected sick population, the proportion of children in elementary schools with revealed phthisis appears to be 1 in 43 (Edinburgh), 1 in 69 (Edinburgh, second series), 1 in 200 (Aberdeen), and 1 in 296 (Brighton). Compare these figures with the estimate of 1 in 333 children based on the national death-rate, and on the assumption that ten non-fatal cases go to every fatal case, I incline to think that there is not, on the average, more than 1 in 300 children in schools showing revealed or diagnosable phthisis.

IS TUBERCULOSIS SPREAD IN SCHOOLS?—To what extent are these children a source of infection? Probably very little. Children seldom expectorate; and a child with a troublesome cough would not be kept long in school. It does not appear likely that there is much spread of tuberculosis from scholar to scholar in schools.

Teachers and caretakers are possible sources of infection. There do not appear to be trustworthy statistics of the amount of phthisis in teachers. Probably it is somewhat more than in the general community, and, judging by my own experience, I should say that it is more often laryngeal than in the averages of consumptives. The medical examination of teachers and of caretakers, as well as of scholars, is obviously indicated as a precautionary measure.

THE AMOUNT OF LATENT TUBERCULOSIS IN SCHOLARS.—The preceding figures deal with revealed tuberculosis. Latent tuberculosis is nearly, if not quite, always non-infectious. Such latent tuberculosis has, however, important bearings on school hygiene. Notwithstanding the small amount of revealed tuberculosis among school-children, such children, if they die of other diseases, show, in a very high percentage, evidence of tuberculosis, especially in the bronchial glands. Thus Naegeli, at Zurich,[1] found in autopsies of children aged 1 to 5 that 17 per cent., and of children aged 5 to 14 that 33 per cent., had tuberculous lesions.

Such latent lesions are undoubtedly very frequent in children. I cannot doubt that the true interpretation of these figures, showing as they do heavy incidence of tuberculosis before as well as during school-life, is that tuberculous infection in children is nearly all domestic and not scholastic in origin.

HOW TO DEAL WITH LATENT TUBERCULOSIS.—The presence of such latent foci is a constant source of danger to the children implicated. Although there is at present no statistical evidence to that effect, it is almost certain that in the children of adult consumptives such lesions are present to a preponderant extent, a fact which supplies a valuable indication for preventive treatment. The children of such parents should be periodically examined by the school-doctor, and the card giving the medical state of each scholar should have a column for family history of consumption, and for entering any cases of this disease that have been or may be subsequently notified in the same household. The general notification of phthisis to the medical officer of health thus forms an essential part of school hygiene.

The course to be adopted in regard to such children is a part of the problem of general public health administration. Two plans are open—the removal of the children from their homes either temporarily or permanently to homes or schools at the seaside or in the country ; or the institutional treatment of the consumptive parent. The former plan has been adopted on a considerable scale in France and elsewhere, and occasionally is the best or the only available line of prophylaxis; the latter plan is the one which has been chiefly employed in England,

[1] Quoted by Dr. H. Méry, *Rapports présentés au Congrès International de la Tuberculose*, Paris, 1905, p. 298.

not intentionally, but incidentally in the relegation of a very
large proportion of consumptives among the poor to the workhouse infirmary and to other institutions. Judging by international statistics, action on the latter line is more effective than
any other. It brings the greatest relief to the family, both from
privation and from infection. Supplemented by earlier treatment and training of consumptives in sanatoria, it will effect
still more good ; and if there is to be a choice of remedies, the
balance of good lies on the side of measures directed towards
removing the patient himself rather than of measures for removing the children from the infected domestic circle. It is
evident, however, that both remedies are excellent, and that
each consumptive family will need to be considered on its merits,
and the most practicable line of action taken. It may be repeated, however, that, given the choice between measures for
increasing resistance to infection, and measures for diminishing
or abolishing exposure to protracted infection, the latter must
always occupy a supreme position.

How to prevent Schools from provoking Latent Tuberculosis to activity.—Both in regard to the children under
special suspicion of tuberculosis, and in regard to all other
children, much can be done to prevent the school from becoming
a place in which latent tuberculosis is brought into activity.
Overcrowding is the rule in schools. A larger floor-space
should be required. Classes are too large, thus straining the
voice of the teacher, and making him much more prone to tuberculosis. Ventilation is usually very defective ; and the methods
of cleansing, involving the raising of dust, need reform. These
are obvious points of hygiene. In school hygiene they are prominent because of the grossness with which they are neglected.
In the boarding-schools of the middle and upper classes we are
familiar with the overwork and over-fatigue due to excessive
games, as well as with the insufficient sleep to which Dr. Acland
has drawn attention. In England the children of the great
majority of the population almost certainly do not suffer from
over-fatigue due to games ; but there is little doubt that many
of these suffer from over-fatigue and want of sleep, due to
domestic and sometimes to industrial demands, and to defective
domestic arrangements. These factors cannot fail to aid in
setting ablaze the smouldering fire of latent tuberculosis. In

each of these particulars, there is much need for detailed medical supervision of our schools and scholars, and for the adoption of preventive measures, on the lines that have been briefly indicated.

If these and similar reforms are secured, the school may be made a most important centre for the prevention of tuberculosis. I think that the principal measures needed for this end may be summarised as follows :—

1. The medical examination of all children on admission to school and periodically afterwards, supplemented as it must be to attain its full value by information systematically acquired in regard to the health conditions of their homes and all living in them.

2. The exclusion of children found to have open or revealed tuberculosis.

3. Special care as to the feeding and general hygiene of children from tuberculous families, including avoidance of fatigue.

4. The frequent wet cleansing of schools.

5. The reduction of overcrowding.

6. The improvement of arrangements for the ventilation and warming of schools.

7. Careful attention to the personal hygiene of all scholars, especially in relation to the removal of adenoids and of carious teeth.

8. The periodical examination of caretakers and teachers, and the avoidance of excessive strain on the voice of the latter, or over-fatigue in general.

THE FORMATION OF PUBLIC OPINION ON TUBERCULOSIS IN THE SCHOOLS.—Public opinion is formed in the schools ; and if each teacher and scholar is taught to practise the laws of health, a much more rapid decline of tuberculosis can be secured. What has been said about the supreme importance of domestic infection illustrates this. The inculcation of good habits as to coughing, expectoration, and scrupulous domestic cleanliness, and of knowledge as to the relative value of foods and the dangers of alcoholic drinks, will go far towards making the school a valuable aid in preventing tuberculosis.

CHAPTER XLV

THE BOARD OF GUARDIANS AND THE PREVENTION OF PHTHISIS

IN previous chapters we have discussed in relation to the prevention of phthisis the functions of the doctor, of his tuberculous patient, and of the Sanitary Authority and the Education Committee as at present constituted in this country. One local governing body remains whose present functions in this connection are not less important than those of the two bodies already mentioned. This is the Board of Guardians, whose duties are to relieve the destitute, giving food, lodging, and medical aid when required. The importance of such aid in preventing phthisis and in helping to diminish the danger of its spread is at once evident. The fact that the help given—especially the domestic medical aid—is ofttimes belated and insufficient (see p. 307) is well known ; while the importance of the institutional relief given by Boards of Guardians has not been sufficiently realised in the past. Its bearing on the past prevalence of phthisis has been fully discussed in Part II. If there is one point that I am more desirous of making common property than another, it is that in the improved and more general institutional treatment of advanced cases of phthisis we have the means ready to hand from which the greatest quickening of the rate of decline of the death-rate from this disease can be expected.

THE INSTITUTIONAL TREATMENT OF ADVANCED CASES.— So long as Boards of Guardians remain a separate local governing body and are hemmed in by present regulations in giving indoor medical relief, this timely and general treatment cannot be obtained. It is to be hoped, however, that ere long sickness will be the sole and sufficient condition of prompt and efficient medical treatment for all requiring it. This will imply the removal of the parochial stigma from treatment in a workhouse infirmary. The infirmary will, in fact, no longer be an annexe,—except perhaps structurally,—of the workhouse. Until this reform is secured, the local problem for administrators is to secure for cases of phthisis in the workhouse infirmary the most abundant and the most efficient use of separate wards consistent with present regulations. There is no compulsory power of removal or detention in these wards. The best policy is, by provision of sufficient and palatable food, by good medical attendance and nursing and general comfort, to make the consumptive patients unwilling to go home. This advice may appear to be contrary to the first principles of poor-law administration. It is, however, actually calculated to diminish|pauperism, which ought to be the object of every one concerned. The return of consumptive patients to small homes, in which due precautions are not likely to be taken, is an effective means of growing a later crop of consumptive paupers. The general conditions of treatment of advanced consumptives in the wards of infirmaries do not differ materially from those in sanatoria. The wards will, however, in view of the more serious illness of the patients, be kept warmer ; lighter and more easily masticated food will be required ; and precautions as to the coughing and expectoration of the bedridden patients will need to be precise and rigidly carried out. Much can be done even for advanced patients to increase their comfort and to smooth their path during progressively increasing weakness.

The medical superintendent of the infirmary occasionally has to deal with another class of consumptive, who is extremely difficult to control. He is not very ill, he has a troublesome cough, and is addicted to indiscriminate spitting. He is occasionally obstreperous, and the temptation then, and even short of this if the patient is dirty in his habits, is to relegate him to the able-bodied part of the workhouse as a punishment. This is obviously unfair to the able-bodied paupers, and some other means, such as separate warding, ought to be devised.

At this stage comes in the difficulty that the patient will probably " take his discharge," and leave the institution, going back to a common lodging-house, where he will continue to disseminate infection. For such patients,—and for such patients only in my opinion,—the power of

COMPULSORY REMOVAL TO AND DETENTION IN AN INSTITUTION

is indicated. We are much more timid on this subject than our cousins in the United States, as shown by the following remarks made by Dr. Knopf at a recent Conference of Sanitary Officers of the State of New York :—

New York was the first city in the world which enacted the compulsory removal law in regard to tuberculosis. That is to say, if in the opinion of the inspector, the physician in charge, or the visiting nurse, the tuberculous patient is a menace to his fellow-men, he is removed to a hospital whether he likes it or not. Now you may think that those patients are refractory and might not do well in the hospital. Not at all. It is my privilege to be on service as attending physician for six months in the year at the Riverside Sanatorium for Consumptives, which is in charge of the New York City Health Department. Half of these patients are there against their will, and you would be surprised what a change it makes in their condition to remove them from the dark, dreary tenement houses—where they have neither light, air, nor decent food—into a clean bed, plenty of air day and night, and give them good food, including eggs and milk. We never lock up the eggs. We tell the patients, " Go and help yourselves." They can drink all the milk they wish. You would be surprised what results we obtain there in spite of the cases being, in the majority, far advanced, and in spite of their being forced to go there. If they recover, in not a few instances they become better men and women. The results as a whole are most satisfactory. Thus I beg of you not to be alarmed when you hear the words compulsory removal. It is the most humane and scientific way of treating the consumptive poor, who are a menace to their neighbours, without food and air, or entirely homeless.

This experience in New York is interesting ; but it would be a mistake to conclude that any such practice would be wise in this country. Resort to compulsion, if it were thought advisable, should undoubtedly be hemmed in by special conditions, such as special investigation and a magisterial decision. There are, however, cases of the nature indicated above, of persons lodged in common lodging-houses or in crowded dwellings who cannot secure proper nursing and attention, and who are suffering to an unnecessary extent themselves, and inflicting suffering and unnecessary danger on those about them ; persons, again, who are already in the infirmary but wish to return to the above conditions ; in whose cases there is need of compulsory removal or detention. In the vast majority of cases there is no need for compulsion, and the power to enforce it against them is undesirable. For them, the one thing necessary is to make the institutional treatment satisfactory to the patient as well as conducive to the public interests. As has appeared so often in considering questions relating to phthisis, this means of protecting the community is identical with the best treatment for the patient, whose cure will usually be the more rapid and more probable if the circumstances in which he is treated are attractive to him.

SANATORIA AND BOARDS OF GUARDIANS.—Liverpool and Bradford have been pioneers in providing for the treatment of comparatively early cases of phthisis through Boards of Guardians. It is to be hoped that other Boards will follow their example. It must be noted, however, that when a patient becomes ill enough to be a pauper, he is usually suffering from well-established or advanced disease, and that the chief medical function of the Board of Guardians under present arrangements is the treatment of patients who are so ill as to be completely unable to work. While infirmary treatment involves the stigma of pauperism, far more patients will struggle against the disease till they are past recovery, in the hope of avoiding the workhouse, than will apply for infirmary treatment at a stage at which it can have a fair chance of producing recovery, and before they have sown widespread infection in their environment. At present, therefore, workhouse infirmaries cannot usually cover so wide a field as the local Sanitary Authority, which may succeed in obtaining patients for treatment at a stage before tuberculosis has produced actual disablement. The Boards of Guardians have, in fact, the accommodation and arrangements for treatment without being able to secure the patients at the most favourable time ; the Sanitary Authority can secure the patients, but seldom or never has the accommodation and arrangements for treating them. This inefficient state of things points to the need for finding a way of combining the resources and functions of the two Authorities in respect to the treatment of the sick. Such a combined Authority would then be able to carry out the complete institutional treatment of this disease among the poor, namely :—

1. The protracted sanatorium treatment of suitable early cases.

2. The shorter treatment of cases of longer duration, among patients still able to earn their livelihood, with a view to temporary improvement, and to training in the management of their illness (pp. 357 and 391).

24

3. The protracted institutional treatment of advanced cases, when the home conditions are unfavourable.

THE HOME TREATMENT OF PAUPER CASES OF PHTHISIS.— The Board of Guardians is frequently faced with the problem of giving outdoor relief to the family of a consumptive patient, to enable medical treatment and nursing of the patient to be continued at home. If any general rule is to be followed in such cases, it should be to the effect that outdoor relief ought never to be given to consumptive patients. Exceptional cases may occur, as, for instance, when the household consists only of the patient and his wife ; but even then it is usually wiser to admit the patient to the infirmary, release the wife from the constant and unrelieved stress of nursing, night and day, and when necessary give her outdoor relief after her husband has been placed in the position of receiving proper medical aid in the infirmary. If there are children in the family, under the domestic conditions in which those needing parochial aid live, such aid ought seldom if ever to be given except on the condition that the patient becomes an in-patient at the infirmary. In the light of the past history of phthisis in this country, and of the important part which has been played by these infirmaries in securing the past decline of the death-rate from this disease, no other course is justifiable either in the public interest or with a view to safeguarding the patient's family.

THE RELIEF OF THE CONSUMPTIVE'S FAMILY.—The fatigue and chronic mal-nutrition in the families of the poor associated with the nursing of a consumptive are powerful influences favouring the active development of tuberculosis ; and there is no doubt that the provision of food, clothing, etc., at the public expense, when required, would tend to diminish this risk for the patient's family ; and would diminish the risk of relapse in patients who have been sent home from a sanatorium after favourable treatment. Dr. Niven has specially drawn attention to the need for a fund from which assistance can be given to households in which the breadwinner is struck down with phthisis while the children are too young to earn wages, and recommends that this fund should be administered in connection with the official scheme of notification.

This is a problem in which Boards of Guardians and private

philanthropy can both bear a part. In my opinion the medical officer of health or his subordinate should not have a direct share in the administration of such relief ; but he should be responsible solely for such relief as can be given by medical and sanitary measures. The most efficient means of relieving the family, and the means which most effectively removes the risk of further cases of tuberculosis, is the provision of satisfactory institutional treatment for the patient, the disinfection of the home, and the removal of insanitary conditions. At the same time the medical officer of health can set in operation both official and private charity for the rest of the household when the need for these is indicated.

CHAPTER XLVI

INSURANCE AND FRIENDLY SOCIETIES IN RELATION TO THE PREVENTION OF PHTHISIS

LIFE insurance and particularly insurance against sickness forms one of the most effective means of combating tuberculosis. The sick-pay received by a member of a friendly society gives him the means of entering a sanatorium, and provides his family with food in his absence, assuming that he is treated without payment. In Germany the system of insurance against sickness has been developed on an enormous scale. All wage-earning workmen in Germany have been compulsorily insured against sickness, employer and workman contributing to provide an annuity to all persons unable to support themselves or over seventy years old. "This insurance is effected (Bielefeldt, 1901) under the supervision of the Imperial Insurance Department, State Insurance Departments, thirty-one insurance institutions territorially limited, and nine special club institutions of the Invalidity Insurance." These offices and institutions have a financial interest in postponing invalidity, as contributions cease when invalidity begins. Hence accurate investigations of causes of invalidity have been made. The results up to 1901 showed that of male workers employed in mining, metal works, factories and the building trades who became invalided up to the age of 30, more than half suffer from phthisis. Of persons engaged in forestry and agriculture, who became pensioners at ages 20–25, 350 out of every 1000 pensioners are consumptive. Death statistics similarly showed that at ages 15–60 in the German Empire, out of every 100 deaths 33 were due to phthisis. Hence it was evident that one of the most important tasks of the officers of the German Workmen's Insurance was to battle successfully against tuberculosis. Obligatory insurance against sickness has been enforced in Germany since June 1883 among industrial employees, the sick employee having the right to free medical attendance and the payment of half his wage for thirteen weeks, or in the alternative to free treatment in a hospital. In January 1891, insurance against chronic invalidity and old age was made obligatory; and six years later it was found that out of 60,000 pensions given, 8500 were given to consumptives. Hospital treatment has been made obligatory in certain cases, and the duration of compulsory treatment has been extended to twenty-six weeks, a fourth of the patient's wages being paid during this period to his family. If the patient relinquishes the treatment without good reasons, and thus incurs the risk of becoming a permanent charge on the pension funds, the pension may be refused either wholly or partially. The extent to which sanatorium treatment has been carried out in Germany is set out on p. 254.

The general system of insurance in Germany has helped to reduce the death-rate from tuberculosis in three ways: firstly, patients are able to afford treatment earlier than was formerly possible; secondly, the importance of keeping down grants for sickness and invalidity has led to assiduous education of consumptive patients and of the entire German public in the means of prevention and cure; and thirdly, there has been institutional treatment on an extended scale, and for a much longer period. A very high proportion of consumptives have been treated in the general hospitals of Germany both before and since the sanatorium treatment was introduced (p. 287). Any measure enabling earlier treatment to be secured by patients, and bringing home to the general population the importance of hygienic precautions against this disease, must greatly aid in reducing its amount.

It is unlikely that any system on the exact pattern of the German system will be adopted in this country. The machinery is complicated and elaborate; and, in part at least, a rate- or tax-supported system of medical attendance for those needing it, on the lines on which " free " education has already been given, is probably more in accord with our national trend of social evolution and with our special needs.

Pending any such great national movement as that suggested by the action of Germany, how can Insurance Societies and particularly Friendly Societies be utilised in the campaign against tuberculosis?

INSURANCE SOCIETIES do their best to eliminate consumptives

from the list of the insured by careful inquiries into family and personal history and by physical examination of the candidate. That they do not completely succeed is shown by the following table, taken from Dr. Muirhead's report on the experience of the Scottish Widows' Fund, 1874–94 :—

Phthisis.—Annual Death-rate per 100,000 Males living at each group of Ages in	Ages.					
	20–25.	25–35.	35–45.	45–55.	55–65.	65–75.
(1) England and Wales, 1881–90 . . .	234	304	358	351	292	182
(2) Scottish Widows' Fund experience, 1874–94 .	104	143	163	115	117	115

The difference between the insured and the general population is partly due to the benefits of selection, though average social condition has also much to do with it. Mr. Hoffman (1901) has discussed whether, especially in connection with the work of Industrial Insurance Companies, it would pay to aid those insured by providing sanatorium treatment, etc., for them. He points out that the financial interest of the companies is limited to the increased duration of the policy-life or the increased premium income in consequence of prolonged life ; and estimating the prolongation of life by sanatorium treatment at five years, and taking as the basis of his computation the experience of his own insurance company among industrial policyholders, he concludes that the additional income secured by prolonged life will not provide by increased premiums one-half of the cost of treatment. In the present state of matters it cannot be expected that private insurance companies should subscribe heavily to sanatoria for consumptive persons whose lives are insured with them. They undoubtedly will gain not only by sanatorium treatment, but also by improved housing, increased cleanliness and temperance, the increasing avoidance of promiscuous spitting, and all the measures of hygiene and education now being pushed forward.

FRIENDLY SOCIETIES are more closely concerned than

Insurance Companies in the diminution of phthisis, for they give sickness as well as burial benefits. About fourteen millions of the population of the United Kingdom belong to such societies, and more than a million and a half belong to Trade Unions which have sick benefits, etc. Many more belong to slate clubs and similar less satisfactory organisations. Mr. J. L. Stead has collected the experience of the Ancient Order of Foresters, with the results shown in Table VIII. p. 16.

Some figures collected by Mr. Garland (1905), based on somewhat scanty data, indicate that the sick pay of consumptive members costs three times as much as (£14 more than) the average sick pay to members dying from other causes. The Friendly Societies are very deeply concerned in reducing the sickness caused by tuberculosis, and even if ultimately they do not find it financially advantageous to provide sanatoria for workers on their own account, they would benefit greatly by active propaganda against tuberculosis, educating their members in every possible way, helping in securing the promptest diagnosis of disease, and in obtaining better conditions of housing and industrial employment for their members.

An interesting scheme has been launched by the National Association for the Establishment and Maintenance of Sanatoria for Workers suffering from Tuberculosis. Mr. Garland and Dr. T. D. Lister, in a description of the objects of this Association and of the sanatorium recently opened in connection with it at Benenden, emphasise the educational aspect of this sanatorium. By the graduated employment of the patient, they hope to avoid the demoralisation which occasionally occurs at the convalescent home and at hospital. They evidently intend the Benenden Sanatorium to fulfil the functions which the Brighton Sanatorium has exemplified since 1902 of being "really a training school for the would-be-well." In their own words—

The palatial building and the liege-halle must give place to the simplest home-like institution and organised training for the resumption of wage-earning. If possible, the patients in whom the disease may be believed to be arrested should be retained in an after-care colony connected with the sanatorium. Here full work and wage-earning can be resumed gradually, while yet not entirely out of touch with the medical authorities of the sanatorium, though not directly under medical control. For the success of such a scheme propagandist work among all the friendly, labour, and trade societies affiliated to the movement must be continuously pursued, and the co-operation of the medical profession in the selection of suitable cases must be anxiously sought. The members of all the affiliated organisations must be taught the means of recognising early consumption as well as the necessity of seeking treatment before being completely incapacitated. The importance of the educational value of a term of residence in a sanatorium is inversely proportional to the magnificence of the buildings and surroundings. Every patient must leave a working-class sanatorium convinced that there is nothing in the accommodation or in the life which he experienced there which is incapable of being copied in his own simple home. If he be of the fortunate majority in whom the disease becomes arrested, he must realise how much his future will depend upon himself, and how much he can do of good to his fellows by inducing them to live the cleanly, sober, busy, regular life of a workers' sanatorium.

If the Association succeeds in training those sent to its sanatorium on the lines here indicated it will be doing admirable work, with which it is to be hoped that Friendly Societies will see the advisability of associating themselves.

Meanwhile, apart from the provision of sanatorium treatment, there is much work for Friendly Societies to do in diminishing the present drain on their resources through tuberculosis. They can ascertain and inform the medical officer of health of any insanitary circumstances, and particularly of any dusty occupations to which their members are exposed. They can start a crusade in every workshop and factory against indiscriminate expectoration. They can encourage and almost insist on any of their members who are losing weight or who have persistent cough being thoroughly overhauled, and having their sputum examined bacteriologically ; and in these and other ways they can help to the early recognition of disease, to its treatment while curable, and to the prevention of infection.

CHAPTER XLVII

DISPENSARIES AND THE PREVENTION OF PHTHISIS

SO far we have been concerned with the measures which the patient himself and his doctor, the different local authorities of the community in which the patient lives, and friendly and similar societies can take in the prevention of tuberculosis. Dispensaries and sanatoria may be either municipal or voluntary in their organisation, and together they hold a high place in the list of measures against this disease.

The French hygienists have especially developed dispensaries and the Germans sanatoria as a means of fighting tuberculosis, and the discussion as to their relative utility has been prolonged and sometimes heated. Thus Dr. Calmette of Lille, with whose name the French dispensary system is especially associated, says that the sanatorium cannot be regarded as a means of prophylaxis, but only as the one great means of cure. Dr. Savoire of Paris, speaking on the same point, minimises the importance of sanatoria because these establishments reject more advanced cases and only isolate tuberculous patients " at the stage of the disease in which they are least dangerous." These and other writers claim that dispensaries, on the contrary, are important means for combating the spread of the disease. The relative value of the two can best be discussed dispassionately after the two institutions have been described.

It is generally agreed that on the Continent Dr. Calmette first realised completely the ideal of a dispensary which would be self-contained, not only treating the patients medically, but watching over their welfare, visiting them at their homes, giving them all the necessary hygienic instructions, and providing material and aid when needed. His dispensary, as described by MM. Courtois-Suffit and Ch. Laubry (1905), consists of a large waiting-hall, two consultation rooms, a dark room for laryngo-scopic examinations, a laboratory, and an office for the assistant investigator.   The chief doctor is assisted by a staff of doctors and bacteriologists.   Their complete medical investigation of each case is supplemented by a social inquiry entrusted to a special officer, who visits the home, inquires into urgent needs, emphasises the hygienic advice already given, and arranges for supplying cod-liver oil, antiseptics, spit-cups, and, where needed, food.   The dispensary is thus a centre of prophylaxis, thanks to its educative work, and to the means of disinfection used by it. Dr. Calmette estimates the cost of an establishment helping 100 families at about 72,000 francs per annum, not including the cost of installation.   The work of the dispensary does not preclude, of course, the recommendation of suitable early cases for sanatorium treatment, and the sending of the children of tuberculous parents to seaside resorts, etc.

The work thus described does not differ materially so far as the homes of the patients are concerned from that carried out under an efficient system of notification of phthisis in England. Such a dispensary as described above does not gather to it all the patients in a town, and almost certainly not so large a proportion of their total number as are notified in an English town to the medical officer of health under a fairly successful system of notification.   The preventive measures that can be taken by a medical officer of health have a wider sweep than those of the dispensary physician or of his domiciliary visitor.   Disinfection is better done, sanitary defects can be effectively remedied, and removal to a suitable institution of patients housed badly for themselves and their families can more easily be arranged.   The chief point in which the French dispensary system appears to be better than the English system of voluntary notification is in the giving of material aid.   This under the English system can be, and is partially in process of being, remedied by co-operation with voluntary helpers, the Charity Organisation Society, etc.

Tuberculosis Dispensaries in England.—The out-patient departments of certain British hospitals and certain dispensaries have for many years past carried on similar work to that of the French dispensaries, apart from the home visits.   Even these have been arranged at Edinburgh in the pioneer work of Dr. Philip.   The Victoria Dispensary for Consumption was founded by him in 1887, and, with the exception of the giving of food, etc., to necessitous patients, the method of procedure is identical with that of Dr. Calmette's dispensary. Dr. Philip (1906) describes the present arrangements of the Victoria Dispensary as follows :—

The Victoria Dispensary, as at present arranged, contains—

Two consulting rooms, a laryngoscopic room, one large waiting-room, two dressing-rooms (male and female), a general office where names are entered, a laboratory for bacteriological examinations, a drug and food store.

The dispensary is open thrice weekly for three or four hours.

The staff consists of—

1. Four qualified physicians who attend when the dispensary is open for the purpose of examining and instructing patients. Three of the physicians are honorary.

2. One of the medical officers receives a salary of £60 a year, and devotes a large amount of time to the work. In addition to examining patients at the institution, along with the honorary physicians, he pays domiciliary visits to the dwellings of patients in co-operation with the trained nurse. He makes bacteriological examinations of expectoration and other suspect discharges. By arrangement with the city authorities, he notifies all cases of tuberculosis which he meets. He advises regarding the disinfection of houses during illness and after the removal or death of the patient. He supervises treatment of patients at their own home when this is desirable. He selects suitable patients for the sanatorium. In co-operation with the city authorities, he drafts the more advanced or dying patients to a hospital now dedicated to such cases in the neighbourhood of the city.

3. A nurse who has been carefully trained in modern open-air methods at the Royal Victoria Hospital for Consumption, Edinburgh—the sanatorium in connection with the dispensary—visits the homes of the patients. She readily wins their confidence by her interest in their welfare. She instructs the patients, or their friends (wives, mothers, etc.), both as to treatment and prevention. In co-operation with the visiting physician, she reports regarding the patient's residence and other conditions according to the annexed schedule of inquiry. The reports, when completed, are vouched for by the signature of both doctor and nurse.

SCHEDULE OF INQUIRY REGARDING DISPENSARY PATIENTS

*No. in Ledger*_____   *Date of Report*_____
Name   Age
Address   Married or single ?
Occupation   Has patient changed occupation ?
Able to work full time ?   Or part time ?
If unable, confined to bed ?
How long ill ?
Situation of house (area, ground floor, first, etc.) ?
Number and ages of inmates ?

Number and description of rooms ?
General aspect of house (clean, damp, dusty, smelly) ?
Number of windows ?   Can they open ?
Are they kept open (a) by day ?
                    (b) by night ?
Have they always been kept open ?
Does patient sleep alone (a) in bed ?
                        (b) in room ?
How is washing of clothes done ?
How long in present house ?
If has moved within two years, previous addresses ?
Have there been illness or deaths in house ?
    (a) In own time ?
    (b) In previous occupancy ?
Exposed to infection (a) at home ?
                     (b) at work ?
                     (c) among friends ?
Present health of other members of household ?
What precaution taken to disinfect ?
T. B. in sputum ?
T. B. in dust of room ?
General dietary ?   Teetotal ?
General condition (well-to-do, badly off) ?
Proximate income of household ?
Assisted by societies, church, friends, rates ?

Signed_____*Reporter.*

_____*Medical Officer.*

4. A volunteer Samaritan Committee of ladies, in conference with the doctors, take charge of more distressing cases, where, through prolonged illness, the financial conditions have been much reduced. In many cases they visit the patients' houses. With the assistance of the numerous charitable and parochial organisations which exist in the city, they are enabled to adapt the relief necessary to the particular case. The members of the Samaritan Committee further occupy themselves with the question of suitable employment for tuberculous persons fit for some effort, although unable to work an entire day. In some cases they arrange likewise for persons who have been discharged from the sanatorium. Attention is also paid to the case of school children affected with the disease, so as to have their education supervised on more physiological lines. The operations of the Committee are regulated at fortnightly meetings, and a minute of the business is kept.

5. An officer—a working-man who gives his entire time to the dispensary—lives on the premises. This man receives and enters the names of the patients on the afternoons when the dispensary is open. When the dispensary is not formally open, he attends to requests from patients or other persons. The officer is conversant with the home and work conditions of many of the patients, and is a valuable lieutenant both to the doctors and nurse.

Dr. Philip holds that such a dispensary as the above "should be, for every city or district, the uniting point of all other agencies." In the strictly medical sense, this is true. The dispensary is the receiving-house, the clearing-house for patients. It feeds the list of official notifications and it enables official preventive measures to be taken. But it does not act—in this country, at least—as a complete receiving-house, and is not likely to do so. A municipal dispensary, and much less a dispensary under the control of private charity, will not draw to itself all the consumptives needing preventive measures as well as curative help, though it may be the largest agent to this end. Many consumptives will remain under the medical care of private practitioners, of club doctors, of private dispensaries, or in the out-patient departments of various public hospitals and dispensaries. Under a system of notification of phthisis the medical officer of health forms the centre from which in a well-governed community the various measures against phthisis start and are co-ordinated and made complete. He is almost certain to know of more cases of phthisis than the physician of the dispensary, and he has the further advantage that he can secure for each patient the removal of insanitary conditions of home and workshop, and the necessary disinfection. He can also provide handkerchiefs and spit-bottles; and we hope shortly will be able in very many towns to arrange for sanatorium treatment and for the hospital treatment of advanced cases. The ideal cannot be better stated than in Dr. Philip's words :—

It cannot be too strongly emphasised that the strength of such a scheme lies especially in its organisation and co-ordination. Each factor is doubtless of value. Each department has its own sphere of operations. As isolated elements their possibilities are relatively limited. In proportion as the various departments are intimately connected and co-ordinated, they each become more serviceable. The key to complete success in the campaign against consumption lies in the harmonious co-ordination of well-directed measures.

CHAPTER XLVIII

THE RÔLE OF SANATORIA IN THE TREATMENT AND PREVENTION OF PHTHISIS

A SANATORIUM, as its derivation indicates, is a place for the cure of disease, in the present connection of tuberculosis. By Trudeau and others the word is used to denote also a hospital or asylum for hopeless cases, in which they can be cared for and treated under conditions preventing infection to others. There is some convenience in accepting this wider meaning of the term, in view of the difficulties likely to be encountered in the future in the institutional treatment of advanced cases of disease. If these are relegated to a separate "hospital," they will probably refuse in many instances to enter ; if only to a separate ward of a "sanatorium," consent to institutional treatment is much more likely to be secured.

It is not difficult to define the respective rôles of sanatoria for early cases and for advanced cases of disease. The former are primarily concerned with the effective arrest, if not actual cure, of the disease ; the latter with the sympathetic care of the progressively sick, and with the prevention of infection. For I quite agree with Dr. Philip's and the general dictum that "there can be no manner of doubt that the far advanced or dying cases constitute the greatest source of infection " (see also pp. 103 and 257). The functions of the two classes of sanatoria overlap, for the effective arrest of disease in the individual is an excellent way of stopping infection ; and for this reason, if for no other, the sanatorium for early cases is also a means of prophylaxis of great importance. Its importance in this respect is enhanced by its educational influence. No self-respecting or even self-regarding patient, after being trained in a good sanatorium, will continue to spit without due precautions, and his general life in regard to cleanliness and ventilation is likely still further to reduce any possible risk of infection. Hence it is a great mistake to regard sanatoria as merely cure-places. They are schools of national importance.

OBJECTS OF SANATORIA FOR OTHER THAN ADVANCED CASES. —1. In early and suitable cases a cure may be expected.

2. Short of cure in a large number of cases, arrest of disease occurs, the patient possibly continuing to have a small amount of sputum daily, but being able to resume his work. In a still larger number of cases, although the disease is not completely arrested, the patient's condition is improved, his sputum diminished, he is able to resume his work at least to a modified extent, and his working life is much prolonged.

3. While the patient is in the sanatorium his home is disinfected, his relatives are free from recurring infection and have time to recover their full measure of resistance to infection.

4. On his return home and to his work the patient is much less likely than before, even though he continues to have sputum containing tubercle bacilli, to be a source of infection to others.

Before considering these points in further detail, it will be well briefly to consider the

HISTORY OF THE OPEN-AIR TREATMENT OF PHTHISIS.—It was an English village doctor named George Bodington who first seriously practised the treatment of this disease by what he called " the natural method." He described his treatment in the following words (1840) :—

> To live in and breathe freely the open air, without being deterred by the wind or weather, is one important and essential remedy in arresting its progress.
> The cold is never too severe for the consumptive patient in this climate ; the cooler the air which passes into the lungs the greater will be the benefit the patient will derive.
> The common hospital in a large town is the most unfit place imaginable for consumptive patients, and the treatment generally employed there very inefficient, arising from the inadequacy of the means at command.

Dr. Henry MacCormac of Belfast, writing in 1855, emphasised the value of open windows and cold air in the arrest of phthisis ; and Sir B. Ward Richardson, writing in 1857, quoted by Dr. Kelynack (1904), used the following words :—

> In a cosy room the consumptive is bound never to live, nor in any room, indeed, for great lengths of time. So long as he is able to be out of doors, he is in his best and safest home.

Stoves of all kinds, heated pipes, and, in a word, all modes of supplying artificial warmth, except that by the radiation from an open fire, are, according to the facts which I have been able to collect, injurious.

If special hospitals for consumptives are to be had, they should be as little colonies, situated far away from the thickly populated abodes of men, and so arranged that each patient should have a distinct dwelling-place for himself. They should be provided with pleasure-grounds of great extent, in which the patients who could walk about should pass every possible hour in the day ; and with glass-covered walks overhead, where the open air could be freely breathed, even if rain were falling.

Opinion gradually grew in favour of an open-air life for consumptives, but the main impetus to systematic sanatorium treatment has come from Germany, especially from the methods employed by Brehmer at Görbersdorf and by Walther at Nordrach. Brehmer, who first began to write on the subject in 1856 and opened his sanatorium in 1859, held that tuberculosis was an infectious disease, and, judging by his experience of the population at Görbersdorf, that high altitude had an inhibitory influence against it. Arguing from this experience, he inferred that anything protecting one person from becoming a victim to tuberculosis must, if properly employed, be able to cure another person of the same disease ; and on these lines he built up his sanatorium treatment, including in it

1. Living in the open air under conditions which appear to give immunity to tuberculosis.

2. Ensuring freedom from debilitating influences or anything likely to cause recrudescence of disease.

3. Methodical exercises, particularly hill-climbing, when the patient's condition permitted it.

4. An abundant diet, especially comprising fatty food, milk, and vegetables.

5. Constant systematic medical supervision, and various hydro-therapeutic measures.

It is unnecessary to follow the recent history of the evolution of sanatorium treatment, or the principles embodied in it. In the words of Dr. F. Rufenacht Walters (1905, p. 41) " the essence of Brehmer's and Dettweiler's methods is the elimination of haphazard treatment and the prescription of absolute repose or of various degrees of exercise according to definite medical indications."

STRUCTURAL CONDITIONS AND ARRANGEMENTS OF SANATORIA.

—A very short summary on this subject must suffice, the reader being referred for details to Dr. Walters' exhaustive work on Sanatoria, and to Dr. Latham's Essay on the same subject. Here we are only concerned with the principles that should guide local authorities in the matter, and with advice as to the avoidance of unnecessary expense. Sanatorium treatment can be carried out successfully in any place where the air is pure, though a position sheltered on the north and east is preferable. If the soil is drained and has a slope, it is unnecessary to select a sandy or other porous soil, though this is preferable when accessible. The main desiderata as to the site are that

1. The air must be free from dust. Hence nearness to main roads is inadvisable.

2. Shelter is desirable to the north and east, and there should be sheltered walks in the grounds.

3. The aspect should be sunny.

The grounds should have shelters suitable for patients to lie out of doors during a greater part of each day, and the walks should suffice for graduated exercise.

The arrangements of bedrooms will vary with the class of patient. It is always desirable to have a number of bedrooms for single patients, but the exclusive provision of single bedrooms in large institutions supported by charity is in my opinion an extravagant use of charitable gifts. My experience is that six or even twelve consumptive working-men can be treated with success in one ward, small rooms being provided for those whose coughs are particularly troublesome. There is the further point that in such wards absolutely complete perflation of air can be secured; whereas in separate bedrooms as usually arranged in sanatoria, a corridor is needed opening from each bedroom door. However well-ventilated is this corridor, it does not permit as good cross-ventilation as in a hospital ward of which the two opposite walls are outside walls with windows between each bed; and single bedrooms on the plan just mentioned are seldom so light and cheerful as a cross-lighted ward. If there is a verandah outside the single bedroom, the defective lighting becomes a still greater detriment for acute cases confined to bed.

Of other structural arrangements it is only necessary to say that they need not be expensive to secure efficient treatment

25

of the patient. A linoleum flooring is as sanitary as parquet and much cheaper. Ledges and corners for dust should be avoided. Furniture should be simple and free from unnecessary coverings and hangings. Walls may be covered with a washable distemper. There is much to be said in favour of these in preference to well-painted cement walls, as the latter favour the condensation of moisture, and clothes hung in the room are on humid days cold and damp. Walls and floor and furniture should be cleansed daily with a damp cloth, a broom or brush only being permitted under special conditions.

Unless in a few special instances for particular purposes, the cost of construction should be kept down to £200 or £300 per patient to be accommodated. It can seldom be justifiable to spend £800 to £1200 per bed, as has occasionally been done.

PRINCIPLES OF TREATMENT.—Some of the essential points have been already indicated, both in dealing with the home treatment of cases (p. 326) and earlier in this chapter (p. 382). In a sanatorium, treatment is more systematic, the patient is removed from temptations to depart from the necessary régime, and he avoids the risks of catarrhal infection and of mental or bodily fatigue or harass which are apt to occur at home. The atmosphere at the sanatorium is usually purer and freer from dust than at his home, and the patient gains the advantages associated with a complete change of environment. Specific treatment by tuberculin, controlled by opsonic testing, is more easily managed at a sanatorium than at home. Hygienic rules can be more easily enforced, rest in bed can be controlled in accordance with exact observations of the patient's .temperature and other conditions ; and, where the appetite is deficient, the more or less forced feeding which is an important part of sanatorium treatment can be efficiently carried out. Although too rapid accumulation of fat is undesirable, the indication is to press feeding sufficiently to ensure in non-febrile cases a weekly gain of weight of at least 1 lb., better 2 to 3 lb. (Walters), " until the natural full weight is reached, and to ensure this being maintained afterwards." The patient can often digest large quantities of meat, even when he is feverish. Many feverish patients begin at once to improve as soon as they sleep out of doors, or at least stay out during the entire day. Complete rest and open-air life give the best prospect of reducing the fever of acute phthisis. The regulation of amount of exercise is one of the most important duties of the sanatorium physician, and it is on this point that the superiority of sanatorium over home treatment is most evident. As Dr. Latham (1906) remarks: "What the patient learns at a sanatorium, and only at a sanatorium, is the fact that *fatigue* kills the majority of consumptives and causes the frequent relapses of the disease. The avoidance of fatigue is therefore of primary importance." This leads to the consideration of the chief practical objection urged against sanatorium treatment for working-men. The problem for them is a serious one. As frequently sent out from sanatoriums they are much improved in health, but their muscles are soft, and they are unable to bear the normal fatigue associated with their daily work. Even when able, they are often unwilling. Dr. Walters (1906) may be quoted here :—

It is justly argued that prolonged idleness is apt to foster lazy habits and to make the patient less capable of steady work. The remedy for this is to substitute other forms of useful occupation as soon as the patients are fit for it. Hard manual labour is unsuitable for something like two years after the breakdown, but many forms of light work are permissible as a rule, such as hoeing, raking, sweeping, pruning, poultry feeding, chopping up thin pieces of food, and some of the work in which hand machinery is used. The spare time should, however, be chiefly employed in education. At Dr. Weicker's sanatorium for artisans in Silesia and in some others the patients have regular courses of instruction in short-hand, foreign languages, cooking, and the like. Many of the applications of science and art to manufacture would also be permissible, such as designing, photography, the reproduction of designs, some methods of decorating pottery, and some of the applications of microscopy and chemistry. A conference of medical men with technical instructors in various branches of handicraft would probably bring to light many useful occupations open to convalescent consumptives. The chief point to bear in mind would be the substitution of delicate for laborious work, brains for brawn. That hygienic teaching bearing upon the disease itself would be given is taken for granted ; but the addition of suitable technical teaching would make the sanatorium a valuable educational centre, would add to the happiness and usefulness of the inmates, and greatly diminish the difficulty in finding work for discharged patients.

Short of the change of occupation wisely advocated above, wherever practicable, much can be done for the industrial patient while in the sanatorium to prepare him to return to his own work. On this point I will quote somewhat fully Dr. Kingston Fowler's (1906) description of the methods adopted at Frimley,

the Brompton Hospital Sanatorium, which have been organised
and successfully carried out under the care of Dr. M. S. Paterson,
the medical superintendent :—

Each batch of patients on arrival from the parent hospital at Brompton
—through which they must all pass—is addressed by the medical superintendent on (1) discipline, (2) fresh air, and (3) feeding. As they have
already been trained at Brompton for the lesson they have to learn, they
find but little difficulty in falling in with the more complete open-air
life followed at Frimley. It was, however, not an easy task to establish
the tradition of absolute obedience to orders which now prevails ; the
conviction as to the wisdom of the regulations came to the patients as
they found themselves steadily improving in health and strength. Now
everyone cheerfully goes about his appointed exercise or work irrespective
of the weather, and if told off to roll the lawn for two hours he does it,
and is not found after five minutes sitting upon the handle of the
roller.

As an illustration of the thoroughness of the treatment, so far as " open
air " is concerned, I may state that the desire of the majority of the
patients whose bedrooms on the upper floor are without a balcony is
to be promoted to a room with a balcony, or to one on the ground floor,
so that they may be able to pull out their beds and sleep in the open
air. I was told when at Frimley in December 1905 that most of the
patients at that time slept in the open air when it was not raining. During
the recent frosty weather the patients were told that they could close
their windows for an hour whilst they were dressing, but it was found
that none of the windows were closed. Hats and caps are not worn except
when walking outside the grounds. The appetite developed by an open-
air life is surprising ; as most of the staff voluntarily lead the same life,
they experience a similar increase of appetite.

Daily Routine.—6.50 a.m. : Rise and turn down beds and proceed
according to " Morning Routine." 8.15 a.m. : Breakfast for tables
1, 2, and 3. 8.30 a.m. : Breakfast for tables 4, 5, and 6. 9.30 to 9.55 a.m. :
Indoor work. 10 a.m. : Outdoor work or exercise. 10.50 a.m. : Lunch.
11 a.m. : Outdoor work or exercise. 12 to 12.45 p.m. : Absolute rest
for tables 1, 2, and 3. 12 to 1 p.m. : Absolute rest for tables 4, 5, and 6.
1 p.m. : Dinner for tables 1, 2, and 3. 1.15 p.m. : Dinner for tables 4,
5, and 6. 2 to 2.45 p.m. : Absolute rest for tables 1, 2, and 3. 2.15
to 2.45 p.m. : Absolute rest for tables 4, 5, and 6. 2.45 to 4.35 p.m. :
Work or exercise in grounds. 5 p.m. : Tea for tables 1, 2, and 3. 5.15
p.m. : Tea for tables 4, 5, and 6. 5.50 p.m. : Temperatures taken for
tables 1, 2, and 3. 6.5 p.m. : Temperatures taken for tables 4, 5, and 6.
6 to 7.45 p.m. : Read papers, write letters, play indoor games, etc.
7.45 p.m. : Supper for tables 1, 2, and 3. 8 p.m. : Supper for tables
4, 5, and 6. 8.40 p.m. : Prayers. 8.45 p.m. : Bed. 9.15 p.m. : Lights
out. 9.30 p.m. : Silence.

A quarter of an hour is allowed for smoking after each meal. A
quarter of an hour is allowed before each meal for washing. Patients
are not allowed indoors except for meals and rest hours until 6 p.m. without

special permission. Patients may use the concert-hall and reading-room from 6 p.m. until prayers.

Sunday Routine.—The routine is the same, with the following differences : There is no work. 9.30 to 10.35 a.m. : Patients walk two miles in all weathers. 11 a.m. : Divine service. 12 noon : Rest hour. 2.30 p.m. : Those patients who have permission may walk outside the sanatorium until 4.45 p.m.

The patient's day is thus so completely occupied that he has little leisure for introspection, and I am informed that the only common complaint is, "We are kept so busy we have no time for anything."

Graduated Labour.—The new feature which Dr. Paterson has introduced at Frimley is graduated labour, a feature which appears to m e to go far to solve the question as to the applicability of sanatoriu m treatment to the poorer classes. County authorities and the public are naturally asking : " Are the patients whom you call 'cured' able to work and earn their own living ? " (I deprecate the use of the word " cure," but the public will have it so.) Upon the answer which we are able to give to this question the provision of adequate sanatorium accommodation for the poor depends. I believe we can state that the patients classed as " arrested " after treatment at Frimley are fit for work.

The gradation of exercise and labour is as follows : Exercise and labour are for two periods daily, each of two hours' duration. (1) Slow walking exercise, beginning at two miles a day and gradually increasing up to ten miles a day. (2) Picking up fir cones and firewood in the grounds and carrying a " half-basket " (weight 11 pounds) to the stack. (3) Carrying a full basket of firewood and cones (weight 16 pounds). (4) Carrying a " half-basket " of gravel or stones from the gravel pit to the place where paths are being made or repaired (weight 21 pounds). (5) Carrying a basket of gravel or stones, the weight of which is gradually increased up to 38 pounds. (6) Rolling the grass or gravel. Sixteen men pull a roller weighing 15 cwt. (7) Digging ground already broken. (8) Mowing grass with a lawn mower. (9) Digging unbroken ground. (10) The same as under (9) but for six hours daily instead of four hours—*i.e.* the hours usually spent at rest are spent in labour.

The indications accepted as evidence of the arrest of the disease are : (1) absence of fever ; (2) absence of adventitious sounds, except such as are indicative of fibrosis ; (3) absence of cough and expectoration ; (4) continuous gain of weight or maintenance of the patient's highest known weight ; and (5) ability to perform labour incidental to grade No. 9 as above.

The point to which I wish especially to draw attention is that no patient is classified on discharge as " arrested " unless for three weeks continuously he can pass one or other of the following tests :—

Test A.—For patients who earn their living by manual labour : To be able on an ordinary diet and without rest hours to use a pick and shovel of the full size and weight for six hours daily and to maintain his health. The shovels and spades are in three sizes, weighing 2, 4, and 6 pounds respectively. The picks vary from 3 to 7 pounds in weight.

Test B.—For patients who do not earn their living by manual labour, *e.g.* clerks, shopmen, or salesmen : To be able on an ordinary diet to perform the labour of grade No. 6 or No. 7 for six hours daily for three weeks and to maintain his health. These patients are, as a rule, gradually brought up to No. 9, and when it is found that they can do this work, they are put back to No. 6 or No. 7. The theory is that a man doing the work described under No. 9 or No. 10 who on discharge will engage in work involving but little bodily exercise, would suffer in health from such an abrupt transition. Further experience is, however, necessary upon this point. In some cases it is found that patients are unfit for No. 9 but that they can be raised to a standard of labour which is equal to their ordinary work. These patients are tested before discharge on the grade to which they have attained, but they are not, as a rule, classified as " arrested."

The system has been gradually evolved and has not yet been in operation for a sufficient time to justify the expression of a final opinion as to its value, but there appears to be every reason for anticipating that it will prove successful.

MEDICAL RESULTS OF SANATORIUM TREATMENT.—After careful consideration, I have decided not to utilise any of the many published statistics as to sanatorium treatment. So much depends upon accurate diagnosis, upon accurate tabulation of figures, and upon the lapse of a sufficiently long and uniform interval before results are tabulated, that I doubt if many of the published figures can be trusted for comparative purposes.

I am completely convinced that the sanatorium treatment is most beneficial to patients, and enables a large proportion of them to resume their ordinary life. This is true even for cases in which there is consolidation, and occasionally also for cases with considerable cavitation of lungs. Although similar cures occur apart from sanatorium treatment, clinical experience indicates that they are more frequent and occur earlier under sanatorium treatment, and I have no doubt that were exactly comparable data available, this would be found to be so. As Professor v. Ziemssen, quoted by Dr. Walters, says :—

The possibility of treatment outside a sanatorium with equally good results cannot be denied, but it requires much more prolonged rest and much more time on the part of the physician, and has by no means so certain a result.

The general results of sanatorium treatment have been well summed up by Dr. J. E. Squire as follows :—

1. It can, he says, be " reasonably expected that of the cases of pulmonary tuberculosis which are recognised sufficiently

early and commence sanatorium treatment without delay, some may be cured and return to work in three months."

2. Three months' treatment being rarely sufficient for the stage in which "early" cases are generally admitted to the sanatorium, "we are justified in stating that early cases of pulmonary tuberculosis may be expected to recover under sanatorium treatment if persisted in sufficiently long," but six or even twelve months may be required.

3. There is a further justifiable expectation that by "sanatorium treatment, even in acute and somewhat advanced cases, arrest may be anticipated provided the patient is able to continue the treatment sufficiently long." This generally means at least twelve months' treatment and a further period under supervision before "cure" can be spoken of.

CLASS OF PATIENTS SUITABLE FOR SANATORIUM TREATMENT.—The great desire of all physicians at sanatoria is to secure patients at an early stage of disease, and their general lament is that this desire is not achieved. Not all the cases with physical signs of early disease do better than cases of disease of longer standing, much depending on the acuteness and febrile reaction of the patient. The three months usually allowed for sanatorium treatment often does not suffice for cure or arrest of disease. The choice of patients in most sanatoria is made from the point of view of the individual. Can the disease be arrested or not? is the question asked from this side. It is not identical with the view of the public health administrator, whose question in relation to sanatoria is, By the sanatorium treatment of what patients, and of these for what length of time, can I secure the greatest amount of prevention of infection? This question is sufficiently important to be dealt with in a separate chapter. Meanwhile, we may add here a few words as to the training of sanatorium patients, and as to their after-care.

THE TRAINING OF SANATORIUM PATIENTS.—An important element in the treatment of each patient is that he should know the nature of his disease, and should receive exact instructions as to the hygienic precautions necessary for aiding his cure, for preventing relapse, and for obviating infection. Whatever differences of opinion there may be as to the economic gain of the sanatorium treatment of wage-earning patients, there can be none as to the great gain to the community secured by this training.   The principles of it are sufficiently obvious, and they have been stated on pp. 348 and 357.   The following card is given to each patient leaving the Brighton Sanatorium :—

Advice to Patients leaving the Sanatorium

1. The spit-bottle should always be carried in the pocket, and daily washed out with boiling water after emptying its contents down the W.C.   At home, if the bottle is not used, spit into paper or rag, and burn this at once.

2. Be careful not to cough directly opposite to any other person. Always hold a handkerchief to your mouth when coughing. Change your handkerchief every day, and put the soiled one into water.

3. In order to maintain a condition of good nourishment, take a glass of milk with each of the three chief meals, in addition to the ordinary food.

4. Keep on taking cod liver oil each day until you have no cough, unless otherwise ordered by your doctor.

5. Do not take beer or other alcoholic drinks.   Money thus spent is wasted.

6. Keep up the practice of sleeping with your bedroom door *and* window wide open.   One of these without the other does not suffice.   To keep warm, wear plenty of woollen clothes.

7. It is imperative that you should sleep in a separate bed, and if possible have a separate bedroom.

8. Do not run the risk of inhaling dust if you can avoid it, either in the house, or when at work, or in the street.   Always insist on the " wet cleansing " of rooms, instead of dry dusting or sweeping.

THE AFTER-CARE OF SANATORIUM PATIENTS.—The permanence of cure or of arrest of disease depends greatly on the training which the patient has received while in the sanatorium, and his intelligence and assiduity in living up to it.   Ofttimes, however intelligent and willing he may be, he cannot live the life best calculated to maintain his ground.   He is obliged, for instance, to return to hard manual labour in a dusty workshop. The general considerations applying in this matter are stated on p. 327.   If alongside these considerations be placed those quoted from Dr. Walters on p. 387, we have a statement of possible alternatives, of which the resumption of previous work most frequently occurs. The difficulty as to subsequent occupation is even greater for patients whose expectoration continues, often fairly abundant, but who have before them several years in which they are still able to work. For these the month's sanatorium training mentioned on p. 395 is particularly indicated. After this, what is to be done with them ?

INDUSTRIAL COLONIES have been advocated for them. During the patient's stay in the sanatorium itself, something may be done in this direction, as indicated on pp. 387-390, and the sanatorium may be arranged so as to merge into the industrial colony. There is little doubt that a year's life on a farm or farm colony after leaving the sanatorium would in many instances which now soon relapse mean permanent recovery. There are, however, difficulties which prevent one from being very sanguine in regard to them. Dr. Jane Walker (1906, p. 365) draws attention to three of these : the patients are mostly town-dwellers, they are often married men, and they have generally learnt a trade, and will not therefore make up their minds to take the wages of an agricultural labourer. The subsequent development of schemes in this direction will be watched with interest, but it cannot be said at present that the establishment of such colonies otherwise than by private charity is to be recommended.

CHAPTER XLIX

THE INSTITUTIONAL TREATMENT OF PHTHISIS FROM THE PUBLIC HEALTH STANDPOINT

THE subject of this chapter necessarily traverses ground already partially covered in previous chapters. It is desirable, however, to summarise from the standpoint of public health administration the question of the institutional treatment of phthisis ; and this chapter may be regarded therefore as an annexe to Chapter XLVIII., as well as an attempt at the practical application of the argument of Part. II.

Three classes of consumptive patients need to be considered : first, those in an early and probably curable stage ; second, those who, though showing marked disease, are still able to work either continuously or with intervals of inability, and who are likely to have several further years of life, whether treated or untreated ; and third, advanced cases, unable to work, commonly confined to the house except in warm weather, and often bedridden.

Which of these is most dangerous to the public health ? Reasons have been already given for the view that the advanced cases do most harm ; for not only are they unable to control so perfectly the disposal of their more abundant sputum, but they require that intimate and protracted personal attention which in the ordinary circumstances of domestic life among the poor especially favours infection. Against this is to be set the fact that the early and the intermediate patients have a wider field for scattering infection. The balance of evidence is nevertheless strongly against their being the chief source of infection. Whatever view be taken on this point, evidently the wise course is to ensure the due disposal of expectoration by each of the three classes of patient. The training of the early patient, when it can be secured, holds good during a longer period of infectivity than that of the intermediate or

advanced patient.   Hence it should be the rule to ensure the training of consumptive patients from the earliest practicable period.

SANATORIUM TRAINING OF EARLY AND INTERMEDIATE CASES.
—Early experience of notified cases of phthisis showed me—
what has been confirmed by later experience—that even when
I had given definite instructions, both verbally and printed
(see p. 324), as to care in spitting, on subsequent visits it was not
infrequently found that these were not being effectually followed.
Sometimes the instructions had been misunderstood, more
often they had been neglected.   The patient's self-interest as
well as his conscience needs to be utilised.   If he can be taught
heartily to believe that his own welfare and that of his family
is favoured by the precautionary measures recommended to
him, we may usually rely on his co-operation.   How to secure
this educational influence became, then, an important question
early in my local experience of the notification of phthisis.   The
plan eventually adopted—the success of which in this respect
has exceeded my anticipations—was the treatment on open-
air principles of all patients who could be persuaded to consent
to such treatment.   This was carried out in a detached pavilion
of our hospital for acute infectious diseases which is locally
known as the sanatorium.   The difficulty in getting patients
to come into the sanatorium was greatly diminished by the
fact that only very short terms of treatment were proposed,
which could in most instances be managed, without the patient
risking loss of his livelihood.   The Fig. on p. 341 shows how
greatly the number of cases of phthisis voluntarily notified
in Brighton has increased since sanatorium treatment became
available.   The details of the system adopted in Brighton
have been regarded with considerable interest, and I therefore
give here certain fuller particulars which may be of assistance
in other towns.

MUNICIPAL SANATORIUM TRAINING AND TREATMENT AT
BRIGHTON.—The earlier details of our local efforts at sanatorium treatment are stated on p. 348 in their relation to the
notification of cases.   Further details will now be given.   The
first point aimed at was to avoid any new capital expenditure
on buildings ; and in order to do so, to utilise an empty pavilion
of our present isolation or fever hospital.   Epidemics of scarlet
fever and diphtheria are intermittent, and of enteric fever are

very rare ; and yet hospital accommodation in most communities is kept ready for the contingency of their occurrence. This accommodation it was proposed to utilise for phthisis patients ; and there did not seem to be any serious difficulty in doing so, as, with the possible exception of an occasional milk outbreak of one of the above acute diseases, plans can be made for several weeks ahead, and phthisical patients can easily be sent home when necessary. Events have proved this forecast correct. Not only has it been unnecessary to cease treating consumptives at the hospital up to the present time, but we have been able to increase our beds for this disease from four to ten and then to twenty-five. This increase is in part owing to a charitable bequest (the Hedgcock Bequest), which enabled the Town Council to devote a yearly income from this source of £600 to £700 to the endowment of further beds. This fund enabled the number of beds for the use of consumptives to be increased from ten to twenty-five, including three beds for paying patients, twelve to be maintained by the Hedgcock Bequest, and ten provided directly by the Town Council. The Town Council provides the entire accommodation for these twenty-five patients in its isolation hospital.

The directly municipal patients are usually admitted for a month each, and are by preference men and women still able to work, and in connection with whom a month's rest, treatment, and training, can effect the greatest good to the patient and to others in preventing infection, both of fellow-workers and of family. No charge is made for the admission of these patients, who are chiefly labourers, artisans, clerks, etc., and their relatives.

The Hedgcock patients belong to the same classes. They must be unable to pay for their own maintenance in the sanatorium. Some of them are very advanced, or even dying cases, for whom continuance at home is undesirable owing to difficulties as to nursing, or because there is a large family and much danger of infection. Where practicable, advanced cases are treated in separate rooms. It is not, in my opinion, necessary to have a separate institution for them ; and the objection mentioned on p. 382 is strongly against this. Hedgcock patients are kept in the sanatorium for several months or for a shorter time, according to individual requirements.

The Method of Using Isolation Hospital Beds [1]

(1) *Accommodation available*

The isolation hospital consists of four main pavilions for infectious cases—an administrative block, the borough disinfecting station, a laundry, and a small destructor. Three of the main hospital pavilions were originally used for scarlet fever, diphtheria, and enteric fever, and the fourth for cases needing special isolation.

In the scarlet fever pavilion (two storeys)		68 beds.
,, diphtheria fever pavilion	,,	56	,,
,, enteric ,, ,,	: .	22	,,
,, isolation ,,	.	14	,,
	Total	160	,,

The population of Brighton estimated to the middle of 1907 was 129,023, the proportion of beds to population being about 1 to 800.

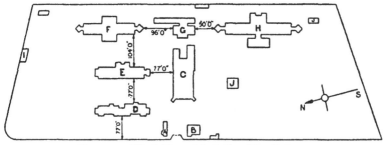

Fig. 39.—Block Plan of Isolation Hospital.

A. Discharge Room; B. Porter's Lodge; C. Administrative Block; D. Isolation Pavilion; E. Diphtheria Pavilion; F. Phthisis Pavilion; G. Laundry and Disinfecting Station; H. Scarlet Fever Pavilion; I. J. Phthisis Shelters

(2) *Isolation of the Consumptive Patients from other Diseases*

Visitors from other towns frequently ask the question : " Do the phthisical patients run any risk of contracting the infectious diseases treated in the hospital ? " The answer is that the possibility of the spread of infection depends on the standard of administration, and that an experience of six years shows a

[1] The following particulars are taken from a joint paper with Dr. H. C. Lecky published in *Tuberculosis*, June 1907.

complete absence of such infection. Infection might be spread in any of the following ways : (a) By contact between patients ; (b) by the carriage of infection by nurses, or (c) by the doctors ; (d) by infection from the laundry or kitchen.

(a) *Contact between patients in different pavilions.*—It being impossible completely to shut off one portion of the grounds from another, the keeping of the prescribed bounds depends upon the supervision by nurses of children and on the honour of patients who have reached years of discretion. Consumptive patients are as desirous not to contract another disease as the doctor is to prevent it, and patients suffering from diphtheria and scarlet fever are under the strictest supervision. In practice, therefore, this difficulty scarcely arises, and the erection of impassable barriers between areas allotted to the different diseases is found to be unnecessary.

(b) *Infection by nurses.*—It is customary in isolation hospitals for the nurses from the various wards for acute infectious diseases to have their meals in a common dining-room in the administrative building. In my experience infection has never been caused by the adoption of this plan. The experience of other isolation hospitals is to the same effect.

The nurses for the consumptive wards use a separate table in the dining-room, and sleep in separate rooms on the first floor of the administrative building. All other nurses dine at another table in the same room. The nurses for diphtheria sleep on the second floor of the administrative building, and those for scarlet fever sleep in the dormitories over the scarlet fever pavilion with a separate means of access. The nurses for different diseases are allowed to go out together, and they occasionally use a common sitting-room.

To enable scarlet fever and diphtheria to be intercommunicated under the above circumstances by the nurses attending these diseases, infection would need to pass through two intermediaries—a highly improbable event. If infection does not spread under these circumstances from scarlet fever to diphtheria, or conversely, it is unreasonable to expect that it would spread from either of these to consumptive patients, and our confidence in this anticipation has been justified by events.

(c) *Infection by the doctor.*—The precautions adopted are those which every careful practitioner adopts in his everyday rounds. The consumptive patients are visited first, and overalls are used when going into the other wards.

(d) *Infection from the laundry.*—The washing from the whole hospital is done in one common laundry. Special precautions are taken with the soiled linen from the scarlet fever and diphtheria pavilions, articles only being sorted after having been in soak for a certain time. A definite routine is maintained, so that when the linen has once been washed no soiled linen is taken into the laundry during the same week. The chances, therefore, of spread of infection in this laundry are less than in an ordinary general laundry, and infection, in fact, has not occurred.

(e) *Infection from the kitchen.*—The food for all the wards is distributed from a central kitchen. Every article to be returned from the various wards is washed first. No food is ever returned.

The above summary of our procedure shows that no risk is involved in the treatment of consumptives in a well-administered hospital, in pavilions properly separated from those for scarlet fever and diphtheria. Experience has justified the advice given as to the à *priori* improbability of such spread, for during the last six years, in which 730 consumptives have been treated for an average period of five weeks for each patient, not a single case of an acute infectious disease has occurred among these patients.

(3) *The Principles on which Beds in the Sanatorium are allocated*

Not every patient notified to be suffering from phthisis is offered treatment at the sanatorium. Since the average time that the patients can afford to stay is from four to six weeks, the main factor determining the admission of patients to other hospitals and sanatoria, namely, the possibility of permanent benefit or cure, obviously is the factor of least importance in deciding as to the admission of patients to our sanatorium. The benefit to be derived from the short treatment of patients has been summarised on p. 349. From the public standpoint it may be summed up in the word *education* or *training*: (a) The patient is taught that he is in part responsible for his own cure, and he is shown the best way of living with this end in view ; (b) he is trained so to manage his cough and expectoration that he is no longer a source of infection to others. These being the chief objects at present attempted, each of the following circumstances is taken into account in considering the suitability of cases for admission :—

(a) *The age of the patient.*—People at the working years of life are those who can derive the greatest benefit from the sanatorium treatment and training. Children, whose home circumstances are in the hands of others, obviously cannot carry out a given line of treatment of their own accord. Furthermore, children are seldom sources of infection to others, owing to the absence of expectoration. Old people suffering from phthisis frequently drift to the workhouse infirmary, and every effort is made to facilitate their admission to this institution, though in the event of their not coming within the legal limits of the poor law they are admitted to the sanatorium if they are likely sources of infection.

(b) *The size of the family.*—If a family consists of a mother and father and several children, and one of the parents has been notified, every inducement is offered to get the patient into the sanatorium. If, at the same time, the cases of a parent and one of the children have been notified, an endeavour is made to get them into the sanatorium together. On several occasions two or more members of the same family have been treated at the same time. If the family consists only of a married man and his wife, past middle age, and one of them is notified, there is less necessity to urge sanatorium treatment than if other and younger people are living with them.

(c) *The occupation.*—This is an important factor. Preference is always given to consumptives working in factories or workshops with a large number of other men or women.

(d) *The stage of the disease.*—As mentioned above, this factor by itself is of minor importance in determining the suitability of notified cases for admission. It is of extreme urgency to educate the young adult, especially if he is a bread-winner and a parent, both from the standpoint of cure and of prevention of infection. Patients with advanced disease are admitted as readily as patients having earlier disease, the one condition of admission being that the possibilities of infection can be reduced by the training of the patient.

(e) *The social position of the patient.*—Under our present

system of voluntary notification information is rarely received of cases where the family has an income of more than £2 a week. Yet, although there is a great difference between the positions of a family with an income of 35s. and one with an income of 25s., the need for sanatorium treatment is almost as urgent for the one class as for the other, and no social distinction is therefore drawn in admitting patients. The only partial exception to this rule is in regard to patients who come within the purview of the poor law. If these patients are possibly curable they are admitted to the sanatorium. If their disease is advanced they are urged to go into the Workhouse Infirmary. The arrangements in the thirty beds of that institution reserved for phthisis are good, and patients who would otherwise be a source of serious domestic infection are well segregated in these beds.

It will thus be seen that the suitability of a patient for admission to the sanatorium depends on the answer to the following questions : (1) " Will the treatment begun at the sanatorium, if subsequently continued, give a reasonable chance of a cure ? " (2) " Even if there is no reasonable chance of a cure, will the treatment and training diminish and possibly prevent the spread of infection to others when the patient leaves the sanatorium ? "

The preceding sketch of local arrangements is given in full not as representing an ideal, but as an illustration of what can, in many districts, be done without expenditure on new buildings. In other districts, if the isolation hospital accommodation is insufficient, new buildings will be required. It is, however, most desirable that local authorities should not unnecessarily incur heavy capital expenditure, when by possible adaptation of already available accommodation the interest on the same money might be utilised for the actual treatment of further patients. It is possible that in a few years interchange of accommodation for consumptives may be possible between the public health and the parochial authorities. If the parochial regulations could be relaxed for the sick, there is in many workhouse infirmaries excellent accommodation for

ADVANCED CONSUMPTIVES WHO ARE NOT PAUPERS.—The provision of accommodation for the patients of this class is the most urgent problem in the prevention of tuberculosis. The way

26

to this provision in most districts will probably lie through the removal of parochial restrictions, and the consequent increase of popularity of the consumptive wards of the infirmary. This question is dealt with to some extent on p. 394.. There can be no doubt, as stated in the admirable circular issued by the Local Government Board of Scotland (March 1906) on the " Administrative Control of Pulmonary Phthisis," that " the isolation of such dangerous cases is a primary duty of the local authority." The view taken on p. 382 is that these cases may properly be treated, though in a separate ward, in the same institution as earlier cases of phthisis. The removal of parochial restrictions in respect of the treatment of the sick, it may be hoped, will ere long remove the chief difficulty in successfully coping with this problem.

The following estimate by Dr. Rushton Parker gives some guidance as to the possible expense involved in the further provision of hospital beds for advanced cases of phthisis :—

As two-thirds (or, strictly, 70 per cent.) of any population usually belongs to the working class, and as during the last ten years there have been about 42,000 deaths annually from consumption in England and Wales, we may assume that 28,000 persons will annually qualify for admission into such homes. At those which already exist the applications for admission far exceed the vacancies ; the duration of stay is about six months ; and the annual cost of maintenance is about £65 per bed. We may assume, therefore, that we shall require 14,000 beds, at an annual cost of £1,000,000 a year. About one-sixth of the cases would be paupers ; so that one-sixth of the cost would be chargeable to the guardians. As it has been calculated that one-eleventh of all the pauperism of the country, costing in England and Wales £11,500,000 a year (1900–1901), arises from consumption, the million pounds a year proposed to be so spent should produce much more profitable results than the million pounds a year already spent in merely relieving the pauperism caused by neglected consumption.

In every population of 100,000, about 120 die annually of consumption, of whom 80 require accommodation in a home of 40 beds, at a cost of £2600 a year, roughly equivalent to a penny rate for such population.

CHAPTER L

THE PREVENTION OF TUBERCULOSIS DUE TO INFECTED FOOD

THE degree of danger from the flesh of tuberculous animals has been already indicated, and it has been seen that on present evidence it is much smaller than that from milk and its products. Both these dangers might conceivably be removed by action along one or, other of the following lines :—

1. The extermination of tuberculous cattle and of other tuberculous animals used for food.

2. The prevention—apart from their complete extermination—of the use of such animals or their products as human food.

3. The sterilisation of food derived from tuberculous animals.

The first of these lines of action is not within the range of immediate practical policy. The Legislature could not be expected to undertake the enormous initial expense of the destruction of all animals found by means of tuberculin testing to be diseased. Short of such wholesale condemnation of diseased cattle, more stringent regulations are undoubtedly indicated, and there is much room for better enforcement of already existing regulations. Thus at the present time it is punishable to sell milk derived from cows suffering from tuberculosis of the udder ; but this power is at present in the hands of authorities who are usually rural authorities, of whose members farmers form a large proportion. If the administration of the powers relating to this disease were in the hands of, or powers of action in default were given to, larger authorities, they would be more likely to be enforced. It is desirable also to increase the power of such authorities, enabling them to test by means of tuberculin if necessary any cow showing symptoms suspicious of tuberculosis, whether in the udder or not. Further power is needed to prevent the same cow from being used for feeding calves or passed on to another farm, after its milk has been stopped on the farm where the disease was first discovered. At present the farmer can evade the results of this discovery, by selling the cow in question. Some unobjectionable method of marking such cattle permanently would be useful in preventing this traffic. Compulsory slaughter is indicated in some cases. Whether limited fractional compensation should be given in such cases may be left open for consideration. It is difficult to devise a local scheme for such compensation which would work equitably.

Apart from specific action in respect of tuberculosis in cattle, much could be done by improved sanitation in cowsheds to diminish the amount of infection from cow to cow.

MEAT FROM TUBERCULOUS CATTLE.—The evidence connecting tuberculous meat with the possibility of infecting man has already been considered (p. 140). In the words of the First Royal Commission (par. 22 of their report, April 1895), "any person who takes tuberculous matter into the body as food incurs some risk of acquiring tuberculous disease." The cooking of meat affords a considerable measure of protection, as all except under-done parts would be sufficiently sterilised. With uncooked meat, which is often given in the form of pounded meat or meat juice to weakly children, there must be considerable risk ; and doctors prescribing such meat should give preference to meat derived from animals known to have been slaughtered at a public abattoir.

The second Royal Commission on the same subject (1898) laid down the following principles in the inspection of the tuberculous carcasses of cattle :—

(a) When there is miliary tuberculosis of both lungs,
(b) When tuberculous lesions are present on the pleura and peritoneum,
(c) When tuberculous lesions are present in the muscular system or in the lymphatic glands embedded in or between the muscles,
(d) When tuberculous lesions exist in any part of an emaciated carcass,

The entire carcass and all the organs may be seized.

(*a*) When the lesions are confined to the lungs and the thoracic lymphatic glands,	The carcass, if otherwise healthy, shall not be condemned, but every part of it containing tuberculous lesions shall be seized.
(*b*) When the lesions are confined to the liver,	
(*c*) When the lesions are confined to the pharyngeal lymphatic glands,	
(*d*) When the lesions are confined to any combination of the foregoing, but are collectively small in extent,	

They add that

in view of the greater tendency to generalisation of tuberculosis in the pig, we consider that the presence of tubercular deposit, in any degree, should involve seizure of the whole carcass and of the organs. In respect of foreign dead meat, seizure shall ensue in every case where the pleura have been " stripped."

These rules, where adopted, give a fairly good guarantee against the entry of tuberculous meat into the market. They are fairly well enforced in all public abattoirs, and possibly in a majority of private slaughter-houses in towns ; but in rural districts there is no efficient control. It is not even obligatory that animals should be slaughtered in a registered or licensed slaughter-house ; and when an animal is killed on the farm, there is no enactment compelling the submission of the carcass to inspection by a competent inspector. Such inspectors often do not exist in rural districts. A large amount of diseased meat is prepared for the market on unlicensed premises in country districts, and is smuggled into towns. The one essential for improvement is that no meat should be allowed to be exposed for sale, or to be conveyed from place to place (except when it is consigned to a clearing house or public abattoir for inspection), unless it is stamped in some way, to vouch that it has been properly inspected.

The following extracts from the above report (1898) emphasise as strongly as is needful the evils of the present state of things :—

So long as private slaughter-houses are permitted to exist, so long butchers, from use and wont, will continue to use them, and so long must inspection be carried on under conditions incompatible with efficiency ; besides other disadvantages and risks to health which lie beyond the scope of our reference.

Nor is there anything lacking in thoroughness in the recommendations of the Royal Commission, which were as follows :—

We recommend that in all towns and municipal boroughs of England and Wales, and in Ireland, powers be conferred on the authorities similar to those conferred on Scottish corporations and municipalities by the Burgh Police (Scotland) Act, 1892, viz. :—

(a) When the local authority in any town or urban district in England and Wales and Ireland have provided a public slaughter-house, power be conferred on them to declare that no other place within the town or borough shall be used for slaughtering, except that a period of three years be allowed to the owners for existing registered private slaughter-houses to apply their premises to other purposes. The term of three years to date, in those places where adequate public slaughter-houses already exist, from the public announcement by the local authority that the use of such public slaughter-houses is obligatory, or, in those places where public slaughter-houses have not been erected, from the public announcement by the local authority that tenders for their erection have been accepted.

(b) That local authorities be empowered to require all meat slaughtered elsewhere than in a public slaughter-house, and brought into the district for sale, to be taken to a place or places where such meat may be inspected, and that local authorities be empowered to make a charge to cover the reasonable expenses attendant on such inspection.

(c) That when a public slaughter-house has been established, inspectors shall be engaged to inspect all animals immediately after slaughter, and stamp the joints of all carcasses passed as sound.

We recommend, further, that it shall not be lawful to offer for sale the meat of any animal which has not been killed in a duly licensed slaughter house.

Up to the present time, however, no legislation has been passed rendering the above practical and important recommendations operative.

MILK FROM TUBERCULOUS CATTLE.—I cannot better summarise the dangers and the remedies for the dangers arising from tuberculous milk than in the words and recommendations of the same Royal Commission (1898). They state their agreement with the opinion of the previous Royal Commission on Tuberculosis, that "no doubt the largest part of the tuberculosis which man obtains through his food is by means of milk containing tuberculous matter." They then go on to say that "even local authorities, which exert themselves to prevent the sale of tuberculous meat, are without sufficient powers to prevent the sale within their districts of milk drawn from diseased cows." It appears clear that the danger of infecting the milk arises chiefly, if not solely, when the tuberculosis affects the udder of the cow ; but inasmuch as "tuberculosis of the udder can rarely be differentiated from other forms of udder disease by the ordinary stock owner or dairyman, . . . all udder diseases should be forthwith notified to the local authority."

Since the above recommendation was made, tuberculosis of the udder has been placed among those diseases of cattle where the sale of the milk for human food is forbidden. It is unfortunate that the recommendations of the First Royal Commission have not been also adopted.

Town dwellers and the local authorities appointed to protect their health are in most instances completely impotent in respect of public measures against tuberculous milk. On this point the report of the same Commission (1898) may be again quoted :—

It will be seen how futile are the restrictions on the sale of tuberculous milk produced within a city in the absence of any safeguard against its introduction from without. Clearly there is the most urgent necessity for powers being conferred on and exercised by local authorities to make periodical inspection of all cows of which the milk is offered for sale within their districts.

They draw attention, furthermore, to the fact already mentioned, that "the spread of tubercle in the udder may be very rapid," becoming manifested "between fortnightly inspections carried on along with a veterinary surgeon." Notwithstanding these facts, they were of opinion, having regard to the extent of prevalence of the disease, that "direct action for the elimination of all tuberculous cows from dairies should proceed tentatively." They recommended at once that

(1) Systematic inspection of the cows in dairies and cowsheds should be made by the officers of the local authorities within whose district the premises are situated ; (2) that the authorised officers of local authorities within whose districts milk is supplied should have power to inspect the cows in any dairy or cowshed, wherever situated ; (3) that power should be given to a medical officer of health to suspend the supply of milk from any suspected cow for a limited period, pending veterinary inspection ; (4) that power should be given to prohibit the sale of milk from any cow certified by a veterinary surgeon to be suffering from such disease of the udder as in his opinion renders the animal unfit to supply milk ; and (5) the provision of a penalty for supplying milk for sale from any cow having obvious udder disease.

The powers enumerated under (2), (3), and (4) remain a dead letter in most urban districts. The nearest approach to them is contained in the " model milk clauses" possessed by a few large

towns in local Acts of Parliament.   It is unnecessary to describe
these clauses in detail ; but subject to tedious regulations they
enable the veterinary inspector and medical officer of health of
the town possessing the above powers to inspect the cattle of a
suspected farm, and if tuberculosis of the udder is found, to
prohibit the supply of milk to that town from the infected cow.
There is no power to prohibit its supply elsewhere, and no power
to prevent the infected cow being sold to another farmer for
milking purposes.   The recommendation of the Royal Commission on this point is that

when, under the certificate of a veterinary surgeon, the sale of milk from
a given cow is prohibited, the local authority should slaughter the
same, and if on post-mortem examination it appears that the cow was
not so affected, the local authority should pay compensation to the
extent of the full value of the cow immediately before slaughter.   If,
on the other hand, the animal be found to be so suffering, the carcase
should be sold by the authority, and the owner thereof should receive
the proceeds of the sale.

This recommendation has not been embodied in legislation.

In the light of the facts described above it seems clear that
the enforcement of much more efficient public health administration in rural districts than has hitherto been the rule is needed.

Failing efficient protection of the public against the supply
of foods which are sometimes contaminated by tubercle bacilli,
the public still have it within their power to protect themselves
by refusing to eat uncooked foods derived from the farm.   They
may at the same time, by bringing pressure to bear on the
purveyors of meat and milk, aid in securing the commercial
protection which is the subject of the next paragraph.

COMMERCIAL PROTECTION AGAINST BOVINE TUBERCULOSIS.—
Apart from the enforcement of public health regulations, public
protection might be entirely secured under the ordinary
conditions of commercial life, if the public were willing to
pay a little more for their milk and milk-products.   There
is in my opinion great scope for commercial enterprise in
this matter ; and it is not unlikely that the additional expenditure at first incurred by the enterprising large farmer, in
eliminating all cattle that reacted to tuberculin, in cleansing
and disinfecting his sheds, and in giving ample light and air in
them, would eventually be recouped by the more permanent

healthiness of his herd. Some doubt may be entertained on this point of expense, in view of the large proportion of the cattle that would in the first instance need to be eliminated (p. 139), and in view of the difficulty in replacing the slaughtered cows by others reacting negatively to the tuberculin test.

The ideal would be that each dairyman should be in a position to issue a guarantee to his customers that all the cows from which his milk is supplied had been proved to be free from tuberculosis by means of the tuberculin test ; and at the same time to certify, by means of expert evidence, that all other sanitary requirements had been fulfilled. It must be confessed that in very few districts is it practicable at the present time to purchase milk under an efficient guarantee to the above effect.

The next alternative is for the dairyman to supply pasteurised milk, and this is now largely done on a commercial scale. Often it is done to preserve stale milk, and the slight taste of pasteurised milk is concealed by mixing the milk with fresh unpasteurised milk. This obviously gives little protection to the purchaser. Furthermore, the dairyman is only concerned in pasteurising at the lowest temperature which will prevent souring of the milk, a temperature which, as will be shortly seen, does not suffice to kill the tubercle-bacillus. If, therefore, commercial pasteurised milk is to be regarded as safe in respect of tuberculosis, the temperature and duration of the heating process must be specified. The following experimental results throw light on this question :—

THE THERMAL DEATH-POINT OF THE TUBERCLE-BACILLUS.— In 1887 Sternberg showed that tuberculous expectoration subjected to temperatures at and above 60° C. (140° F.) was rendered harmless. From this date onwards there has been considerable disagreement as to the exact temperature fatal to the tubercle bacillus. Theobald Smith in 1897 found that the variable results as to the death-point of the tubercle bacillus in milk were probably due to the formation of the milk pellicle in which bacilli were caught, and thus artificially protected against further heat. Russell and Hastings in 1900 found that exposure of tuberculous milk to 60° C. (140° F.) in a tightly closed commercial pasteuriser for ten minutes always destroyed tubercle bacilli, while, when milk was heated under conditions allowing a pellicle to form, exposure to the same temperature (60° C.) for considerably longer times did not kill the bacilli.

DOMESTIC PROTECTION AGAINST BOVINE TUBERCULOSIS.—As domestic pasteurisation is not likely to be carried out under scientific conditions, it would not be safe to adopt a temperature lower than 85° C. (185° F.) in domestic life. Probably, although home sterilisers are to be obtained, the safest plan for most households is to boil the milk in accordance with the following directions given in a pamphlet issued by the National Association for the Prevention of Consumption. If these are carried out exactly, the " cooked " flavour objected to by many individuals will be found to be comparatively slight, and little if any surface scum will be formed.

1. Use a double milk saucepan ;[1] if, however, this cannot be obtained, put the milk into an ordinary covered saucepan and place it inside a larger vessel containing water.

2. Let the water in the outer pan be cold when placed on the fire.

3. Bring the water up to the boil, and maintain it at this point for four minutes *without removing the lid* of the inner milk pan.

4. Cool the milk down quickly by placing the inner pan in one or two changes of cold water *without removing the lid*.

5. When cooled down, aerate the milk by stirring well with a spoon.

THE PROTECTION OF OTHER DAIRY PRODUCTS.—Butter and cheese may also contain tubercle bacilli. The first is the more important, as it bulks more largely in the dietary of children. Some of the results as to the presence of tubercle bacilli in butter may be exaggerated, owing to possible confusion with other acid-fast bacilli. They are, however, sometimes present, and the only safe protection is by partially cooking the butter; which, however, loses much of its palatability by this process.

[1] Obtainable from any ironmonger.

CHAPTER LI

THE CO-ORDINATION OF MEASURES AGAINST TUBERCULOSIS

REFERRING to the tabular statement on p. 317 it will be seen that preventive measures against tuberculosis must have regard to the receptivity of the patient, as well as to the prevention of infection. The measures against receptivity have been almost sufficiently indicated in previous chapters. Every improvement in cleanliness and ventilation, every approach towards better nutrition, every avoidance of excessive fatigue and of other depressing influences undoubtedly tends to diminish active infection. Whether to these should be added measures directed against the marriage, and especially the inter-marriage, of those with a strong family history of phthisis is a subject of much greater difficulty. As already indicated (p. 189), each family history would, in the event of advice on this point being given, need to be considered as a separate problem ; and the opportunities for infection in the family, as well as the possible inheritance of innate weakness, would need to be carefully weighed.

In this chapter, we propose to endeavour to summarise and obtain a conspective view of all those measures against tuberculosis which public authorities and the governing bodies of hospitals, dispensaries, and friendly societies may be able to adopt. Evidently the greatest efficiency of result is likely to be secured by first obtaining a complete view of the measures which are practicable, and then by bringing the scattered efforts *in posse* as well as *in esse* into active relationship with each other.

The following schemes, which to a certain extent overlap, show the main official measures and the operations of hospitals and dispensaries in the prevention of phthisis. In each scheme I have placed the medical officer of health as the agent for originating and co-ordinating preventive measures ; and although

SCHEME I

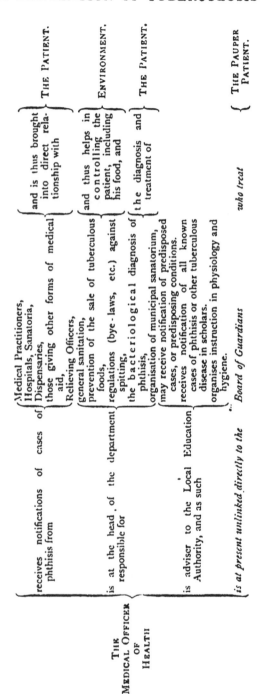

THE MEDICAL OFFICER OF HEALTH

receives notifications of cases of phthisis from {Medical Practitioners, Hospitals, Sanatoria, Dispensaries, those giving other forms of medical aid, Relieving Officers,} and is thus brought into direct relationship with } THE PATIENT.

is at the head of the department responsible for {general sanitation, prevention of the sale of tuberculous foods, regulations (bye-laws, etc.) against spiting, the bacteriological diagnosis of phthisis, organisation of municipal sanatorium, may receive notification of predisposed cases, or predisposing conditions.} and thus helps in controlling the patient, including his food, and } ENVIRONMENT.

is adviser to the Local Education Authority, and as such {receives notification of all known cases of phthisis or other tuberculous disease in scholars. organises instruction in physiology and hygiene.} the diagnosis and treatment of } THE PATIENT.

is at present unlinked directly to the Board of Guardians who treat } THE PAUPER PATIENT.

personal, domestic, and industrial measures of prevention are practicable, and are occasionally practised, apart from notification of cases to the medical officer of health, it is none the less true that they are commonly neglected and cannot in the completest sense be carried out apart from such notification.

The second scheme indicates from the point of view of the individual patient as well as of the public health what is practicable under present conditions.

SCHEME II

PATIENT WITH
PHTHISIS
NOTIFIED
TO THE
MEDICAL OFFICER
OF HEALTH.

I. *Patient is treated at* HOME.
  (1) Under the charge of his own doctor, the dispensary, out-patient department of the hospital, etc.
  (2) Home visits are made by the medical officer of health, or his assistant, in connection with which
    (*a*) Cleansing and disinfection are arranged.
    (*b*) Instructions are given as to general hygiene, and as to the special hygiene of the disease.
    (*c*) Handkerchiefs and spit-bottles are provided as required.
    (*d*) Material aid is given in conjunction with voluntary agencies, friendly societies, and the poor-law organisation.
    (*e*) Regular visits to the doctor or dispensary are urged.
    (*f*) Dispensary or hospital tickets are given to other members of the same family who appear to be failing in health.
    (*g*) Free bacteriological examination of sputum from these or from any other suspected patients is provided.

II. *Patient is admitted to a* SANATORIUM.
  (1) Disinfection of the patient's home is arranged.
  (2) Aid is organised as required for the patient's family, hospital tickets provided for suspected cases, etc.

III. *Patient is admitted to a* HOSPITAL FOR ADVANCED CASES.
  At present in most districts the only hospital available for advanced patients is the workhouse infirmary, which is only available for pauper patients.

The preceding schemes display the imperfections of our present official measures and the reforms which are indicated. Thus there are insufficient encouragements to early treatment of this most curable disease. We have no system of sickness insurance of a national character as in Germany, and medical aid is not so readily obtainable as to compensate in part for the absence of this. Friendly Societies do not completely fill the gap here indicated. We have no universal system of compulsory notification of phthisis, nor, it may be added, is public opinion—without which it would be inoperative—completely ripe for such a measure. Sanatorium accommodation for early cases among wage-earners is very deficient. There is a still more serious deficiency of institutional treatment for advanced patients who are not paupers, but who cannot afford to provide suitable treatment at home. The arrangements for providing suitable occupation, or part-time employment, for patients discharged from a sanatorium partially cured, need to be organised on a larger scale, and the practicability of industrial colonies will require to be considered.

But even under present conditions a study of the two preceding schemes indicates how much admirable work—beyond what is done in most communities—can be done under present conditions by the full employment of official machinery and by its co-operation with voluntary agencies. By proceeding on the tried lines described in the preceding chapters, by further experimental advance from the points of vantage already reached, and above all by the earnest and combined efforts of voluntary and official workers, there is, in my opinion, no reason why, within a relatively short period, tuberculosis should not follow the closely allied disease of leprosy towards extinction.

BIBLIOGRAPHY

ABRAHAM, P. (1896). Discussion on Latency, etc. *Proc. Med. Chi. Soc. Lond.*, 1896.

ALLBUTT, CLIFFORD (1899). On the Preventive and Remedial Treatment of Tuberculosis. *Brit. Med. Journ.*, Oct. 28, 1899, pp. 1149–1151.

ANNETT, H. E. (1902). Tubercular Expectoration in Public Thoroughfares. Vol. iv. pt. ii. *Reports of Thompson Yates Laboratories*.

ARLIDGE (1892). Diseases of Occupations, p. 246.

ARMSTRONG, H. (1902). A Note on the Infantile Mortality from Tuberculous Meningitis and Tabes Mesenterica. *Brit. Med. Journ.*, vol. i. p. 1024.

BARTHET AND STENSTROM (1905). The Action of Heat on the Virulence of Tuberculous Milk. *Le Bulletin Vétérinaire*, 1905, p. 510, and *Journal of Compar. Pathol. and Therapeutics*, vol. xix. pt. i. p. 62.

BEEVOR, H. (1899). Hunterian Oration on the Declension of Phthisis. *Lancet*, April 1899, p. 1008.

—— H. (1900). Sex Constitution and its Relation to Pulmonary Tuberculosis. *Med. Magazine*, June 1900.

—— (1901). Maps, Charts, and Tables illustrating the Associations of Phthisis in England. *Descriptive Catalogue, Brit. Congr. on Tuberculosis*, 1901, p. 158.

—— (1905). Discussion on Paper by A. Newsholme. *Epidem. Soc. Trans.*, p. 130.

BIELEFELDT, PRIVY COUNCILLOR (1901). The Battle against Consumption . . . by means of the German Workmen's Insurance. *Trans. Brit. Congress on Tuberculosis*, vol. ii. p. 336.

BIGGS, HERMANN (1903–04). First Ann. Rep. of the Henry Phipps Institute, p. 191.

—— (1903). Tuberculosis: its Causation and Prevention in a Handbook on the Prevention of Tuberculosis (Charity Organisation Society, New York, etc.).

BODINGTON (1840). The Treatment and Cure of Pulmonary Consumption; reprinted in Selected Essays, etc., New Sydenham Soc., 1901, p. 125.

BOWDITCH, H. I. (1862). Paper on the Topographical Distribution and Local Origin of Consumption in Massachusetts. Read before the Mass. Med. Society, May 28, 1862.

BROADBENT, Sir WILLIAM (1905). Discussion on A. Newsholme's Paper. *Trans. Epid. Soc.*, p. 118.

BROUARDEL (1901). Address to the British Congress on Tuberculosis, vol. i. p. 66 and p. 48.

BUCK (1879). Manual of Hygiene and Public Health, vol. ii. p. 29.

BULSTRODE, H. T. (25, vii. 1903). Milroy Lectures. *Lancet*, ii. p. 208.

BURTON-FANNING, F. W. (1902). On the Etiology of Pulmonary Tuberculosis. *Practitioner*, vol. 68, pp. 317–326.

—— (1904 ?). The Open-Air Treatment of Pulmonary Tuberculosis.

CALMETTE AND GUÉRIN (1905). Origine intestinale de la tuberculose pulmonaire. *Annales de l'Institut Pasteur*, tome xix. No. 10, p. 601.

CHEYNE, WATSON. *Practitioner*, April 1883.

COATES, J. (1891). Tuberculosis viewed as an Infectious Disease : its Prevalence and the Frequency of Recovery from it. *Sanitary Journal*, No. 189, p. 343.

COHNHEIM (1890). Lectures on General Pathology. *New. Syd. Soc.*, vol. iii. p. 1030.

CORNET, G. (1904). Tuberculosis in Nothnagel's Encycl. of Practical Medicine.

COURTOIS-SUFFIT ET CH. LAUBRY (1905). Rôle des Sanatoriums et des Dispensaires dans la Lutte Anti-Tuberculeuse. *Rapports présentés au Congrès Internat. de la Tuberculose*, p. 503.

DEBOVE AND ACHARD. Manuel de Médecine, tome ix. p. 271.

DELÉPINE, S. (1898). Tuberculosis and the Milk Supply. *Lancet*, vol. ii. p. 736.

—— (1899). Prevention of Tuberculosis in Cattle. *Veterinarian*, July and August 1899.

FAGGE (1886). Medicine, vol. i. p. 983.

FAGGE AND PYE SMITH. Principles and Practice of Medicine, 3rd ed., vol. i. p. 639.

FARR (1885). Vital Statistics, p. 513.

FLINT, AUSTIN (1882). The Self-limited Duration of Pulmonary Phthisis. *Brit. Med. Journ.*, Sept. 30, 1882.

FLÜGGE C. (1898). Die Verbreitung der Phthise durch staubförmiges Sputum und beim Husten versprizte Tröpfchen. *Ztsch. f. Hygiene u. Inf. Kr.* xxx. 107.

FOWLER, J. K. (1896). Discussion on Latency, etc. *Proc. Med. Chi. Soc. Lond.*

FOWLER, J. K. (1906). The Therapeutic Value of Sanatorium Treatment in Pulmonary Tuberculosis. *Lancet*, Jan. 6, 1906.

—— (1898). Diseases of the Lungs, p. 305.

FOX WILSON (1891). Diseases of the Lungs, p. 563.

—— Treatise on Diseases of the Lungs and Pleura, ed. 1891.

FRÄNKEL (1906, Mar. 1). *Deutsch. Med. Woch.*, quoted in *Brit. Med. Journal Epitome* (1906), p. 53.

GANGHOFNER, F. (1905). Préservation Scolaire contre la Tuberculose. *Rapports présentés au Congrès Internat. de la Tuberculose, Paris,* p. 315.

GARLAND, C. H. (1905). Assurances et Mutualités dans la Lutte contre la Tuberculose. *Rapports preséntés au Congrès Internat. de la Tuberculose, Paris,* p. 495.

GRAY, E. G. (1906). An Unusual Case of Typhoid Infection. *Lancet,* July 1906.

GREENHOW (1869). *Path. Trans.,* vol. xx. p. 57.

GREENHOW, KNAUFF. Archiv für path. Anat. und Physiol. und für Klin. Med. von Virchow, Bd. xxxix. S. 442.

GUTHRIE, L. G. (1899). The Distribution and Origin of Tuberculosis in Children. *Lancet,* vol. i. pp. 286–290.

HARRIS, T. *Brit. Med. Journ.,* vol. ii. p. 1385.

HAYWARD, T. E. (1904). On the Construction of Life Tables, p. 27. *Victoria University Reports,* edited by Professor Delépine.

HENSCHEN, S. E. (1905). La Lutte contre la Tuberculose en Suède. *Ouvrage dédiè au Congrès Internat. de la Tuberculose à Paris,* 1905.

HEYMANN (1901). Versuche über die verbreitung der Phthise durch ausgehustete Tröpfchen und durch trockenen Sputum. *Zeits. für Hyg. und Infektionskrankheiten,* xxxviii. 20–93.

HILLIER, A. (1903). The Nature of the Infectivity of Phthisis : A Study of the Views of Koch, Flügge, and others. *Brit. Med. Journ.,* vol. i. p. 593.

HIRSCH. Geographical and Historical Pathology, vol. iii. p. 203. *Syd. Soc. Trans.*

—— vol. iii. pp. 197–198.

HOFFMAN, F. L. (1901). Industrial Insurance and the Prevention of Tuberculosis. *Trans. Brit. Congr. on Tuberculosis,* vol. ii. p. 348.

HUTCHINSON, JONATHAN (1896). Discussion on Latency, etc. *Proc. Med. Chi. Soc. Lond.*

KELYNACK (1904). The Sanatorium Treatment of Consumption, p. 7.

KINSFORD, L. (1904). The Channels of Infection in Tuberculosis in Childhood. *Lancet,* vol. ii., Sept. 24, 1904.

27

KNOPF. Pulmonary Tuberculosis : its Modern Prophylaxis, p. 55.

KOCH, R. Etiology of Tuberculosis, translated by Stanley Boyd, vol. cxv. *New Syd. Soc.*

—— (1901). Address to British Congress on Tuberculosis. *Trans. Brit. Congr. on Tuberculosis*, vol. i. p. 52.

—— (1906). Nobel Lecture on "How the Fight against Tuberculosis now stands." *Lancet*, vol. i. pp. 1449–1451.

KOSSELL, H. (1905). A Report on Human and Bovine Tuberculosis. *Brit. Med. Journ.*, 1905, vol. ii. p. 1445.

LARTIGAU (1901). On Tuberculosis. Twentieth Century Practice of Medicine, vol. xx.

LARTIGAU AND NICOLL. *Amer. Journ. Med. Sciences*, June 1902.

LATHAM, A. (1900). Pulmonary Tuberculosis in Early Childhood. *Lancet*, 1900, vol. ii. pp. 1785–86.

—— (1903). Prize Essay on the Erection of a Sanatorium for the Treatment of Tuberculosis in England. *Lancet*, Jan. 3, 1903.

—— (1906). The Economic Value of Sanatoriums. *Lancet*, Jan. 6, 1906.

LECKY AND HORTON (1907). Revealed Tuberculosis in Children at School Ages. *Lancet*, Dec. 28, 1907.

LISTER, J. (1868). Address on the Antiseptic System of Treatment in Surgery. *Brit. Med. Journ.*, vol. ii. p. 55.

LOUIS, P. C. A. (1844). Researches on Phthisis. *Sydenham Society.*

MACFADYEAN, J. (1901). Address on Tubercle Bacilli in Cows' Milk as a possible Source of Tuberculous Disease in Man. *Trans. Brit. Congr. on Tuberculosis*, vol. i. p. 83.

MARFAN, A. B. (1905). Préservation de l'Enfant contre la Tuberculose dans sa Famille. *Rapports présentés au Congrès Internat. de la Tuberculose, Paris*, p. 255.

MATHESON, R. E. (xi. 1903). The Housing of Ireland during the Period of 1841–1901. *Journ. Statist. and Social Inquiry*, vol. xi. pt. lxxxiii.

MEMORANDA, etc., prepared by the Board of Trade. Cd. 1761, pp. 215 and 224.

—— Second Series. Cd. 2337.

MORGAN, G. (1899). Remarks on Tuberculous Adenitis. *Brit. Med. Journ.*, Aug. 19, 1899.

MOTT, Report of Pathologist to London County Council for year ended March 1904, p. 1.

MOXON (1885). *Brit. Med. Journ.*, vol. i. p. 130.

MÜLLER, D. (1905). Milk and Dairy Products as Sources of Infection in Tuberculosis. *Journ. Compar. Path. and Therapeutics*, vol. xix. pt. i. p. 19, and *Proc. 8th Internat. Vet. Congress*, Budapest.

NEWMAN AND SWITHINBANK (1903). Bacteriology of Milk, p. 268.

NEWSHOLME, A. (1896). On the Study of Hygiene in Elementary Schools. *Public Health*, vol. iii. p. 135.

—— (1901). The Influence of Soil on the Prevalence of Pulmonary Phthisis. *Practitioner*, New Series, vol. xiii. p. 206.

—— (1903). Public Health Authorities in relation to the Struggle against Tuberculosis in England. *Journal of Hygiene*, vol. iii. p. 461 ; also *Compt. rend. XIIIᵉ Congrès International d'Hygiène et de Démogr., Bruxelles*.

—— (1904). Protracted and Recrudescent Infection in Diphtheria and Scarlet Fever. *Med. Chi. Trans.*, vol. 87.

—— (1905). A Study of the Relation between the Treatment of Tuberculous Patients in General Institutions and the Reduction in the Death-rate from Tuberculosis. *Reports to Internat. Congr. on Tuberculosis*, Paris, p. 427.

—— (1905). The Relative Importance of the Constituent Factors involved in the Control of Pulmonary Tuberculosis. *Trans. Epidem. Soc.*, New Series, vol. xxv. p. 32.

—— (1906). An Inquiry into the principal Causes of the Reduction in the Death-rate from Phthisis during the last Forty Years, with special Reference to the Segregation of Phthisical Patients in General Institutions. *Journal of Hygiene*, vol. vi., No. 3, p. 304.

—— (1907). The Co-ordination of the Public Medical Services. An Address given at the Meeting of the State Medicine Section of the Meeting of the British Medical Association at Exeter, July 1907. *Brit. Med. Journ.*, Sept. 14, 1907.

—— (1907). Poverty and Disease as illustrated by the Course of Typhus Fever and Phthisis in Ireland. Presidential Address, Epidemiological Section, Roy. Soc. Med., Oct. 1907.

OSLER, W. (1901). The Principles and Practice of Medicine, pp. 258, 338.

PARKER, W. R. (1903). Sanatoria *plus* Homes for Consumption. Mar. 14, 1903.

PEARSON, KARL (1907). A First Study of the Statistics of Pulmonary Tuberculosis. *Drapers' Company Research Memoirs*.

PHILIP, R. W. (1906). The Public Health Aspects of the Prevention of Consumption. *Brit. Med. Journ.*, Dec. 1, 1906.

POWELL, DOUGLAS. Lecture on the Prevention of Consumption. *Journ. San. Inst.*, Aug. 1904, vol. xxv. pt. ii. p. 353.

QUAIN's Dictionary of Medicine. Ed. 1894, vol. ii. p. 414.

RANSOME, A. (1890). The Cause and Prevention of Phthisis, p. 50.

—— (1895). Consumption a Filth Disease. *Lancet*, Jan. 1, 1898, p. 15.

—— (1902). The Intercommunicability of Human and Bovine Tuberculosis. *Proceedings Patholog. Soc. of Philadelphia*, May 1902.

—— (1905).¹ Comparative Study of Various Forms of Tuberculosis. *Rapports au Congrès Internat. de la Tuberculose*, Paris, pp. 135–148.

RINDFLEISCH (1875). On Chronic and Acute Tuberculosis, in von Ziemssen's System of Medicine, vol. v. p. 649.

ROBERTS, F. T. (1902). On the Comprehensive Study of Thoracic Phthisis. *Lancet*, vol. i. pp. 867–874.

RUCHLE (1875). Pulmonary Consumption. Von Ziemssen's Medicine, vol. v. p. 508.

SANTOLIQUIDO (1903). *Compt. rend. XIIIᵉ Congr. d'Hygiène et de Démogr., Bruxelles*, vol. vii. p. 45.

SHADWELL, A. (1905). Industrial Efficiency, vol. ii.

SMITH, THEOBALD (1904). A Study of the Tubercle Bacilli isolated from Three Cases of Tuberculosis of the Mesenteric Lymph Nodules. *Amer. Journ. of the Med. Sciences*, Aug. 1904.

—— (1905). Studies in Mammalian Tubercle Bacilli : III. Description of a Bovine Bacillus from the Human Body. *Journ. of Med. Research*, vol. viii. No. 3, pp. 253–300.

—— (1905). The Reaction Curve of Tubercle Bacilli from Different Sources in Bouillon containing different Amounts of Glycerine. *Journ. of Med. Research*, vol. xiii. No. 4.

SQUIRE, J. E., C.B. (1906). A Lecture on Pulmonary Tuberculosis in Children. *Brit. Med. Journ.* 1906, vol. ii. p. 133.

—— (1906). The Results of Sanatorium Treatment of Consumptives. *Tuberculosis*, vol. iv. No. 3.

STENGEL. Manual of Pathology, p. 255.

STILL, G. F. (1901). Tuberculosis in Childhood. *Practitioner*, vol. 67, pp. 91–103.

TATHAM, J. W., Report of Royal Commission on Tuberculosis, part. ii. Appendix C., and Annual Reports of Registrar-General of Births and Deaths.

THOMSON, ST. CLAIR (1901). Tubercular Infection through the Air Passages. *Practitioner*, 1901, vol. ii. pp. 80–90.

THOMSON, ST. CLAIR AND HEWLETT (1895). *Path. Soc. Trans.*, vol. lxxviii.

—— (1896). The Fate of Micro-organisms in Inspired Air. *Lancet*, vol. i. pp. 86–87.

THORNE, R. T. (1888). The Progress of Preventive Medicine during the Victorian Era, p. 51.

TYNDALL (1876). The Optical Deportment of the Atmosphere in relation to the Phenomena of Putrefaction and Infection. *Phil. Trans. Roy. Soc.*, vol. clxvi. pt. i. p. 27.

VALLEE, M. H. (1905). De la Genèse des lésions pulmonaire dans la Tuberculose. *Ann. de l'Institut Pasteur*, tome xix. No. 10, p. 649.

VON BEHRING (1904). The Suppression of Tuberculosis. Cassel Lecture, September 1903, American Translation, p. 14.

WALKER, J. (1906). Employment of Consumptive Patients. *Tuberculosis*, Jan. 1906.

WALSHAM, HUGH (1904). The Channels of Infection in Tuberculosis, p. 6.

WALSHE, W. H. (1871). Diseases of the Lungs.

WALTERS, F. R. (1905). Sanatoria for Consumptives.

—— (1906). *Lancet*, Jan. 6, 1906.

WASHBOURNE (1896). Discussion on the Latency of Parasitic Germs or Specific Poisons in Animal Tissues. *Proc. Med. Chi. Soc. Lond.*, 1896.

WATSON, A. W. (1903). An Account of an Investigation of the Sickness and Mortality Experience of the I.O.O.F. Manchester Unity.

WEBER, H. (1874). On the Communicability of Consumption from Husband to Wife. *Clin. Soc. Trans.*, 1874, vol. vii. p. 144.

WEST, S. (1902). Diseases of the Organs of Respiration, vol. ii. p. 436.

WILLIAMS, DAWSON. *Trans. Path. Soc.*, vol. xxxv. p. 413.

WOODHEAD. Report of Royal Commission on Tuberculosis, 1895, p. 145.

INDEX OF PLACES

INDEX OF NAMES OF PERSONS

(See also under Bibliography)

INDEX OF SUBJECTS